Governing Health

Governing Health

The Politics of Health Policy

Third Edition

Carol S. Weissert

LeRoy Collins Eminent Scholar Chair
Professor, Department of Political Science
Florida State University
Tallahassee, Florida

and

William G. Weissert

Professor, Department of Political Science
Faculty Associate, Pepper Institute on Aging and Public Policy
Florida State University
Tallahassee, Florida

The Johns Hopkins University Press
Baltimore

© 1996, 2002, 2006 The Johns Hopkins University Press

All rights reserved. Published 2006
Printed in the United States of America on acid-free paper
9 8 7 6 5 4 3 2 1

The Johns Hopkins University Press
2715 North Charles Street
Baltimore, Maryland 21218-4363
www.press.jhu.edu

Library of Congress Cataloging-in-Publication Data

Weissert, Carol S.
  Governing health : the politics of health policy / Carol S. Weissert
and William G. Weissert.—3rd ed.
      p. ; cm.
  Includes bibliographical references and index.
  ISBN 0-8018-8431-4 (hc. : alk. paper) — ISBN 0-8018-8432-2
(pb. : alk. paper)
  1. Medical policy—United States.   I. Weissert, William G.
II. Title.
  [DNLM: 1. Health Policy—United States. 2. Politics—United
States. WA 540 AA1 W433g 2006]
  RA395.A3W45 2006
  362.10973—dc22

                                          2006001805

A catalog record for this book is available from the British Library.

Contents

I. Health Policy and Institutions

II. Health and the Policy Process

Acknowledgments

WE THANK our editor at the Johns Hopkins University Press, Wendy Harris, who through all editions has graciously accepted our delayed deadlines for turning over the manuscripts. We also thank students at Michigan State University and Florida State University, including Paul Burton, Shunta Matsumoto, and John Radziewicz, for their help in locating articles for our use in preparing the manuscript. As usual, our colleagues in the political science and health policy fields have offered kind compliments and useful suggestions for which we are most grateful. Now that we've both moved to the political science department at Florida State University and our kids are out of the house, only our cocker spaniel, Bailey, is left to accept responsibility for errors and omissions in this third edition. This he has done. Of course, for a doggie treat, he'll accept anything.

Florida State is a great place to pursue our health policy and politics interests, and our colleagues and students have been warm and welcoming, as is the beach, an easy drive away and a great place to finish chapters. Finally, we're especially appreciative of Congress and President George W. Bush for passing the Medicare Prescription Drug, Improvement and Modernization Act, which, besides at least partially solving a problem, gave us an excellent case study for chapter 7 and proved, as much as anything, our point that health policy change happens in every Congress regardless of which party is in control. Now if the Democrats will just figure out how to cover the uninsured, control rising health care expenditures, and finance long-term care, there will still be plenty to write about.

Governing Health

Introduction

THIS BOOK explores how government makes health policy. Most health care in the United States is delivered by the private sector, but because public policy pays for and regulates so much of it, health policy is vitally important. Moreover, private payers for health care tend to mimic the payment approaches of public policy, so public policy's reach extends even further into the private portion of health care policy. For this reason, and because so much of health care is outsourced and becomes the income stream of private sector providers, claims processors, makers of health care products, and others, private interest groups have a huge stake in public policy and find it a good bargain to spend rather lavishly on lobbying and other strategies aimed at influencing public health care policy.

One result of this lobbying for private health care delivery is that public health, which has few dollars to fund its advocacy, tends to be neglected. Over the decades since the passage of Medicare and Medicaid, the nation has witnessed the slow shrinking of the reach, scope, and funding of public health. When disasters such as the events of September 11, 2001, hurricane Katrina in 2005, periodic outbreaks of influenzas, and continuing threats of bioterrorism are considered, the nation sees the downside of such heavy reliance on private health care delivery at the expense of public health policy, but this doesn't seem to change our commitment to heavy reliance on the private market. Hence, health care policy in the United States is largely the process of trying, through payment policy, regulation, and sometimes information and education, to influence private health care delivery and health care consumption. These are more limited strategies than might be employed by government if we had a publicly managed delivery system and emphasized public health over private health.

Despite its complexity and fragmentation (or perhaps because of these features), few issues have the personal, social, and economic significance of health policy—which is, by the way, responsible for one-seventh of the nation's gross domestic product. And few problems have so persistently demanded public action from presidents, congresses, legislatures, bureaucracies, and courts, and the interest groups that want to influence their decisions. This no doubt reflects the reality that health policy problems are never really solved; rather, they are only managed better (or at times worse).

The nation continues to face a plethora of health policy problems, some new (the obesity epidemic) and some very old (medical errors and patients' safety). A persistent one, getting worse for many rather than better, is access to care. Indeed, in recent decades this lack of access has gotten worse at faster rates as more and more employers reduce the scope of their health care coverage or give it up altogether, leaving much of the workforce uninsured. Most Americans enjoy health care that at times, for some conditions, is the best (and most expensive) on the planet, but 45 million or more of us go without health insurance, and nearly as many more have inadequate or intermittent coverage, thanks to our nation's incomplete, uncoordinated, and very expensive health policy approaches. Even more Americans go without any or adequate coverage of their prescription drugs, although beginning in 2006, elderly people—especially poor elderly people—have some level of coverage under the Medicare Prescription Drug, Improvement and Modernization Act of 2003 (or, in brief, the Medicare Modernization Act, MMA). Mental health coverage, dental coverage, and long-term care are particularly lacking, even for middle-class Americans. Those who have access to insurance are not always able to get appropriate care within a reasonable time or within a convenient geographic area. Rural and inner-city areas suffer shortages of facilities and specialty medicine.

Mainstream health care for most Americans is now delivered by managed care organizations. Even Medicare beneficiaries, who have generally shunned managed care, have begun to embrace it. Incentives in the MMA are encouraging more firms to enter (and stick with) the senior health care market, as they take advantage of the increased public subsidies afforded by the new act.

The Centers for Disease Control and Prevention has as its mission the responsibility for helping Americans curb unhealthy lifestyles and behaviors, but that agency's budget is tiny next to those of the Centers for Medicare and Medicaid Services and the National Institutes of Health, which focus on cures rather than prevention. Teen smoking persists as a problem, and low birth weight and out-of-wedlock births, while showing some improvement, are problems of epidemic proportion in some subgroups. HIV/AIDS and other infectious agents continue to spread through risky behaviors and lack of adequate progress toward vaccines and cures, often bouncing back as affected populations relax their vigilance with the availability of improved life-sustaining treatment regimens. Again, there have been some improvements but also some backsliding.

No one can be sure that the care he or she receives will be free of errors, omissions, or excesses. The quality of care delivered in the United States has come under broad attack for high rates of medical errors, inappropriate and ineffective treatments, periodic reports showing little relationship between higher quantities and costs of health care and better health outcomes, and lack of any systematic mechanism for defining, monitoring, reporting, and working to correct patterns of inadequate care. Privacy of medical records and timely accessibility to these records by those who should appropriately have access to them are far from assured, despite decade-old changes in public law. In general, improvements in technology have come much more slowly to health care administration than to health care delivery. There seems to be little political will to confront the medical care delivery system with a broad demand to heal itself.

Health care is very expensive in the United States. Health care research into understanding diseases and finding cures has seldom been better publicly funded than it is now, but public and private health care costs continue to rise at alarming rates, especially the cost of prescription drugs. It is not uncommon for drugs to cost twice as much in the United States as in many other industrialized countries, sometimes even more. Many new drugs cost five and ten times as much as older treatments but treat more effectively the conditions of only a small fraction of patients who switch to the newer form. New drugs approved by the federal agency that attempts (sometimes unsuccessfully) to protect the public from adverse side effects often require testing only against a placebo, not against existing treatments.

For these and other reasons, per capita spending for health services vastly exceeds that of any other country. Though most other industrialized countries pay for much more of their citizens' health care publicly while in the United States we rely more heavily on private sources, health policy choices nonetheless dominate our public budgets, federal and state, even when policymakers try to make other issues their priority. States have always played a major role in health policy, accepting responsibility for basic health and safety laws, innovating in everything from care for the poor to control of prescription drug costs, and paying nearly half of Medicaid costs. Now, with the MMA, the role of states as innovators in prescription drug policy is diminished, yet the law forces states to continue to pay a considerable share of the expenses for drugs for poor Medicare beneficiaries. Businesses of all sorts have now figured out that they can put a stop to pesky state restrictions on their behaviors by seeking federal preemption of state law.

Federal health policy harkens back to the earliest days of the nation, when the federal government extended its reach up the rivers and into port cities to control infectious disease. Current times have seen both an expansion of the federal role (the MMA's coverage of some prescription drug costs) and some efforts to pull back (reducing entitlements by trying to shift from guaranteeing a set of benefits to paying a fixed "premium support" regardless of costs). Health savings accounts—a fixed contribution of funds (from employer or government) that the consumer uses tax-free for health care—may come to replace employers' previous commitment to pay for a set of health care benefits. The great benefits of these accounts for employers are that the payments are fixed, predictable, and potentially not adjusted to health care cost-inflation, which is almost always higher than general inflation. But the people who choose these savings accounts are likely to be those who enjoy good health status. When they withdraw from the common insurance risk pool, they leave behind a population likely to face higher insurance premiums, because the average risk in the remaining risk pool is now higher.

Proposals for comprehensive national health insurance coverage have been particularly important public policy concerns in decades past. With rare exceptions, these proposals have failed to become policy. Democratic and Republican presidents since Harry Truman have moved onto the national agenda one or more proposals to expand Americans' access to health insurance or improve their coverage. Yet each saw his proposals radically scaled back or rejected. All proposals tend to stumble over the same concerns: the role of the public sector versus the private sector; who will pay the enormous costs; whether the plan will be means-tested, so that those who can pay more do pay more; and the potential burden on employers of the paperwork that tends to be associated with most plans.

So the debate goes on and stays interesting because the users of health care—the patients—are real, their problems are serious, and the stakes are quite high. Absent any clear vision, or consensus on solutions, or sustained interest in the issue, the U.S. policy process is designed to default to inaction. And so it does on most major reform options. Yet seldom does a Congress adjourn without having made important changes in health policy. There is always something interesting happening.

This book examines the United States' experience with governing health. It is a political science book about health care policy. As such, it presents health care policy as the product of the U.S. system of government, combining several forces:

— the persistent power of ideological polarization and party politics;
— the dominant need for members of Congress to constantly seek reelection, claim credit, trade votes, and overcome uncertainty in their policy choices;
— the waxing and waning persuasive power of the presidency, promising much, sometimes delivering, but more often disappointing;
— the discretion exercised by the bureaucracy in its role as agent of the president, Congress, the courts, its clients, and the public;
— the pervasive and well-financed influence of the burgeoning army of health interests, the coalitions they form, and the strategies they employ to frame issues and shape health policy to their liking;
— the continuing struggle of the states, torn between sovereigns and supplicants in their wish to call on the federal government for more financial support but desperate to control their own health policy destinies; and
— the challenge of effective problem definition, the choice of solutions, and various models of the policy process, all incomplete but each capturing an aspect of the insights we need if we are ever to predict policy outcomes.

In addition, we use a chronicle of the MMA to demonstrate the longitudinal dimension of health policy, the critical roles of presidents, commissions, foundations, bureaucrats, researchers, committee chairs, party leaders, and interest groups.

The book originally grew out of a frustration at the absence of a text written by political scientists for use in health politics classes. Sociologists and economists have authored or contributed to a small number of worthy volumes bringing their own disciplines' perspectives to the topic of health politics and policy, and though they have much to offer, a gap remains. Politics is more than the sociology of institutions or economic self-interest. And health care policy is politics at its richest and fullest. Politics is about power, and the making of health policy is nothing if not the wielding of power. Institutional rules endow some actors with more power than others, differential endowments of other types give some interests more power than others, and the fleeting saliency of the issues themselves sometimes gives one side more bargaining power than the other. This book illuminates how the institutions and the policy-making process work to wield power over health policy.

The intended audience is health policy analysts who want to become more adept at gauging the political feasibility of their proposals; health professionals who seek a better understanding of how policy is made and how they might alter and change it; health system managers who are savvy enough to see that in a system in which nearly half the money and most of the paperwork burden come from government, they need to understand how government makes its policies; and finally, political scientists who seek illustrations of how the principles of government work in a policy arena with all the magical ingredients of political conflict: saliency, huge financial stakes, powerful interests, and venues in all the institutions of government. The book presents a comprehensive synthesis of political science research on the institutions of government and the policy process and an extensive review of the policies that have governed health care for more than a generation.

The book is divided into two parts. Part I describes the institutions of government, reflecting the insights of political science research into the interaction of structures and motivations influencing their members. Part II then describes the policy process, including an illustration of how the theories worked to produce the MMA. A conclusion pulls together the political and policy components of the book.

A central focus of the book is on documenting change in the nation's chief political institutions over time. In part I, we use the device of beginning each chapter with a comparison of how different the institutions under study looked during the various periods, beginning in the mid-1960s, when new presidential administrations began their policy-making quest that ushered in a new era of public health policy:

— President Lyndon Johnson in 1965, riding the crest of a Democratic wave of power and ideas and a growing consensus that the poor elderly, at least, deserved public health care subsidy, only to stretch the compromise by eliminating means testing from his Medicare proposal;

— President Ronald Reagan in 1981, ushered in with a mandate to shrink and constrain government-supported health care, welfare, and social services, overseeing the passage of a major Medicare expansion program to cover catastrophic events and costs;

— President Bill Clinton in 1993, quite inexpertly misinterpreting Americans' concerns that their insurance might be canceled as a mandate for employer-subsidized universal coverage, only to have his congressional supporters punished at the next election, sweeping in the first Republican-dominated House in 40 years; and

— President George W. Bush in 2005, unable to build, or uninterested in building, on the successful passage of the MMA, the largest expansion of Medicare since its inception.

Each chapter in part I relates changes in the institutions to these touch points and others, reflecting the conviction that only through a longitudinal view of policy making can one accurately identify trends and chart the enduring progress of ideas and changes in ideologies and political positions.

Chapter 1 describes the structures and functioning of Congress and the motivations of its members. Its theme is that Congress was intended as, and has continued to be, the dominant branch of government. The chapter begins with a review of the motivations and sources of ideas of the framers, who conferred on the legislative branch enormous powers and many binding constraints. We describe shifts in power of party and institutional leadership relative to committee and subcommittee chairs in the context of their roles and responsibilities and sources of power, including personality and institutional rules. Committees and subcommittees of special importance to health care policy receive the most attention. We discuss conference committees, a central source of policy making in health care but little understood, and give examples of how they rewrite legislation, often on the fly.

Budgeting, the increasingly dominant task of a deficit-swelling Congress, is closely examined; we step carefully between the concepts that are likely to continue to characterize the process and the changing rules and terms that complicate its understanding. A chapter section devoted to legislative parties addresses the paradox of their uncertain importance in the nation at large but their increasingly powerful role in Congress. Incumbency and its benefits and persistent reelection statistics highlight the discussion of congressional motivations, and this discussion introduces a review of the considerable political science literature on congressional behavior and its evolution. This chapter illustrates the growing importance of partisanship and its implications for strengthening the hand of party leaders.

Chapter 2 examines the presidency, starting with the sources and scope of presidential power and the high-stakes but sibling-like rivalry that characterizes the relationship between the presidency and Congress even in the best of times. Focused as the book is on health care policy making, the subject of this chapter is the domestic president and how he makes choices about proposals and solutions for domestic problem solving. While his role in setting the agenda and proposing initiatives in his state of the union addresses and other forums, and his monitoring of the progress of proposed solutions, are closely examined, a theme of the chapter is that there is much truth to the axiom that a president proposes but Congress disposes. The president is much more influential than any of the 535 members who work for or against him, but he is not, in the final analysis, a legislator. We examine the measures of presidential legislative success, though their validity becomes somewhat equivocal when the president's party controls both houses. Clearly he would be less successful if he could not count on the strong support of congressional leaders to add to or subtract from his proposals in whatever ways prove necessary to pull support from the wings of his party, manage the conference committee, and discipline recalcitrant party members.

Bureaucracy nominally reports to the president, too, though few presidents have found effective ways to use it, leaving its direction much more to Congress than is suggested by government manuals' organization charts. But when the president and both houses are controlled by the same party, bureaucrats find that they have fewer opportunities to resist their political leaders. That other bureaucracy, the White House staff, has shown itself likely to consume the managerial talents of many presidents, though less so with a president who sees his role as CEO of an organization largely run by those to whom he has delegated power and responsibility.

In chapter 3 we describe the zealous hucksterings of that diverse congeries of niche groups, coalitions, political action committees, and groundswell participants that engage in lobbying, campaign financing, and grassroots organizing to try to keep things off the public agenda or shape them to their liking when they cannot. A theme of the chapter is that interest groups are extremely influential—and in many instances, the controlling influence—in health care policy making. With their money, organizing skills, and singularity of purpose, they are altogether competent and only too happy to show a legislator the correct path toward constituent service and comfortable reelection margins. Another theme is that interest groups have always been one of the key institutions of government. We do not suggest that groups always or even usually act in the public interest. Much of President Bush's success in passing the MMA can be attributed to party leaders' willingness to remove from the bill or greatly modify those provisions that key interest groups found offensive—whether or not the public strongly supported those provisions.

We examine how interest groups form and stay together, including the role of economic self-interest, selective benefits, and entrepreneurs, the dominant role of occupational alliances, and the deliberate or inadvertent role of government itself in sometimes spawning groups. The interest-group world of today is much more complex than that of the 1960s or earlier. It is now characterized by permanent and temporary coalitions that share and complement one another's strengths and resources. Counts show a hugely increased number of interest groups. Their unglamorous daily ardor for monitoring legislation and providing information is the essential ingredient in that magic elixir of influence—access—which must precede their ability to provide a pearl or two of information that may sway a critical decision. We describe the ways in which these groups alter strategies as they move through the many venues of government, as well as the strategies they employ in campaign giving and grassroots campaigning. The link, or lack of it, between the giving of money and casting of votes is examined, but there seems little doubt that coupled with features of congressional decision making described in chapter 1, the role of interest groups makes health reform all that much harder.

Chapter 4 takes a sympathetic view of public bureaucracy. Bureaucracy here is viewed as a repository of expertise, of detail people who bring the long view to the policy process and stand ready to serve their multiple masters—Congress, the president, the courts, their beneficiary constituents, and their regulatory foes—but who suffer as much when pulled in multiple directions as when they are ignored. The differences between careerists and politicos, the nature of an agency's political environment, and the importance of its mission are highlighted in a comprehensive review of the fascinating literature that describes how bureaucrats function, their relationship to the other branches of government, and the incentives and constraints that govern their behavior.

Both sides of the argument over whether bureaucrats are getting weaker or stronger are advanced, and though we choose neither side as more correct, a rich array of examples from health care policy leaves the clear impression that bureaucrats influence all aspects of the process, especially their own particular province: implementation. There is no question that bureaucracy is more effectively controlled by political leaders whose partisan ideology is shared by the president and leaders of both houses when government is not divided by party. Under such circumstances, it is unlikely that complaints to key committees by bureaucrats who feel pressured to bend to presidential will are likely to result in the launching of congressional investigations to haul a secretary before an unfriendly committee hearing.

A substantial portion of chapter 4 is devoted to regulation and the factors that modulate the degree of success agencies enjoy or suffer in gaining industry compliance. An overarching point is that no matter how green the eyeshades, regulation is political and agency performance is evaluated with a political yardstick. We examine the health agencies, describe their turf, and weigh their political fortunes in the light of past performance and as viewed by important beholders.

Chapter 5 traces the evolution of state governments from the good old days of the good old boys of the 1950s and 1960s through their own awakening and federalism's many redefinitions. The case is easy to make that most states today are modern, savvy, lean, innovative, socially responsible, and politically independent power centers—with huge differences in resources to be sure, but determined to regain their autonomy and not to lose their identity. They still want all they can get from the federal domestic budget, but they have grown weary of the federal government's presuming that Washington knows better how to spend the money to solve problems.

A theme of the chapter is that while no one was watching, the states reformed their governance and became important players in health care provision and policy. One major section recounts the long list of state health innovations, suggesting that most ideas about health policy reform offered by the federal government began as a state initiative. One message we want to convey is that the future is likely to see more of the same, especially if the federal government removes some of the barriers it has erected to state innovation. Unfortunately, interest groups have figured out that when state innovation begins to cut into their profits too substantially, they can appeal to Congress to preempt state law by going forward with a federal program.

Institutions are again a central focus in chapter 5, highlighted by a close examination of state-to-state differences and similarities and comparisons with the federal government in the areas of budgets, spending, revenues, and documentation of the rapacious effects of Medicaid and other health spending on states' ability to set their own agendas. We examine the unique state feature known as direct democracy—initiative, referendum, and recall—and consider its benefits and liabilities. Also discussed is the impact of legislative term limits in more than a dozen states—including several of the nation's largest.

Beginning the discussion of the policy process in part II, chapter 6 defines public policy, its evolution, unintended consequences, and demands. We describe various attempts to categorize public policies and their value in understanding the effect of the type of policy on its politics, and vice versa. We also describe several frameworks of the policy process, including David Baron's model, new to this edition, and provide a compendium of examples of the political ways in which health care problems get defined as part of the effort to widen the scope of conflict and to interest the uninterested so that topics move to the public agenda. Problems do not just emerge; they are carefully nurtured, defined, framed, and often exaggerated to promote a desired policy solution. Ultimately, a decision must be made on whether a problem augurs for a public or a private solution, a choice inevitably tied to the often controversial concern about the role of government. Finally, theories of policy change are presented and analyzed.

Chapter 7 chronicles the passage of the MMA, tracing its policy legacy to the 1980s and showing that ideas shaped in one Congress become the starting point for negotiations in the next. The problem of drug costs became a rallying point in the presidential campaigns and a focus in the 2000 debates, and ultimately perceived by the new Republican president as a chance to rip a key plank from the Democratic Party's platform. Armed with the reality that budget deficits growing at rapid rates would probably make the Congress of 2003 the last chance for a drug bill, groups such as the AARP and health policy advocates such as Sen. Edward Kennedy (D-MA)—who might otherwise have opposed such a limited improvement in coverage—relented and threw their weight behind the GOP proposal. Traditional opponents such as the Pharmaceutical Research and Manufacturers of America (PhRMA) decided they would be better off supporting a program that specifically avoided their worst nightmares—firms having to negotiate Medicare drug prices with the federal bureaucracy, or drugs being imported from abroad. Committee chairs, especially the chair of the powerful Senate Finance Committee, demanded and got what was good for their districts. Party leaders made the concessions to interest groups needed to win their support, bent congressional rules to the point of breaking, controlled the conference committee to the point of excluding most minority party members, and used pork-barrel promises in the bill, and in others that came later, to buy the votes of their party members. When the vote was finally taken in the wee small hours of the morning, after a record-setting delay, Republicans won by a narrow margin.

We conclude the book with a prognosis for health care policy, predicting an era of vigorous efforts by both federal and state governments to control their financial obligations through much tougher payment and subsidy policies.

For those comparing the first, second, and third editions, we offer the following guide to changes:

— Our first priority was to update examples and theory perspectives, keeping older examples only when they were too good to lose and favoring more recent incarnations of theory perspectives over more dated presentations of what may be classic ideas.

— We updated all statistics.

— We replaced the case study of the 1997 Balanced Budget Act in the second edition with a case study of the MMA in this edition. It focuses attention on, and illustrates the critical importance of, party leaders and also provides an opportunity for making use of the theories and concepts advanced and summarized in the previous chapters.

— We added information on changes in the institutions over the years since the second edition, and we updated our prognostications, which, wisely, we had made for the coming 10 years, so that in most cases we were either right or not yet wrong.

Part I

Health Policy and Institutions

1

Congress

A LOOK BACK

1965

DEMOCRATS SEEMED to be everywhere when the first roll of the 89th Congress was called on January 4, 1965. So tightly squeezed in were House members that many found it more comfortable to stand at the railing around the back of the chamber. There were 155 more Democrats than Republicans in the House, and 36 more in the Senate, the product of a Democratic landslide victory that would make possible feats of legislative legerdemain seldom seen in the almost always fractious Congress. There was the usual splintering of Democrats, which typically separated Northerner from Southerner and big-city from small-town Democrat, but when sufficient numbers of Democrats stuck together, they could pass almost anything. Their newly elected president, Lyndon B. Johnson, meant to take full advantage of the majority held by his party to tackle a huge legislative agenda: Medicare, Medicaid, maternal and child health programs, health planning, regional medical programs, physician training programs, programs aimed at specific diseases (including cancer and heart disease)—not to mention civil rights, education, economic opportunity, model cities, urban mass transit, nutritional programs for the poor, and more. Though some of these subjects—civil rights and Medicare, for example—were among the most divisive issues in American politics, this Congress would tackle them all and pass legislation on most of them.

In 1965, John McCormack was the Speaker of the House, and Mike Mansfield the majority leader of the Senate. While both were well-respected and talented legislators, their powers were constrained by the strength of the committees, headed by Southerners. The North-South split was the greatest source of conflict in the Democratic Party. The 1964 Johnson landslide brought 42 new Northern Democrats into the House and forced a change in the balance of party power. The Ways and Means Committee was transformed; a bare majority of curmudgeons had steadfastly refused to allow a payroll tax to finance Medicare. Legislative leaders, urged by the president, took every opportunity to replace them one by one.

Medicare, usually in its broader incarnation called "national health insurance," had been the subject of bitter debates, media fear campaigns, and committee-blocking tactics for some two decades. But with its decisive majority, the 89th Congress would (after considerable bargaining and compromises aimed at splitting interest-group opposition) roll over its opposition. As the final vote on Medicare was being tallied and the outcome became clear, one member of the Republican leadership stormed out of the House center-aisle doors and in exasperation turned to the pages and house doorkeepers gathered there to watch the show, and exploded: "We've got Goldwater to thank for this." He was referring to the fact that the defeat of the 1964 Republican presidential candidate, Barry Goldwater, had been so decisive as to sweep in the large Democratic majority, which could now run roughshod over the shrunken Republican minority.

1981

Contrast the bold, decisive, ideologically unalloyed Democratic juggernaut of 1965 and its massive show of party strength with the Congress of 1981—a time when the seeds of conservatism and antigovernment sentiment, growing in the late 1970s, had flourished to produce a Republican landslide presidential election and the first Republican majority in the Senate in a quarter-century (table 1.1).

Republicans picked up 34 seats in the House and 12 in the Senate. An

Table 1.1

Congressional Parties and Leaders in 1965, 1981, 1993, and 2005

Year and Congress	House of Representatives	Senate
1965, 89th Congress	295 Democrats	68 Democrats
	140 Republicans	32 Republicans
	Speaker: John McCormack (MA)	Majority leader: Mike Mansfield (MT)
1981, 97th Congress	243 Democrats	46 Democrats
	192 Republicans	53 Republicans
	Speaker: Thomas P. "Tip" O'Neill (MA)	Majority leader: Howard Baker (TN)
1993, 103th Congress	258 Democrats	57 Democrats
	176 Republicans	43 Republicans
	Speaker: Thomas Foley (WA)	Majority leader: George Mitchell (ME)
2005, 109th Congress	201 Democrats	44 Democrats
	232 Republicans	55 Republicans
	Speaker: Dennis Hastert (IL)	Majority leader: Bill Frist (TN)

Source: Office of the Clerk, U.S. House of Representatives, 2005.

Note: Excludes independents and vacancies, typically one or two of each per Congress.

oppressed minority for a quarter-century, they relished their new leadership role in the Senate. Liberal critics said Republicans had been put in charge only because voters were dominated by the "me" generation, yuppies who had lost faith in—or could no longer see themselves benefiting from—public programs. Republicans retorted that liberals had had their chance. Health care reforms would take the shape of reduced spending, prospective budgets, and narrowed eligibility rules for subsidized services. This was nothing short of a sea change in the role of government, made possible by the Republicans' majority in the Senate, a large enough minority in the House to forge a majority with Democrats who strayed from their party's dominant positions, and, for a time, Democrats' fear that the popular Republican president could hurt them in the next election.

But the Democrats had a few resources of their own. They were not so easily split as in the old days, when quarrels over racial policies sent Southerners across the aisle looking for allies. Party leaders were stronger. No longer could they be held hostage by feudal committee chairs who bottled up legislation they didn't favor, snubbing their noses at their party's majority. Leaders had been given their own weapons by a series of reforms in the early 1970s, which were gleefully used by the large first-year class of 1974 elected on the heels of Watergate (named for the site of the attempted burglary of the Democratic National Party Headquarters in 1972, which led two years later to the resignation of President Richard Nixon). The party's leaders now appointed members of the Rules Committee, which set the rules for floor debate on most bills; leaders could refer bills to multiple committees, virtually ensuring that at least one committee would report a bill; and leaders played a crucial role in awarding committee assignments by appointing a majority of the members of the steering and policy committee—the committee that made appointments. Leaders were more aggressive and more willing to use institutional resources to a greater extent than those who had served in previous Congresses (Herrick and Moore 1993).

But one price of clipping the wings of committee chairs was fragmentation. Subcommittees had filled the power vacuum, and, with their own staffing and considerable autonomy, subcommittee chairs and members could become expert in health policy and use their influence to profoundly shape the legislative proposal that went to the full committee (Bowler 1987). House Energy and Commerce Health Subcommittee chair Henry Waxman embodied this new entrepreneurial subcommittee chair. Accepting the reality that no comprehensive health care program would see the light of day in the near term, he adopted an incrementalist approach: gradual expansion of Medicaid, the federal-state health care program for people who are poor or disabled, to cover more and more near-poor individuals, starting with children and their mothers. This approach worked for eight years. Every year between 1984 and 1991, at least one federal law expanding Medicaid eligibility and/or services was enacted, until opposition from state governors finally persuaded the powerful Senate Finance Committee chair to put an end to Medicaid mandates in 1991 (C. Weissert 1992).

1993

The Congress faced by President Bill Clinton in 1993 was again different. The 1992 elections brought in the largest first-year class in the House since 1946: 76 Democrats and 54 Republicans. But these newcomers were not political neophytes. Many had come up through the political ranks, including state legislative stints. Along the way they had lost the patience and humility usually expected of first-year representatives. After five months of toeing the line, they began showing their independence. With 82 more Democrats than Republicans in the House, the president's hallmark budget and tax package passed with only two votes to spare. Was this the party that would try a year later to overhaul a health system comprising more than one-seventh of the economy, and potentially displace 3.1 million workers?

Leadership had also changed. Though powerful on paper, the current crop of leaders had a more mellow style than their predecessors. Rather than commanding their troops, modern leaders had learned to act as "agents in pursuing the party's legislative agenda" (Rohde 1991, 35). Their job had become more collegial, using the powers granted to them to accomplish goals they held in common with other members of Congress. Rather than raw power, leaders counted on homogeneity of values. Where it existed, leadership could be granted discretion and expect to be followed; where it did not, members would go their own way. Since the late 1970s, Speakers had relied heavily on the party whip organization to enhance morale, build support for party positions, and poll members. Since the 1980s, around 20 percent of Democratic House members had been part of the whip "organization," which met weekly with the leadership to "enhance their two-way communication with members" (Rohde 1991, 93) and make the leadership more effective in advancing its program.

House Speaker Thomas Foley (D-WA) showed his distaste for bare knuckles early in the session. Eleven Democratic subcommittee chairs voted with the Republicans against the administration's budget. Some in the party wanted to "strip" the chairs of their subcommittees, but Speaker Foley demurred, preferring instead to share the task of reprimanding recalcitrants by forcing caucus elections of all subcommittee chairs.

The president had even less power to force compliance with his program. Thanks to independent candidate Ross Perot, President Clinton had been elected with only 43 percent of the popular vote—a smaller margin than any member of either House. He would be of limited use at reelection time. This would become important when members of his party splintered in their support for health care reform: one gaggle demanding complete government takeover of financing while, at the other extreme, another group pressed for everything to be voluntary. In a word, the Democratic Party controlling the House lacked the discipline required to produce a legislative program.

2005

By January 2005, the Republicans had held control over the House of Representatives for a decade. The number of Republicans in the 109th Congress beginning that month was higher than in any of the previous five Congresses, but it was still relatively small—232 of 435 seats. But the numbers were never a problem for the Republicans. For most of the decade, they had operated boldly and confidently, continuing to push forward a conservative domestic agenda that included two major tax cuts, a faith-based initiative, and a major new federal program in education. The early years of Congress in the twenty-first century were defined largely by nonhealth issues, indeed nondomestic issues, as the country recovered from the September 11, 2001, attacks and launched major military action in Afghanistan and Iraq. However, in 2003 the Republicans in Congress followed the lead of their Republican president, George W. Bush, and enacted a major health program—adding a prescription drug benefit to the popular Medicare program.

The early reign of the Republican Congress was a political and policy tour de force. Led by the visionary but sometimes abrasive Speaker Newt Gingrich (R-GA), the Republicans took control of the House in 1994 for the first time since 1952. After making several structural reforms, including increasing the power of the leadership (and reducing the power of committees), the Republican majority overreached and underestimated the popularity and steadfastness of Democratic President Bill Clinton, and lost in several well-publicized public relations disasters. But with George W. Bush in the White House, in 2003, the House, Senate, and president were all Republicans—the first unified Republican regime since Dwight D. Eisenhower was in the White House.

The House in 2005 was notably different than it was 10 years before—under the last Democratic majority. Changes included term limits for party chairs and selection of committee chairs (and appropriations subcommittee chairs) by a leadership-dominated steering committee. Minority party members were barred from conference committee participation, and an omnibus appropriations measure replaced traditional appropriations bills. (However, in 2005, Congress voted to return to the individual spending measures.) Speaker Dennis Hastert (R-IL), mild-mannered and reluctant to take on visible, aggressive positions or appearances, was nonetheless stalwart and determined to pursue a conservative Republican agenda without the assistance of Democrats. This required near lockstep allegiance from party members—a situation he achieved much more often than not. Partisan voting was at an all-time high for Republicans and Democrats alike, in a Congress where turnover was extremely low. Even following the 2001 redistricting in all 50 states, 98 percent of incumbents in the House were reelected, and, of the few who were not (a paltry 16), half were in contests pitting two incumbents against each other (Dodd and Oppenheimer 2005).

The Senate, too, was a different place in 2005. Still the more staid and less partisan of the two bodies, the Senate was more partisan and less civil than in recent memory. The traditional gentlemen's agreement between majority and minority leaders was dashed in the 2004 election when Republican majority leader Bill Frist (TN) actively campaigned for the Republican who was trying to unseat Democratic minority leader Tom Daschle (SD). Offering amendments on the Senate floor increased over the decade, and voting became more partisan. Senate and House Republicans complained about each other in the media as the Senate successfully stymied House-passed legislation that senators considered too strident or simply misguided.

Both congressional parties relied on communication techniques to keep their own members in line and to help "frame" issues for the general public. Distinctions between campaigning and policy making blurred as media consultants, blogs, focus groups, and message boards came to play major roles in the election and in informing constituents. Howard Dean, Democratic governor of Vermont, was early and highly successful in raising money for his short but meteoric presidential campaign in 2004, and both political parties, interest groups, and members of Congress followed suit in using the Web for raising money, encouraging participation, sharing information, and shaping public discourse (in English and Spanish).

Finally, the Republican president, George W. Bush, emboldened by his reelection, proposed an ambitious recasting of the popular Social Security program and, less robustly but similarly important, proposed a revamping of Medicaid. In his first term, the president had almost always had his way with a Republican Congress in which party leaders cast the party's electoral future with this president. It was much less so in his second term.

POWERS AND CONSTRAINTS

Many people forget that for its first 13 years, the United States operated under the Articles of Confederation, which set up a weak national government and strong states. The experiment failed, and a convention ostensibly called only to modify the Articles of Confederation took the opportunity to rewrite the institutional power structure in significant ways. When the debate ended, a national government had been designed that placed primary power in a legislative body that was split between a popularly elected House of Representatives and an elitist Senate elected by the state legislatures, and was further checked by the powers of an energetic executive with veto power and a strong appointed judiciary. Any tendencies central government might have to wield power with a heavy hand would be checked internally by its own structure. In turn, democracy running amok in the states could be restrained by the powers granted to the national government.

The Constitution, like the country it reflects, is far from static, however, and the carefully balanced power relationships of 1789 have been skewed over the years. Thanks in part to some key Supreme Court decisions, the national government is the most important player in federalism. (Although the Court in the late 1990s rediscovered and reinvigorated federalism by ruling against broad federal power in a number of cases; see for example, Schram and C. Weissert 1999.) Congress is the dominant player among the three coequal branches. Such dominance would have suited at least one of the Founding Fathers, James Madison, just fine: "In republican government, the legislative authority necessarily predominates" (quoted in Oleszek 1989, 1). Two hundred years have proved him correct.

CONGRESSIONAL STRUCTURE

The bicameral nature of the congressional structure, carefully designed by the framers, is an important element in national policy making. Political scientists have studied the effect of bicameralism and concluded that the presence of a second chamber does tend to provide a check on potentially volatile and misled majorities in one house and that bicameralism is central in shaping policy outcomes (Hammond and Miller 1987; Janiskee 1995). In 1995, Americans witnessed what has been dubbed "cooling the coffee" as the Republican-led House passed 27 of 29 elements of the Republicans' "Contract with America" in the first 100 days of the session; the Senate, in contrast, passed only 3 and expressly rejected 1 contract measure. Two more provisions were later included in the 1996 welfare reform act (Temporary Aid to Needy Families) and the 1997 Balanced Budget Act. In recent Congresses, the Senate has continued to apply its brakes on House policy preferences. Sinclair (2005) reported that over the 103rd, 104th, 105th, and 107th Congresses, some 33 major measures were passed by the House but not by the Senate. Over that same period, only 3 major measures were passed by the Senate but not by the House.

The institutions and those who serve in them are vastly different. U.S. senators serve six-year terms, are elected statewide (thanks to a 1913 constitutional amendment), and tend to have a broader, more long-term focus than their colleagues on the other side of the Capitol. The Senate has 100 members, 2 from every state regardless of population. The House has 435 members, allocated on a state's relative population. Delegation sizes vary from 1 member representing each of the Dakotas, Alaska, Montana, Wyoming, Delaware, and Vermont to 53 from California. Since the size of the House membership remains stable, population shifts cause changes in the distribution of members every 10 years following the census. For example, in 1992, among other changes, Michigan lost 2 members; California added 7. Ten years later, in 2002, New York and Pennsylvania each lost 2 seats, Michigan and other Midwestern states and Mississippi and Oklahoma each lost 1 seat, while California, Nevada, Colorado, and North Carolina all gained 1, and Arizona, Texas, Georgia, and Florida all gained 2 seats. The population was shifting south and west, and so was the House.

In an unusual move, in 2003 the newly Republican Texas legislature redrew congressional districts that had been in place for only one election. The redistricting was the result not of court rulings but rather of the desire of the Republican congressional leadership to increase its margin in the House by drawing lines that would help ensure Republican victories by pitting popular Democratic members against each other. It was clearly a power play, fully acknowledged by House majority leader Tom DeLay from Texas, the mastermind of the plan. He said simply, "I'm the majority leader, and we want more seats" (Riddlesperger 2005). And he got them. The 2005 Texas congressional delegation added six new Republicans (increasing from 15 to 21).

In recent years, the Senate has attracted extremely wealthy people, often without prior political experience, who use their own resources to fund their campaigns. For example, a candidate spent more than $35 million in the 2000 Democratic primary in New Jersey to capture the nomination from a far better-known former governor. About one in four senators are millionaires. Few are women, and far fewer are African American or of other minority groups. The House is more representative, but only in comparison to the Senate. In good years, 10 to 15 percent of representatives may be women, and perhaps another 10 to 15 percent members of a minority group. In 2005 there were 65 women (voting members) in the House (3 other women were nonvoting delegates), or 15.6 percent of the membership, and 14 in the Senate (14 percent)—an all-time high. The banner year for election of women to the House remains the 1992 election, when 23 women were elected. The November 2004 election brought only 7 new women members.

Senators and House members in 2005 are older than in earlier years and have been in office longer. In the 108th Congress (2003–4), 32 House members were 70 years old or older, compared with only 19 in the 99th Congress in 1985; in the Senate, 24 senators were 70 years old or older, compared with only 6 in 1985. In 2004 there were 7 senators who had served 30 years or more, compared with only 2 in 1985. House seniority showed a less dramatic difference. In 1985 there were 10 members who had served 30 years or more; in 2004 there were 13 (U.S. Census Bureau 2005).

Newspaper columnist and commentator David Broder (1993) contended that the compromise that made the Senate a smaller and more lordly body than the House has run amok in recent years. A majority of senators come from states that collectively elect only 20 percent of the members of the House, and Senate leaders typically come from smaller states such as Maine, Kansas, Kentucky, Wyoming, West Virginia, and Mississippi. In 2005, the chairs of the powerful Appropriations, Finance, and Budget committees were from Alaska, Iowa, and New Hampshire. The Senate majority leader for that session was from Tennessee, and the minority leader from Nevada. The leaders of the House tend to come from large and medium-size states such as Texas, Illinois, Michigan, Washington, Missouri, and Georgia. A similar disparate domination of state legislatures by rural legislators in the 1950s made it impossible to pass progressive legislation for cities and suburbs until the U.S. Supreme Court ruled that state legislators had to be apportioned on the basis of population, not geographic area (*Reynolds v. Simms* 1964). Is such a reform possible for the Senate? No: the Constitution precludes amendments that strip away the geographic basis of Senate membership. Perhaps populous states should seek permission to split into two or more states to gain more equitable representation. Or the nation might follow the extreme remedy of one prominent congressional scholar, whose advice regarding the Senate was "Close it down. Put it out of its misery. It's just a bunch of egomaniacs looking around for people to fawn over them."

And no wonder they feel important. Senators have a greater chance of serving on desirable committees and achieve chair status more quickly than their House counterparts. Wording of legislation is hammered out in full committees, instead of subcommittees, and the Senate has fewer rules of procedure to restrict members' individuality. Amendments do not have to be germane to the subject of a bill. A senator can put a "hold" on a bill, requesting consultation before a measure is scheduled, and the common use of unanimous consent agreements (similar to rules issued by the House Rules Committee) requires extensive consultation and negotiation. One senator can temporarily halt floor action with a filibuster, which can be stopped only with 60 votes. And senators are no longer shy about using it.

Once a rarity, the filibuster has been used increasingly in recent years. In 2003, liberal Democrats filibustered against the Medicare Prescription Drug, Improvement and Modernization Act, arguing that it would privatize Medicare. However, 22 of the Senate's 48 Democrats voted with most Republicans to break the filibuster (Pear and Hulse 2003). Threats of filibuster have become even more frequent than actual filibusters, with some votes for cloture (to end the filibuster) taken before any filibuster actually occurs (Sinclair 2005). In 2005, the Democrats' use of filibusters on judicial nominations so angered the Republican majority leader that he threatened to abolish the use of the filibuster for judicial nominees. On the eve of the vote for the "nuclear option" to eliminate this use of the filibuster, a compromise was reached, preserving the judicial filibuster for extraordinary circumstances.

Unless a bill has 60 aggressive supporters who are willing to stay up late, a small group can defeat it in the Senate. No wonder that less than one-fourth of the bills introduced in a given two-year Senate session pass, compared with more than half of all bills in the middle of the last century. The House passes an even lower percentage—around 15 percent—but about twice as many bills are introduced in the House as in the Senate—around 5,000 per session in the House (and dropping), compared with fewer than 3,500 in the Senate (and also dropping in recent years). Bills take longer to consider nowadays than 50 years ago. Both houses' daily sessions are longer than in years past—close to 8 hours or more. Time in committee and subcommittee session has fallen over the years but is still substantial—around 2,000 hours in the Senate and more in the House (Ornstein, Mann, and Malbin 2002).

Many factors go into explaining why Congress may be working harder and producing less, including divided government, sharp partisan differences, budget constraints, and rules changes such as permitting cosponsorship of bills (which should produce fewer introductions and more passages per introduction, but may not). An increasing complexity of the content of bills is also a factor. Over the past 50 years, the number of pages of statute per Congress has nearly tripled. In recent years Congress has averaged 9 pages of law per statute, compared with only 2.5 pages in 1950 (Ornstein, Mann, and Malbin 2002).

Leadership

Both houses are organized by the political parties. The majority party selects a leader (Speaker in the House, majority leader in the Senate), who makes the decisions on scheduling, committee membership, the committees that bills get referred to, membership of "conference committees" to resolve differences in legislation passed by the two houses, and more (see box 1.1).

Not surprisingly, the strength of party leadership is affected by party unity and the personality of those chosen as leaders. Where party leadership is weak, committee chairs often gain in power. Congressional history is replete with pendulum shifts in the predominant source of power. In the 1890s, the Speakers were so strong as to be dubbed "Czar" Reed and "Boss" Cannon. The Speaker's powers were curbed shortly after the turn of the century, and for decades the power of committee chairs, and later subcommittee chairs, increased.

Information is important to party leaders—both providing information to rank-and-file members about the party position and obtaining information on the preferences of the rank and file. Information sharing takes place through (1) the activities of the party whips, whose job it is to serve as liaison for the rank and file; (2) the views of party whips who represent different "factions" of the party; and (3) regular caucus meetings (M. Jones and Hwang 2005).

However, as Speaker of the House (1995–98), Newt Gingrich reminded us how a dedicated and resourceful Speaker can make an enormous difference in both process and policy. Under Gingrich, House rules changed to strengthen the Speaker and to expedite passage of desired legislation. Informal rules changed as well, including an increasing role of some interest groups in policy development, manipulation of the media, reliance on task forces rather than committees, and extensive use of political consultants to chart legislative strategies and to gain public support. The Republican Speaker following Gingrich, Dennis Hastert, has continued the strong Speaker role, but in a much less public and egocentric manner. Under Hastert, committee chairs continue to have four-term limits, although the term limits for the Speaker were lifted. Committee chairs must meet the approval of a steering committee dominated by party leadership. In a new development, appropriations subcommittee chairs must also be approved by the steering committee. Members who support the party leadership will be rewarded, and those who do not will be punished. The Speaker has not hesitated to skip over senior members to install loyal party members as committee chairs. Decisions on most major bills are made in party caucuses or in leaders' offices, limiting

Box 1.1
Party Leadership in the U.S. Congress

The main leadership positions in the Congress are the Speaker of the House, the House majority and minority leaders, the House majority and minority whips, and the Senate majority and minority leaders.

The House of Representatives

The Speaker of the House is formally elected by the chamber as a whole, though really chosen by majority caucus. The Speaker presides over the House, shapes the agenda by deciding which bills have priority and on which calendar they appear, refers bills to appropriate committees, and designates members of joint and conference committees. The Speaker is the majority party spokesperson in the House, assisted by a number of party leaders, including:

— the majority leader, who formulates that party's legislative program in cooperation with the Speaker and other party leaders, helps steer the program through the chamber, and assists in establishing the legislative schedule;

— the minority leader, who has the top leadership position for the minority party, formulates the party's legislative program in conjunction with other leaders, helps steer the program through the chamber, and serves as the party spokesperson for that chamber;

— party whips, who assist both the majority and the minority leaders, mobilize party members behind legislative positions that the leadership has decided are in the party's interest, and keep an accurate count of the votes and preferences of members on bills.

The Senate

According to the U.S. Constitution, the vice president of the United States assumes the post of president of the Senate and presides over it. In the vice president's absence, the president pro tempore (a powerless, honorific position) generally presides over the Senate.

The primary leadership duties are performed by the majority leader, who is the spokesperson for the majority party. He schedules floor action, formulates the party's legislative program, schedules bills, works with committee chairs on actions of importance to the party, and directs strategy on the floor. The minority leader is the spokesperson for the party, mobilizes support for minority party positions, and directs the minority party's strategy. He does not appoint committee chairs. Until 1995, seniority dominated chair selections. When the Republicans became the majority party, they changed the rules, permitting members to select their chair by secret ballot, regardless of seniority.

The role of Senate whips is similar to that of House whips: aiding party leadership in developing a program, transmitting information to party members, conducting vote counts, and persuading members.

the role of committee discussions and markup (a process in which the committee makes changes in the bill's language). Finally, the House Committee on Rules is not shy about rules that limit or deny Democrats the opportunity to offer amendments.

Hastert has also used the Speaker's powers on the House floor to good advantage—holding roll-call votes open for long periods of time, calling tough votes at a very late hour to minimize media attention, and keeping certain issues off the floor entirely. He has orchestrated efforts to keep Democrats out of committee deliberations until a consensus among Republican members has been fashioned. And he has used the resources of a Republican president to help rein in possible Republican hold-outs (Dodd and Oppenheimer 2005).

The Republican leadership has not always won—particularly in the early years of Hastert's leadership when he lost on several important bills, including a patients' bill-of-rights measure. To ensure the success of his proposal, he virtually shut down the work of the House health committees and shifted the debate to the House floor—where his own provision withholding the right of patients to sue their self-insured health maintenance organizations (HMOs) went down to defeat (Rogers 1999). However, in the early 2000s, the House Republicans were increasingly successful in getting their way, generally by marshalling every possible Republican vote. Although bipartisanship was initially promoted in the early years of the George W. Bush presidency, it was quickly abandoned in the House. The Republican strategy in 2004 was to win 218 votes (of 229) from House Republicans, thus obviating the need for Democratic crossovers. Leadership put pressure on members (threats of loss of committee chairs and earmarked district funds; promises of votes on cherished bills and of funding for a family member's congressional campaign) and bent the rules to get what it wanted. A case in point was the MMA of 2003, a major change in the Medicare program and one that was desired by Congress and the president. In a vote beginning at 3 a.m. (unusual in its own right), Republican leaders held the floor open for votes for nearly three hours, until the initial vote of 215–219 became 220–215 (Schickler and Pearson 2005).

On "party votes," or those votes important to party leadership, both Republican and Democratic leaders often expect their members to vote the right way. Failing to do so can lead to future problems. In the last few years, the House Democratic leadership has become tougher—punishing members who do not vote with the party. In the vote on the MMA in 2003, nine Democrats voted for the measure in spite of strong opposition from the party. While those nine were not threatened with losing any positions (they are, after all, the minority party), they were faced with possibly being passed over for plum committees or travel opportunities. Even more problematic was possible loss of money for their districts. Rep. David Obey (D-WI), ranking member on Appropriations, told colleagues that he would "not give a red cent" to any Democrat who "voted against us on Medicare" (Pershing, Billings, and Pierce 2003). In 2003, Democrats voted unanimously on 27 percent of roll calls, compared with around 10 percent in the 1970s and 1980s. Democrats have also been more active in stalling action via discharge petitions, appeals of rules, and motions to instruct. They have been more vocal in accusing Republican leaders of ethical violations (Schickler and Pearson 2005). Oleszek (2004) calls these actions "ad hoc lawmaking," in which each party finds new uses for old rules, employs innovative devices, or bypasses traditional procedures and processes to help its cause.

The strengthening of party leadership is to be expected, say Aldrich and Rohde (2005), when the policy preferences of party members become more homogeneous and the differences in ideology between the parties widen. In 2005, party voting was strikingly more common than in earlier years, and few failed to recognize the strong allegiance to ideology in both parties.

Committees

To Woodrow Wilson, writing in 1885 (1913, 79), "Congress in its committee-rooms is Congress at work." More than a century later, Wilson is still correct. Standing committees, about 20 in each house, are "the main paths along which Congress moves [and] all lead through the committee system" (Keefe 1984, 92). They are the "workhorses" of the legislature: considering legislation, holding hearings (often outside Washington), amending legislation, and supporting their product on the House floor. Conference committees are temporary, created to adjust differences between the chambers when the two houses pass different versions of legislation. Conference committees are crucial in resolving remaining issues but also serve as additional venues for lobbyists and others whose proposals failed to pass one or both houses.

Standing committees are those with stated jurisdictions, created by the rules of the House, permanent (unless rules are changed), and responsible for screening, examining, and reporting on the legislation referred to them. Committees are where ideas are debated, deals are cut, and interest groups ply their trade, and where partisanship is paramount. The stakes are high in committees, and members know it.

The influence of committees extends beyond Congress itself. They also wield considerable clout over the bureaucracy, conducting oversight or congressional review of the actions of the federal departments, agencies, and commissions and of the programs and policies they administer. When the party that is in the minority in a chamber is in the White House and charged with overseeing administrative agencies, the committees turn up the heat. But even a president of their own party does not go unwatched. Cabinet officers say they spend one-third of their time on Capitol Hill testifying before committees and meeting informally with congressional staff. One cabinet secretary serving under Clinton said he was "astonished at the degree to which Congress is present in my daily life and shares at every level" in the direction of his department (Broder and Barr 1993, 31).

There are clearly checks on the power of committee chairs. When House Appropriations Committee chair Robert Livingston removed a first-year member from a subcommittee in direct retaliation for his defection on a floor vote on that subcommittee's conference report, fellow first-year members protested to the party leadership. The ousted subcommittee member was granted a seat on the prestigious Budget Committee in compensation (Aldrich and Rohde 1995). Of course, the revolt and restitution were noteworthy for their rarity. Committee chairs more often than not get their way. However, under the Republicans, the power of committee chairs has declined relative to party leadership, since selection is no longer based on seniority. Instead, chairs can be deposed or members with less seniority installed as committee chairs—particularly if the lower-seniority members have agreed to be loyal to the party leadership goals.

Committees are not equal in power or popularity among members. House Ways and Means, Senate Finance, House and Senate Appropriations, House and Senate Budget, and House Rules are typically referred to as power or prestige committees. Membership on these committees is very competitive and highly prized by legislators who want to make a name for themselves in Congress. Leaders usually get their training there, learning to cut deals, avoid minefields, and work to balance the conflicting pressures of other committees, lobbyists, and the broader house membership.

Policy committees are responsible for authorizing legislation and are organized by subject area. Some policy committees are more attractive than others. Popular House policy committees are Energy and Commerce, Education and the Workforce, and Financial Services. Constituency committees are those that provide electoral benefits to members, including Agriculture, Transportation and Infrastructure, and Veterans' Affairs committees. Committee attractiveness can wax and wane with changing policy priorities and the recent esteem or repute in which a committee is held. During the 1980s, the House Judiciary Committee's popularity plummeted, and in the 1990s, following its embarrassing racially and gender-bias tainted hearings on the Supreme Court nomination of Clarence Thomas, found itself for a time unable to find enough members to fill all its slots.

Not surprisingly, there is more conflict on power committees than on policy and constituency committees. In the 104th Congress, there was conflict on 76 percent of the bills in the policy committees (excluding Rules and Budget), compared with 34 percent and 24 percent for policy and constituency committees, respectively (Aldrich and Rohde 2005).

Box 1.2 lists the eight committees and six subcommittees that have the most impact on health legislation. Only two are policy committees—the Senate Health, Education, Labor, and Pensions Committee and the House Energy and Commerce Committee—yet these two are extremely important in defining health policy. These committees plus a few others try to carve out a piece of any major health care reform proposal. The House Rules Committee and the leadership must then find a way to put the pieces together.

In recent years, with the rise of party leadership power, the importance of committees has diminished—especially compared with the 1950s and 1960s when committee chairs could single-handedly stop legislation desired by most of their colleagues and the nation. Party leaders can bypass committees by setting up independent task forces, attaching legislative riders to

---

Box 1.2
Committees and Subcommittees on Health

Senate Committee on Finance, Subcommittee on Health Care

House Committee on Ways and Mean, Subcommittee on Health

Senate Committee on Health, Education, Labor, and Pensions, Subcommittee on Bioterrorism and Public Health Preparedness

House Committee on Energy and Commerce, Subcommittee on Health

Senate Committee on Appropriations, Subcommittee on Labor, Health and Human Services, Education, and Related Agencies

House Committee on Appropriations, Subcommittee on Labor, Health and Human Services, Education, and Related Agencies

Senate Committee on the Budget

House Committee on the Budget

appropriations bills, having the House Rules Committee bring bills to the floor without committee hearings or markup, or adding provisions to conference committee reports. Nevertheless, the committee chairs are key players in the legislative process—especially for legislation that does not have high party interest. Committee chairs continue to control the staff and name subcommittee chairs (Oleszek 2004).

Theories of Committees

Political scientists have developed three theories to explain congressional organization: gains for trade, or distributive theory; information theory; and partisanship. All have an important element in common: they explain the institution's structure as the result of individuals pursuing their self-interests to solve collective-action problems. All members seek reelection, constituent benefits, and policy outcomes. The actions they take to achieve these individual ends more or less coincidentally serve the collective ends and explain why the institution is structured the way it is.

Gains for Trade

Legislatures can be viewed as a collective of members acting together to allocate public benefits. However, since legislators seek to please their constituents in order to be reelected, they must seek selective benefits for their constituents. To link these selective benefits with collective action, legislators seek to capture gains from trade or cooperation. Legislator A agrees to help legislator B by voting for B's bill, in exchange for B's help with A's bill. As long as the help A provides is worth less than the reward she gets from achieving her objectives, there is a net gain. This happy circumstance occurs more often than not, because legislators are heterogeneous in their preferences and priorities. Some care deeply about health policy, while others care little about it but have strong constituent or personal motivations for an interest in agriculture or international trade. Votes on health policy issues can be traded at little cost by the legislator with interests in agriculture in exchange for votes on agricultural issues, again, at low cost to the giver but high value to the receiver. This heterogeneity of preferences and priorities is an essential element of the gains-for-trade model. But one more element is needed to make the model work: that is, some way to enforce the deals—to make them "stick" over the months of congressional decision making. With some votes taken early in the session and others late in the session, legislator B needs a way to guarantee that legislator A does not renege or strike a new, better deal with legislator C. The body needs a way to institutionalize the exchanges so that a large number of decisions can be made efficiently and with the assurance that deals will be honored. Enter committees.

Those who care about health policy self-select onto health committees, for example, while those more concerned with agriculture or other issues choose one of those committees. Each committee is given disproportionate control over its issue by virtue of jurisdiction. Health committees control the agenda by receiving all health-related bills and deciding which ones they will kill and which they will hold hearings on, mark up, and send on to the full chamber. These "institutional endowments" related to agenda-setting authority are *a priori* because they precede the legislative process (Shepsle and Weingast 1994). Other endowments are called *post hoc* because they come after the house has acted (such as the high likelihood of serving on the conference committee, or oversight responsibility for the agency implementing the law). Together these endowments assure the committee that it will have disproportionate influence over policy in its area. This assures members interested in health policy that no one else has much of a chance of breaking the implicit deal these members made when they gave up similar disproportionate influence over other issues such as agriculture. Committee membership seals the deal because all members agree to give the committees disproportionate power over a set of issues within their jurisdiction.

The upside is that everybody gets rewarded by being able to influence the policies of most importance to them. The downside is the potential for moral hazard: raiding the treasury by writing policies that serve committee members' own districts outrageously at the expense of everyone else. To prevent this, more generalist committees such as Ways and Means and Rules were structured by leadership to be more representative of the whole party. Bills giving too many benefits to specialty committee members (health committee members, for example) will be rejected by the power committees. If not, they may be rejected on the floor. Fearful of such rejection, the specialty committees are well served by not being too selfish in the bills they write.

Information and Expertise

In contrast, the informational approach argues that committees form because of the need of individual members to ensure that the entire legislative body acquires and disseminates information. Information is vital because it reduces uncertainty. Expertise is essential because it helps members choose policies most likely to accomplish their policy goal and enhances their reelection prospects. Committees generate and provide information and expertise (Krehbiel 1992). Committee members who bear the high transaction costs of gathering information become experts and share their knowledge, not from altruistic motivations, but because they are rewarded by the organization. Transaction costs are lowered because only members with special interest and perhaps special background join the committees whose jurisdictional property rights give them incentives to become experts in such arcane fields as Medicaid policy. Free riding is discouraged because members' self-interest is served by gaining enough expertise and working hard enough on bill drafting to be able to cash in on the disproportionate influence that accompanies committee membership: agenda-setting power, bill drafting, hearings, the likelihood of conference committee membership, and oversight of the law's implementation. Committees that include a broad range of ideologies and views best serve the information needs of the body. Leadership, in this view, serves the party's interests by shaping committee membership to represent all the views of the party.

Partisanship

The third model explains congressional structure by focusing on legislative parties: it is the parties that provide the means for cooperation by which gains can be made for trade. Committees are the best way to organize, but committees require oversight and orchestration by party leaders to ensure that legislative efforts benefit party members (Cox and McCubbins 1993). Leaders serve as the agents of the membership, knowing that if the party is ill served, they will lose their power positions following defeat at the polls. Leaders thus face incentives to protect the membership by making sure committees represent party views; free riders are punished with loss of committee membership; bills not representative of the party preferences don't make it to the floor; and party priorities are helped along by exercise of the leadership's prerogatives, including power to control the calendar, interpret the rules, and make deals with the minority that help the party achieve its policy goals.

Forgette and Scruggs (2005) quantified anecdotal reports that the committee selection system is more partisan than in earlier years. They found that party loyalty, as measured by a member's attendance rate at Republican Party conferences, was a better predictor of Appropriations Committee and Ways and Means Committee assignments after the 1994 Republican takeover of Congress than before that time. They also found that traditional norms of key committee assignment behavior, including restrained partisanship, decayed in the wake of Republican House reforms. "Claimants today recognize that party fundraising and party fidelity on key floor votes are more important now compared to the old-school tactics of regional and state alliances," concluded Forgette and Scruggs (2005, 14). "As this trend continues, the committee system will increasingly function as an organizational means for party caucus governance . . . [and] will function less and less as bodies for mediating partisan and ideological conflict, crafting bills that are informed by diverse committee members' policy expertise and compromises."

Balancing Committee Interests

In the gains-for-trade perspective, one result of the passion and district-interest motivations of committee members is that they are not typical of Congress as a whole. Shepsle and Weingast (1984, 345) called committee and especially subcommittee members "preference outliers." Not surprisingly, this puts committee and subcommittee members in a difficult position. If they draft legislation to their own liking, it may not be approved by the larger, more general committees through which it may have to pass, or by the whole house. The result: committees are often constrained in their actions by the expected reception on the house floor. They risk rejection if they report bills that deviate substantially from the majority's values. Hence, one of the jobs of an astute representative or senator is to become expert at anticipating chamber reactions (Shepsle and Weingast 1987; Kiewiet and McCubbins 1991). Committees that too frequently do not correctly adjust to the prevailing political winds lose power (Fenno 1973). That some committees are more responsive to outside forces than others is usually explained by the salience or visibility and level of conflict of the issues assigned to them (D. Price 1978).

Some committee members are especially vulnerable to self-interested behavior, and this makes clear that an old adage also applies to Congress: money isn't everything, but it can be exchanged for everything. The House Appropriations Committee usually takes the lead on budget actions, and, even though its power was reduced in the 1970s with establishment of the Budget Committee and the consolidated budgeting process, it is still a highly desirable committee. It offers opportunities for legislators to "bring home the pork" in the form of appropriations targeted to benefit programs and projects in their home districts.

The fiscal year 2005 omnibus appropriations bill contained thousands of special projects, including funding for the Country Music Hall of Fame, a municipal swimming pool in Kansas, a paper-industry international hall of fame, and even fitness equipment for a Pennsylvania YMCA (Citizens Against Government Waste 2004). Though the nation at large might be well served if these kinds of deals were better held in check by the whole house, often they are not, because deals are struck to make sure that everyone or nearly everyone is getting enough for her district to encourage her to go along with the special benefits going to others.

While "pork" is often contained in appropriations bills, it finds its way into other bills as well. For example, the House-passed MMA of 2003 contained a number of elements called "rifle shots" for their narrowly targeted effects. In a high-profile bill such as the 2003 Medicare bill, these components can help build support for the bill and provide interest groups with a mechanism for passage of provisions that might not make it alone. Among the rifle shots in the House bill were higher Medicare payments to physicians in Alaska, four two-year pilot projects to determine whether Medicare should pay for more chiropractic services (sought by the American Chiropractic Association), and a measure to extend the existing moratorium that prevented the Saginaw (MI) Community Hospital from being designated an "institution for mental disease" (Lee 2003).

This tension between, on the one hand, protecting the body from failures of the commons (raiding the treasury for pork projects) and, on the other, ensuring that the powers granted to committees, and particularly to committee and subcommittee chairs, are protected, explains why so many veterans' hospitals are built in the districts of Veterans' Committee and subcommittee chairs while defense plants go to the districts of Defense Committee and subcommittee chairs. But those districts do not get all the veterans' hospitals or defense plants. Self-interest must be balanced with the public interest if committee power is to be maintained. When it is egregiously abused, chairs may be replaced when the next Congress is formed, or a committee's jurisdiction may be narrowed or shared with another committee, or an entire committee may be abolished by the next Congress, or the house membership may gather the simple majority of votes for a discharge petition, forcing a committee to give up a bill so that it can be considered by the whole house.

Committees are powerful, and members and chairs surely do wield disproportionate influence over their issues, but there are limits, even if at times they get stretched. In recent years, the party leaders in the House have claimed more control over Appropriations Committees—naming chairs and subcommittee chairs and, in 2005, proposing a change in organization: eliminating three subcommittees, including the popular Veterans Affairs' Housing and Urban Development Subcommittee (Taylor 2005a).

Appropriations Committees, especially in the House, have become more partisan as well. Before the mid-1990s, decisions by these committees were based on consensus, and bipartisanship was the norm. Former House Speaker Newt Gingrich recognized that appropriations were crucial to his vision and to the Republican agenda, so the type of member appointed to the committee was changed—from someone willing to work across the aisle to someone closely tied with the leadership agenda.

The nature of the Appropriations Committee has also been affected by the choice of its members. With the increased role of leaders in making appointments came different criteria for choice of those appointments. Appointees are now more party-loyal and more electorally challenged than in earlier years, when members of the committee were known for their bipartisanship and were chosen largely from "safe" districts as a way of ensuring long-time members with appropriations expertise (Gordon 2005, 278). Today's members are increasingly from marginal districts (where both parties are well represented in the electorate) and can use their position to help solidify their importance to their district.

Another change has been the increase in riders—or legislative language in appropriations bills. Exceptions to allow riders can be made by the House Rules Committee, largely controlled by party leaders. Thus, more and more appropriations bills now carry substantive riders (Aldrich and Rohde 2005). Finally, the number of appropriations earmarks has increased in recent years. In fiscal year 2002, some $46.6 billion was earmarked in a total of 10,631 separate earmarks (Taylor 2005a). According to Gordon (2005), over the past 10 years earmarks have increased by more than 640 percent. The problem was not simply the increasing amounts being earmarked but also the way they were added—often in the middle of the night in a conference committee report without the knowledge of other committee members. One example was a California road project in a highways appropriations bill that ballooned from $30 million in the original proposal to $750 million when it came to the final vote (Abrahms 2006).

Writing the Rules

Bills that make it out of Senate committees go directly to the floor, but most major House bills need an additional stop: the House Rules Committee. This committee decides the rules of floor debate for the bill, including time for debate, whether or not amendments will be allowed, the level of detail at which sections of the bill must be voted up or down, and other aspects of the amendment process. Two political scientists compared the House

Rules Committee to the "crossroads of the legislative process," where most members must come at one time or another to ask for favored treatment or protection with special rules (Bach and Smith 1988, 12). At one time the Rules Committee was a formidable barrier to a bill's progress. Democrats on the 1965 Rules Committee—over the objections of the Republicans on the committee—allotted only 10 hours to debate the original Medicare bill, permitted no amendments, and required an up or down vote on the entire complex bill rather than allowing section-by-section votes. Disallowed by that rule were votes on amendments that might have passed, such as relating premiums to income. Members who wanted to support the bill but with changes had to vote for it "as is" or go home and explain during reelection campaigns why they had voted against a popular bill.

The authority of the Rules Committee has ebbed and flowed a bit—ebbing in the 1970s and 1980s, but strengthening again in recent years. Ironically, the Republicans had complained vociferously under the Democrats about the iron hand of the committee. But in 1995, when they took over the House and Senate, they too used the rules to stymie debate and waylay Democratic proposals. Aldrich and Rohde (2005, 259) recount one angry Democrat complaining in 1995 that "the Republicans came to power promising change, open rules . . . [but] they are no more fair than the Democrats." What Rep. Gene Taylor (D-MS) was angry about was the Rules Committee barring a substitute amendment for a Medicare reform bill.

The more homogeneous the majority party, the more likely it is that the rules changes will be used to tighten the party's agenda control—and stymie the other party (Cox and McCubbins 1997). In 2003, 76 percent of all rules governing debate on the House floor were restrictive (Schickler and Pearson 2005).

The Rules Committee is often used by leadership to shape legislation to enhance its chance of passage, but leaders can also use both the committee and existing House rules to block issues that they do not want coming to the floor.

For example, to facilitate passage of a $50 billion deficit-reduction package that the leadership wanted in order to placate angry party conservatives, leaders arranged for the Rules Committee to remove from a reconciliation bill a provision that would have raised co-payments for Medicaid recipients. The change made the package acceptable to Republican moderates, who without removal of the offensive provision would have opposed the whole package. Conservatives regretted the change but were willing to accept it as the price of moving the bill (Cohn 2005).

A final example from 2005 deals with the war in Iraq. Leadership did not want the Iraq war debated on the floor; but as casualties mounted and national discontent grew, a bipartisan group of six members introduced a House joint resolution, H.J. Res 55, which would have forced President Bush to set a time-table for withdrawing U.S. troops. Though tension over the breach with the White House and leadership raised awareness of the growing impatience that had even spilled into Congress, leaders refrained from engaging the debate or even showing much concern, confident that their control of the House Rules Committee would prevent the resolution from seeing the floor and that the committee would reject a Democratic amendment to the defense spending bill that would have forced the president to define his criteria for deciding when troop withdrawal could commence (Donnelly 2005).

Subcommittees

Since the mid-1970s, subcommittees have played an increasingly important role in congressional decision making, especially in the House. There have been as many as 140 or more subcommittees in each house in some Congresses, but recently the totals have dropped to around 85 in the House and fewer than 70 in the Senate (Ornstein, Mann, and Malbin 2002). Appropriations Committees in both houses have the most subcommittees.

The two houses vary in the ways they use subcommittees. The House subcommittees are heavily involved in legislating: holding hearings and marking up bills. Full committees conduct their own markup but generally do not hold additional hearings. Senate subcommittees often hold hearings but frequently do not mark up (or write) bills; markup is usually the province of the full committee. The Senate Health, Education, Labor, and Pensions Committee retains jurisdiction over two dozen major health programs at the full committee level. It does not have a health subcommittee.

In the House, the responsibility for health care policy lies mostly with Energy and Commerce's Health Subcommittee, not the full committee. That subcommittee traditionally sets it own agenda, picks its own battles, and usually wins them. One exception was the major health care reform initiative of the Clinton years. Neither the subcommittee nor the full committee was able to reach consensus on a bill.

The larger clout of House versus Senate subcommittees can be quantified. S. Smith and Deering (1990) found that 85 percent of measures brought to the House floor were first referred to subcommittees, compared with only

42 percent in the Senate. Sinclair (2005) noted two reasons that the Senate does not use subcommittees to write legislation. First, senators have a larger workload, since they deal with the same issues as the House but with less than one-fourth of the members; second, the individualistic nature of the smaller Senate is to give all committee members the opportunity to participate in decision making—thus favoring a committee, rather than a subcommittee, decision-making venue.

Conference Committees

Conference committees are ad hoc congeries of representatives from both houses charged with the responsibility of reaching a compromise version of a bill. Conference committees are older than Congress itself: state legislative bodies used them to resolve differences before the U.S. Constitution was put in place (Oleszek 2004). Membership in conference committees, dubbed by scholars the "penultimate power" (Shepsle and Weingast 1991) or the "third house" of Congress (Oleszek 2004), is prized because the decisions made in conference are usually final. Conference committee language cannot be amended: the houses must vote the whole bill up or down. Conference committees can rewrite or change the legislation (for example, by choosing to "give up" items passed in their own house in favor of the other house's language). Sometimes they add provisions out of whole cloth or delete measures that were included in both House and Senate bills. "It is elementary," said Sen. Mitch McConnell (R-KY), "that if you get a bill to conference, you have wide latitude to produce a bill the majority is comfortable with and the president is comfortable with" (Oleszek 2004, 270).

Conference committees are lobbied hard by the president and interest groups, because even if these interests lose in one house (or both), they can recoup victory in the conference committee. Particularly effective is a president of the majority party, who can invite conferees to the White House for a pep talk, have staffers show up at conferences, and threaten a veto. In the 1997 Balanced Budget Act, the Democratic president was an active participant, bargaining with Republican leaders in both houses—often without close consultation with Democrats in Congress. Party leaders also know the power of the conference committee. House majority leader Tom DeLay actively opposed a drug importation bill that passed the House floor in 2003, but he won when it was excluded from the final conference report (Schickler and Pearson 2005).

Conferees are named by the House and Senate leaderships based on recommendations from committee chairs, and the conferences are usually dominated by members of the committees that originated the legislation. On major bills, the party leaders often serve on the conference committees themselves. A conference on the 2003 Medicare prescription drug bills had both the Senate and House majority leaders as members (the latter was the lead negotiator for the House). The House and Senate can adopt motions instructing the conferees, but the conferees can disregard their instructions. Party leaders can—and do—box out members with views they do not support. For example, Sen. John McCain (R-AZ), sponsor of the bill to repeal the Medicare catastrophic coverage program in 1989, was not named to the conference committee reconciling his bill with its House counterpart. Rep. Charles Norwood (R-GA), sponsor of the House-passed patients' rights bill, was not named as a conferee in the 1999–2000 conference committee trying to settle differences between House and Senate bills, because he had rammed the House bill through over the leadership's objections. In fact, only 1 of the 13 House members appointed to that conference committee had actually voted for the final version of the bill the House had passed (Rogers 1999).

In recent years, the role of the minority party in conference has been minimized. For example, the MMA of 2003 was written by 10 Republicans and 2 moderate Senate Democrats. Although named to the conference committee, 5 Democratic conferees were not permitted to participate in the process. Schickler and Pearson (2005, 211) concluded that "the degree to which Republicans exclude Democrats from conference deliberations is unprecedented in the modern era, though Democrats at times sidelined Republicans during key points of the negotiations when they were in the majority." The authors noted, however, that the Democrats did hold public conference committee meetings with all conferees, at least providing Republicans (then in the minority) with a forum where they could voice their displeasure publicly.

Conference committees can be quite large, especially when bills were considered by more than one committee. In 1971, the average number of House conferees was 8; in 1991, it was 25. The average number of Senate conferees increased from 8 to 12 over that period of time (Oleszek 2004). Since any agreement must have the majority vote of both houses, such a mismatch in numbers is not problematic. However, sheer mechanics may be difficult. Subconferences sometimes are named to deal with specific issues; sometimes conferees are limited to discussing only certain parts of the measure on which they are most knowledgeable; sometimes informal rump groups evolve into preliminary negotiating panels. In the Balanced Budget Act of 1997, which made major changes in Medicare and Medicaid, there were 13 subconferences. On large conference committees, much of the work is done by staffers who conduct major negotiations among members on key issues.

Sometimes conference committees bring out "power" issues between the House and Senate or simply between powerful representatives of those bodies. A case in point was the conference committee for the MMA in 2003. Sen. Charles Grassley (R-IA), chair of the Finance Committee, and Rep. Bill Thomas (R-CA), chair of the Ways and Means Committee, clashed over who would chair the conference committee (both wanted to do it) and later over provisions increasing Medicare payments to rural areas (wanted by Grassley but not by Thomas). At one point Senator Grassley and his staff boycotted the sessions when his issues were not on the agenda (Pear 2003a).

Most Americans do not appreciate the formidable power of conference committees. Few are aware, for example, that the conference committee on the Employee Retirement Income Security Act (ERISA) of 1974 inserted a preemption clause that has proved a major impediment to state-level health care reform. A few House conferees inserted language that preempted state laws relating to "any employee benefit plan" to replace language that prevented states from legislating about subject matter regulated by the act. A second phrase was then added stating that no employee benefit plan shall be deemed an insurance company. The result: state insurance regulation of self-insured or corporate health insurance plans was prohibited. Together, the two provisions—added 10 days before final passage of the law without the knowledge of many health insurers, the Department of Labor, or the state government associations—have withstood efforts in Congress and the courts to make changes and have played a powerful constraining role in state health care innovations (Fox and Schaffer 1989).

Similarly, a last-minute "surprise" in the 1988 catastrophic health insurance conference bill was a mandate that state Medicaid programs must pay all Medicare premiums, deductibles, and co-payments for beneficiaries with income below the federal poverty level (Torres-Gil 1989). This provision for the "dually eligible" was one of only two major initiatives not repealed the following year. Ironically, dually eligible beneficiaries became major users of the program—accounting for 35 percent of total Medicaid spending in 2003 (Ryan and Super 2003).

It is not uncommon for bills to languish and often die in conference committee—the fate of the patients' bill of rights noted above. Though the bills were passed by the House and Senate in October 1999, by August 2000 the conference committee was still stymied over major issues such as which patients should be covered under the new law and whether or not to allow patients to sue their self-insured HMOs. Since the issue was one of high visibility, there were many efforts to disgorge a bill from the conference. President Clinton met with conferees at the White House to try to resolve issues. The American Association of Health Plans launched a two-week, $200,000 television ad campaign aimed at the conference committee. Both Republicans and Democrats thought the issue was important to the upcoming congressional elections. So, seven months after floor passage, the conferees began a marathon series of meetings that included late-night sessions. As a sign of desperation, a House leader on the issue who had been excluded from the conference committee (Rep. Charlie Norwood) was brought into the conference negotiations in their seventh month (and four months before the election). Republicans wanted a bill passed before the election, because the issue gave Democrats a popular claim to use against them. But the differences were too great, and, even with the election just days away, conferees went home with no agreement, leaving the bill to be reintroduced in the next Congress. The bicameral process, said House Ways and Means Committee chair Bill Thomas, is "akin to mating a Chihuahua with a Great Dane" (Oleszek 2004, 269). No wonder, then, that it is often unsuccessful.

BUDGETING, WASHINGTON STYLE

Under the U.S. Constitution, Congress has the "power of the purse," embodied in the language that gives it the power to "lay and collect taxes . . . to pay the debts and provide for the common defense and general welfare of the United States." Congress can also borrow money. The congressional allocation of resources gets to the basic political question of who gets what and who pays. Further, the budget not only represents a document of government operations but also is a statement of government priorities.

The legislative process is defined by two types of bills: authorizations, which establish or continue an agency or program and describe its operations, and appropriations, which provide the funding for the agency or program. The two-part system is designed to separate the policy from fiscal decision making. The process is generally sequential, with the authorization preceding the appropriation. There have traditionally been 13 annual appropriations bills, considered by the 13 appropriations subcommittees in each house. These appropriations are generally specific about the money to be provided and the use to which that money is to be put. Unless a program is funded by appropriations, it ceases to exist. Congress must vote affirmatively to increase the funding level of a program each year; the funding cannot grow automatically (entitlements are an exception).

Traditionally, the appropriations bills were processed and enacted separately—involving 13 different votes. In recent years, however, a new approach has emerged, in which the measures are combined into an omnibus appropriations bill. In 2004, for example, the omnibus spending bill appropriated a staggering $388.4 billion and included all of the discretionary spending except defense and homeland security. It was the third multi-bill package in three years and the eighth since 1995 (Taylor 2004). Even more staggering, at least for some House members, was that the vote on the House floor took place just hours after the measure made it through conference at midnight the previous day. The speed backfired in the Senate, where embarrassed members had to strike from the measure passed the day before a provision allowing the chairs of Appropriations Committees and their aides to view individual tax returns (Taylor 2004). Sen. Kent Conrad (D-ND) complained that "this stack of paper was dropped on people's desk about 2 p.m. on Saturday, and we were voting about six hours later. What else is in this? What else is in this stack of paper that nobody knows about?" (Taylor 2004, 2778). Perhaps this negative experience helped force Congress to return to the usual approach of separate appropriations, because, in 2005, the House finished approval of the 11 annual spending bills in July.

Entitlements

Entitlements are guaranteed services that will be provided to all beneficiaries who meet the specified qualifications for the program. Entitlements are funded automatically and do not require appropriations. Entitlement spending makes budget control difficult: there is no overall limit on spending, but rather the spending is determined by the number of eligible beneficiaries, those legally entitled to the program funds. The largest entitlement programs are Social Security, Medicare, Medicaid, and Food Stamps. Social Security alone accounts for more than one-fifth of total federal spending; Medicare and Medicaid are the next largest spending category, at 20 percent (fig. 1.1).

The growth in entitlement spending has eclipsed other domestic spending over the past 20 years. Between 1993 and 2003, nondefense discretionary spending grew at annual rates of 5.5 percent, compared with annual growth rates of 6.7 percent for Medicare and 7.8 percent for Medicaid. The Congres-

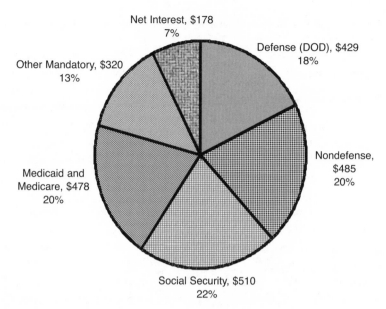

Net Interest, $178
7%

Defense (DOD), $429
18%

Other Mandatory, $320
13%

Medicaid and
Medicare, $478
20%

Nondefense,
$485
20%

Social Security, $510
22%

Figure 1.1.
Federal Spending, in Billions.
Source: Data from Budget of the United States Government, Fiscal Year 2006.

sional Budget Office (CBO) is predicting an even larger differential for fiscal years 2005–15. They estimate that nondefense discretionary spending will grow 2.1 percent annually over this period, compared with 9 percent for Medicare and 7.8 percent for Medicaid (CBO 2005a). Stanley Collender, Price Waterhouse's budget expert, summed up the role of Medicaid and Medicare in the entitlement picture as follows: "When you look at entitlements, controlling Medicare and Medicaid are the top five priorities, period" (Ratan 1993, 102). While Social Security is growing as well, its growth is much slower than that of the two health entitlements. The escalation of entitlement spending can be attributed in part to demographic factors, including the aging of the nation's population, to increased utilization, and to automatic cost-of-living adjustments.

Once an entitlement program is enacted, it can escape yearly evaluations. Further, many entitlements are indexed to the cost of living, so payments are increased automatically without congressional action. Entitlements can be curbed only by changing the law that set up the program or the regulations governing its implementation. Other "uncontrollable" elements of the budget are interest on the debt and outlays from prior obligations (largely related to defense spending).

Cutting entitlements is extremely difficult. Entitlements are popular programs—especially to the recipients. Elderly people, a major category of recipients, are well organized and are quick to fight any possible cut in their programs. Another House member, Rep. Kevin Brady (R-TX), described the power of Medicare this way: "A good Medicare solution is more difficult than the war on terrorism, education, Social Security and homeland security combined" (Roth 2005). Nevertheless, entitlements were once again in the congressional and presidential cross-hairs in 2005. The chair of the Senate Budget Committee targeted entitlement programs for possible cuts, and entitlement spending reductions were central to fulfilling President Bush's promise to cut the deficit in half by 2010 (Taylor 2005b). Robert D. Reischauer, president of the Urban Institute and former CBO director, put it this way: "Those who are interested in reducing spending to lower the deficit . . . are going to focus on Medicare and Medicaid" (Adams and Schatz 2004, 2695). It is noteworthy that President Bush's 2005 efforts to significantly change one popular entitlement program—Social Security—ran into a political buzz saw.

The Congressional Budget Process

For the country's first 150 years, there was a surplus of funds; and federal spending, with the exception of military pay, equipment, and supplies, was relatively low. But in the 1930s, the federal budget began to grow as the government assumed new domestic responsibilities, including regulating business and providing for those temporarily or permanently disadvantaged. Presidential control over the budgetary process dates back to 1939, when the Bureau of the Budget (BoB) was made part of the executive office. In 1970, the BoB became the Office of Management and Budget (OMB) and its responsibilities expanded (see chapter 2). The presidential budgetary power peaked in the early 1970s, when President Nixon aggressively "impounded," or refused to spend, funds appropriated by Congress for programs he did not support. The Congressional Budget and Impoundment Act of 1974 (Public Law 93-344) was passed in part as a response to congressional unhappiness over this increased presidential role. It was also enacted as a way to improve congressional control over the federal budget, thus allowing it to set fiscal policy and make choices among programs (Ellwood and Thurber 1977). The law set up the House and Senate Budget committees and the Congressional

Budget Office. It also mandated a concurrent budget resolution setting forth aggregate federal spending, which serves as a fiscal blueprint to guide the actions of authorizing, appropriating, and taxing committees. Finally, it established a process known as reconciliation, designed to bring existing law into conformity with the budget plans.

The budget process has evolved since it was set up, with the focus changing from the process of priority setting, to controlling the size of the federal budget and federal budget deficits, to controlling domestic spending. In the early 1980s, it became clear that something was needed to control government spending and reduce the burgeoning deficit. Though it had taken more than 200 years for the deficit to get to $1 trillion, it took only four more years to get to $2 trillion and little more to pass $5 trillion, before it started back down as annual surpluses replaced deficits. The deficit doubled (from $1 trillion to $2 trillion) in the first term of the Reagan administration, thanks largely to a $600 billion reduction in taxes ($150 billion a year) and a $115 billion increase in defense spending.

The first major move toward fiscal responsibility was in 1985 with the Balanced Budget and Emergency Deficit Control Act, known as the Gramm-Rudman-Hollings Act, which used the budget process to limit spending. It mandated that some $36 billion be cut yearly from deficit ceilings until the deficit—it was fondly hoped—would be zeroed out in fiscal year 1991. Of course, this was easier to hope for than to make happen, as targets were set and then not met.

The budget process has been reassessed and revised several times since 1985, with presidential-congressional summits and several new provisions, including the Budget Enforcement Act (BEA) of 1990, which established a binding five-year deficit-reduction plan, capped three areas of spending (domestic, defense, and international), and set up "pay-as-you-go" rules governing mandatory spending (including entitlements) and revenues. In 1993 the process was strengthened with the enactment of a "hard freeze" on spending, rigidly setting the amount of money that could be spent on non-entitlement, nondefense programs until 1998. In 1997 a bipartisan balanced budget act extended the spending limitations. But the squeeze of these pay-as-you-go rules was politically smothering and, given the budget surplus in the late 1990s, seemingly unnecessary. While many citizens might welcome such constraint, members of Congress find that the budget rules dramatically restrict their room to negotiate and their ability to respond to their constituents' needs. When the Republicans wanted to enact a major tax-reduction initiative in both 1999 and 2001, they had to find cuts in existing programs. Thus it is not surprising that in 2000, Congress began a search for new ways to handle the budget process—ways that would allow it to enact new programs. The BEA expired in 2002, and the fiscal constraints of pay-as-you-go with it (although the Senate opted to maintain it for several more years).

President Bush has argued for reinstating the pay-as-you-go rules, but only for domestic spending. Even a persuasive president often does not get his way, and such was the case on this issue. A handful of moderate Senate Republicans supported a Democratic amendment that would extend pay-as-you-go rules to tax cuts or new entitlement spending unless 60 senators voted to skirt the rules. House Republicans were opposed to including tax cuts under such constraint, and no agreement between the two houses was reached.

During the years of the Republican-controlled Congress and Democratic president, the budget, constrained by the spending limits, became a major battlefield. It culminated in 1995 when the federal government was shut down because of a budget dispute between the White House and Congress. The rancor subsided a bit with the emergence of a surplus in the fiscal year 1998 budget. But the disappearance of the spending caps, major new tax cuts, and continued federal spending soon led Congress back to its deficit ways.

In short order, Congress, encouraged by the president, went through the surplus, and by 2005 the federal deficit was a staggering $400 billion (Taylor 2005b). Further, the budget process has changed considerably in the twenty-first century. In 2004, for the third year, there was an omnibus appropriations bill rather than the 13 separate spending bills. Discretionary spending was held in check in 2004, with both houses abiding by a White House–supported cap on spending (Taylor 2004).

In 2005, the budget again was an issue. President Bush's proposed budget called for zero growth in nonmilitary, non–homeland security discretionary spending over the next five years (similar to his earlier call in 2004). Given that domestic spending had been the target of cuts over the past five or so years, some observers thought there were no substantial savings to capture (Taylor 2005c). In contrast, spending for defense increased 7 percent in the same fiscal year, and for homeland security increased 9 percent. Domestic discretionary spending accounts for only around 16 percent of the total budget.

Some political scientists have harkened back to the blueprint of Ronald Reagan's budget director, David Stockman, as a way of understanding current political rationales for cuts. Called "starve the beast," the idea is that taxes should be cut so much that insufficient money is available for spending programs (Rudder 2005, 329). Indeed, in 2005, both tax cuts and spending cutbacks were making the Stockman dream of two decades earlier a reality.

The Reconciliation Process

As it has evolved over the years, the budget process has weakened the power of authorizing committees and given more power to party leaders. Authorizing committees rarely have the opportunity to launch new programs, but rather must work hard to protect established programs from budget cuts. The Appropriations Committees—once viewed as the "cardinals" of the appropriations process—now have control over only about one-third of federal spending. This is because so much spending is in the form of entitlements, not subject to appropriations. Further, the party leaders and Budget committees often make key decisions about what programs to fund and how much to alter entitlement programs to produce savings or increase the amount of spending they will require to cover new benefits or newly eligible beneficiaries.

Beginning in the early 1980s, the reconciliation bill, a compilation of legislative committee recommendations implementing the concurrent budget resolution, began to be used as a vehicle to enact new provisions and programs and otherwise change policy. Its attractiveness was clear. Measures could become law with minimal attention and no hearings and would likely sail through both houses, which were eager to vote to reduce the deficit. Importantly, reconciliation bills cannot be filibustered in the Senate and permit actions to be taken in tandem that arguably would never survive separately.

The reconciliation bill is important to health policy. In the 1980s, virtually every major piece of health legislation was included in that bill, including four new health block grants, changes in physician payment systems, expansion of home and community-based care, and nursing home reforms. Although measures in the reconciliation bill were often justified as a way to reduce spending, some provisions in reconciliation actually increased spending—especially Medicaid mandates to states to qualify women and children above the poverty level for the program. Rep. Henry Waxman (D-CA), chair of the Health Subcommittee of the Energy and Labor Committee, was a master at using the reconciliation process to achieve his goal of providing health care to near-poor women and children. Called variously the budgetary time bombs or, more alliteratively, the Waxman wedge, the strategy called for stretching out the spending so that it would fall mainly in later years, not included in the budgetary ceilings (Morgan 1994, 8). It was a precedent that came back to haunt the Democrats in years to come.

Most major changes in Medicare and Medicaid over the past 20 years have been in the reconciliation bill—with the sole exception of the 2003 MMA. The 1997 reconciliation bill, called the 1997 Balanced Budget Act, was designed to save $115 billion in Medicare over seven years. Later CBO projections showed the savings to be even larger, or $192 billion more than what might have been spent without these changes between 1998 and 2002 (Gardner 1999). The cuts were scattered across the major health care providers: hospitals, physicians, home health agencies, nursing homes. In the 2000s, the emphasis in reconciliation bills was on tax, not spending, cuts.

While consideration in reconciliation bills is given special treatment, rules have been made along the way—particularly in the Senate—to curb excesses in the reconciliation process. For example, reconciliation provisions cannot contain non-revenue-related items and cannot incur revenue loss beyond 10 years—provisions that can be waived by a three-fifths vote of the Senate (Oleszek 2004). However, rules can be skirted. For example, the 2001 reconciliation bill, the Economic Growth and Tax Relief Reconciliation Act, contained provisions set to expire before the end of 10 years, carefully timed cuts in the estate tax to occur gradually so as not to "cost" too much, and some cuts selectively allowed to start immediately but others phased in (Rudder 2005). The 2003 reconciliation measure, the Jobs Growth Tax Relief Reconciliation Act, contained tax cuts set to end in one year to make the cost seem lower (Rudder 2005).

Although the 2003 Medicare prescription drug bill was not part of the reconciliation process, the costs were of paramount concern to members of Congress, especially some Republican members who did not want to increase deficit spending. The ceiling agreed to by the White House and Congress was $400 billion over 10 years. The measure's expected spending was held to that figure only by "backloading" expenses (full benefits accrued four years after passage) and underestimating costs. Only four months after passage of the MMA, the administration admitted that costs were closer to $534 billion over 10 years. One year later, those costs were estimated to exceed $720 billion over 10 years, an increase in part reflecting the shift of the 10-year horizon to 2015, when more and more baby boomers would become eligible for Medicare (Citizens Against Government Waste 2005a).

LEGISLATIVE PARTIES

Few people argue with the statement that political parties in the United States are fairly weak. Crossover voting, split tickets, and the growth in number of voters calling themselves independent provide evidence that voters can no longer be considered stalwart partisans. Direct primaries, growth in political action committees (PACs), and the increased role of the media in campaigns have contributed to a weakened position of parties in recruiting candidates and in funding and guiding their campaigns. The party in government—the role of the political party in organizing and overseeing legislative action—has also often been characterized as weak (Burns 1984; J. Schlesinger 1966; Scott and Hrebenar 1979). In comparison with their counterparts in the British House of Commons, for example, members of Congress do not vote in unified blocks to enact policies espoused in the previous election, majorities that coalesce are fleeting and ad hoc, and action can be stymied by small groups of strategically placed opponents.

Nevertheless, there is evidence that parties play an important role in defining and shaping the legislative product. Parties help facilitate communication among members, members of the other house, the president, and the states. Legislative parties provide a place to air issues, collect support, and broker compromise. Importantly, the legislative party reduces information overload by providing cues to members (which is especially important to new members). Finally, the legislative party facilitates the identification of issues that differentiate it from the other party. Most members' daily activities are much more dominated by party activities than they were in the 1970s, when committee work occupied most of their time.

Party leadership picks its battles, staking out positions on bills most important to the party ideology and to future elections. These "party" bills or issues are the ones that party leaders expect their members to support. If they do not get that support, some retribution may result. One estimate is that in recent Congresses (103rd, 104th, and 105th), the party played a role in the votes of about 40 percent of roll calls (Ansolabehere, Snyder, and Stewart 2001).

Party leaders can also play an important role in "framing" issues to appeal to voters "back home." One example of such framing was when Senate Republicans stopped pushing the "Patients First Act of 2003" and in its place began talking about the "Healthy Mothers and Healthy Babies Access to Care Act." Both bills were actually tort reform measures designed to cap the size of awards in medical malpractice court cases. The second bill, targeted only at obstetricians and gynecologists, was then cast as a measure to improve women's access to care. "This is about women," said Sen. Judd Gregg (R-NH), sponsor of the bill. The renaming and retargeting of the tort reform bill in 2004 may well have been part of a Republican effort to lessen, if not eliminate, the advantage Democrats usually have among women (Martinez and Carey 2004).

Rick Wilson (1992) described three problems, inherent in the congressional structure, that political parties can help solve: problems of coordination, collective action, and collective choice. Parties and leaders can be focal points to coordinate individual members following sometimes similar, sometimes dissimilar, interests. They can bind individual members to collectively desired goals that without parties would not be articulated or achieved. They can provide the stability necessary to prevent domination by individual members bound to highly variable districts. In short, parties can transform the actions of 535 independent agents into a workable, more focused institution that has the opportunity to act in the public interest.

Increased Party Loyalty

A crucial factor in how effective parties are is how homogeneous they are. Do they speak with one voice or many, divergent voices? For years, the parties, particularly the Democratic Party, have fallen at the divergent end of the spectrum. In recent years, first the Republicans, and then the Democrats, have become more homogeneous and are voting more in line with the party.

Figure 1.2 provides a longitudinal look at House party loyalty as evidenced by legislative voting—called party unity scores—since 1965. Party unity scores, the percentage of votes on which a majority of Democrats opposed a majority of Republicans, are a measure of conflict or interparty disagreement. As figure 1.2 illustrates, party loyalty in the House has risen substantially since 1965. In 2004 a majority of voting House Democrats opposed the majority of voting Republicans on 86 percent of the votes; voting House Republicans opposed the majority of voting Democrats on 88 percent of the votes. House Republicans' unity scores saw an uptick in the mid-1990s—coinciding with their majority status and strong party leadership by Newt Gingrich. Democratic unity scores lagged, but increased in 2002 to the point that the two parties had roughly the same unity scores by 2004 (Poole 2004). The Senate unity votes are more variable but show the same trend toward more party voting, especially for the Republicans. In 2004, Senate Democrats' unity scores were 83 percent; the Republican unity scores were 90 percent (Poole 2004).

While these unity scores are useful, especially in their ability to mark trends, they are not without critics. Political scientists have developed other measures to quantify partisan pressure (Ansolabehere, Snyder, and Stewart 2001; Binder, Lawrence, and Maltzman 1999; Snyder and Groseclose 2000), but it is difficult to separate out the party influence from the ideological proclivity of the member of Congress and the preferences of her constituents. What seems to be clear is that party influence is greatest on procedural issues—such as votes

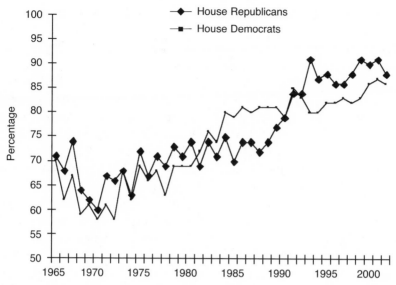

Figure 1.2.

Party Unity Scores in the House of Representatives, 1965–2004. Party unity scores reflect the percentage of Democratic votes and Republican votes when a majority of Democrats oppose a majority of Republicans.

Source: CQ Weekly, Dec. 11, 2004.

on rules—that are key to shaping the legislation but are not as transparent to voters (except, perhaps, when politicians try to "explain" apparently contradictory votes, as did the Democratic presidential nominee in 2004).

Nevertheless, most observers agree that allegiance to party is strong in the modern Congress and that differences between the parties are notable. One reason often cited is the loss of many members in the middle or moderate stream of both parties. While a few moderate Republicans remain in the Senate, conservative Southern Democrats who once voted with Republicans (called "Blue Dog" Democrats) are a dying breed.

Increasing party unity can also be attributed to other factors, including the increasing homogeneity of the voting population, the effects of legislative reforms that strengthen the role of party leaders, and the personalities and persuasiveness of party leadership. In fact, an argument can also be made that voters' disdain for electoral party loyalty might well lead to strengthened parties in the House and Senate, because "candidates need all the help they can get; they are finding that the best place to get it is from their fellow partisans"

(J. Schlesinger 1985, 1168). Rohde (1991, 170) argued that the two are related in that members of Congress are linked to their party through their constituency. Where these party constituencies are similar across the country, the positions taken by their representatives become more similar.

At the same time that parties are becoming more homogeneous, the conflict between the parties is growing. This has led to more acrimony in committees and on the floor and to stronger party organizations. In 1995, when the Republicans took over Congress, the Democrats who retired or were not reelected were primarily moderates, and the newly elected Republicans were mainly conservatives (Aldrich and Rohde 2000). The new leadership—headed by Speaker Newt Gingrich and strongly supported by the new members—put in place a series of reforms to strengthen its position. Under these reforms, the Speaker named committee chairs, the tenure of chairs was capped at three two-year terms, leadership staffs were increased while committee staffs were cut, appropriations subcommittee chairs were asked to sign an agreement that they could be removed if they failed to follow the GOP conference agenda, and one-party task forces replaced committees as the vehicles for crafting salient, substantive policies.

In part the changes were made to push a legislative agenda encapsulated in the Contract with America, a list of policies that the House Republicans pledged to enact when they were in the majority. The leadership promised that the legislative goals in the contract would be passed in the first 100 days of the session. This could be achieved only under a party-centered, leadership-directed model. As one Republican legislator put it, "You can't depend on the committee system to make bold changes. The leadership needs to pick up the slack" (Davidson 1995, 2). While the centralization of leadership under Newt Gingrich was striking, it was nonetheless part of a trend in which House and Senate party leaders have become increasingly important in setting the policy agenda (Taylor 1998). Later Congresses have tried to be bipartisan, but bad memories and an unwillingness by the majority to give up power to the minority have kept partisanship strong.

Today's parties have been characterized as legislative cartels, which use procedural powers—including naming committee members, using the legislative calendar, and spawning favorable rules—to produce outcomes favorable to the party (Cox and McCubbins 2002). These cartels work best in a majority party that has near-complete control over the procedural powers, particularly in the House.

What is the effect of this party resurgence? The effect is probably at the margins—but the margin is important, since parties tend to take positions on major bills, and votes on those bills are more important than those on more narrowly construed, less salient measures (Sinclair 1989). In recent years Congress seems to be best described by conditional party government, in which legislative parties are cohesive and polarized in large part because the policy preferences of party members have become more homogeneous and ideologies more divergent. In such a situation, party leaders become very important (Aldrich and Rohde 2005). Although Republican margins in Congress have been small, the leadership has operated in a unified fashion, eschewing bipartisanship and often achieving goals through maintaining strong party unity.

There is evidence that partisan differences in the House and Senate—more so than differences between the parties of Congress and the president—increase legislative "gridlock," with a low percentage of legislative output produced in proportion to the policy agenda (Binder 1999). Partisan differences also resulted in increased bickering and finger-pointing. In the second session of the 106th Congress, before the 2000 congressional elections, the partisanship was particularly heated, even in the Senate, the traditionally more sedate body. At one point, both floor action and committee hearings were shut down by party leaders miffed at each other and at other party members (Preston 2000). Rival House party leaders no longer meet regularly, and in one well-publicized incident, the Capitol Hill police were called to roust Democrats from the Ways and Means Committee library where they were protesting the call for a vote on an important bill that they had received only hours before (Schickler and Pearson 2005, 212).

Funding Legislative Elections

Particularly in the House, party leadership has become much more active in raising funds. Of course, congressional campaign support has a long history. Rep. Lyndon Johnson of Texas was among the first to see the value to the party in actively seeking funding for congressional candidates. However, even his enthusiastic and persuasive efforts pale compared with today's campaign juggernaut.

In 2004, the average Senate candidate spent $2.6 million on his or her campaign, and the average House candidate spent more than $520,000. Interestingly, members seeking reelection spent more than their challengers. The average amount of money raised by Senate incumbents was $8.6 million, compared with less than $1 million by their challengers. Similar differentials were found in the House, where incumbents raised more than $1.1 million, compared with $192,00, on average, raised by challengers. Perhaps most interesting is that for open seats, which one might expect to engender the most money, less money was raised in both the House and Senate. On average, open seats in the House saw $563,000 raised, and in the Senate $3.0 million, in the 2004 election (Center for Responsive Politics 2005).

The 2004 election was the first following a major campaign finance law, the Bipartisan Campaign Reform Act, commonly known as McCain-Feingold for its Republican and Democratic champions. The law sought to close loopholes in campaign finance laws, particularly those related to soft money—contributions to national political parties from corporations, labor unions, and wealthy individuals. The law banned soft money and prohibited labor unions and for-profit corporations from funding "electioneering communications" or issue advocacy. Nonprofit corporations can make such ads as long as they use only individual contributions and provide certain disclosures. McCain-Feingold doubled the amount of "hard" money individuals could contribute to state parties and to individual candidates. Indeed, in the 2004 election, House general election candidates raised 16 percent more money than in the 2002 cycle (Herrnson 2005).

With the ban on soft money came the launch of another, related effort—funding through Section 527 political organizations that can engage in voter mobilization efforts, issue advocacy, and other activities as long as they do not expressly advocate the election or defeat of a federal candidate. There are no limits on how much money Section 527 organizations can raise and spend. In the 2004 presidential election, "527 committees" played a key role—mostly negative. For example, Swift Boat Veterans for Truth, a 527 group organized against the Democratic presidential candidate John Kerry, garnered considerable media attention (in addition to paid advertising) by questioning the actions of Lt. John Kerry while he was commander of a swift boat during the Vietnam War. Overall, 527 committees raised and spent more than a half-billion dollars during the 2004 campaign (Center for Responsive Politics 2005).

LEGISLATIVE BEHAVIOR

Fenno's research on congressional motivations (1973) found that members of Congress strive to meet three goals: reelection, influence within the house, and good public policy. Individuals differ in how much importance they place on each. Someone secure in her district may prefer to try to gain influence or promote her idea of good policy. Mayhew (1974) argued that of the three goals, reelection underlies everything else. It keeps members accountable, and without reelection the other goals mean nothing. Members can, if they choose, focus on producing particularized benefits to their districts in the form of casework and federal funding for projects ("pork"). Or they can take the high road: trying to help enact good public policy that produces collective or generalized benefits. They can choose committee membership that best meets their electoral needs, either a constituency-responsive, reelection-oriented committee (Agriculture or Resources, say), a policy committee (International Relations or Energy and Commerce), or a power committee (Appropriations, Rules, or Ways and Means).

For most, reelection is their proximate goal, in Mayhew's terms (1987), a goal that must be achieved over and over to make everything else possible. Incumbency helps make that happen. Incumbents are overwhelmingly reelected, with margins that have increased markedly in most elections in recent decades. From the mid-1960s through the early 1990s and beyond, members were rarely defeated, and changes were usually instigated only by retirement—reminiscent perhaps of Robert Audrey's dictum: "Where there's death, there's hope." Table 1.2 shows the percentage of incumbents elected in the House and Senate and the margins of victory since 1964. Compared with the mid-1960s, reelection was increasingly the expected outcome of House races—and with larger margins—until a downturn in the early 1990s, probably as a result of redistricting, anti-incumbent feelings, and fewer contested seats (Ornstein, Mann, and Malbin 2002). Even the 1994 election, which turned the House over to the Republicans for the first time in 40 years, defeated only Democratic incumbents. Not a single Republican incumbent was defeated, so the percentage of incumbents reelected was still quite high. In 2002, the percentage of incumbents reelected remained 96 percent—despite the national redistricting that had taken place following the 2000 census. In fact, most of those who were defeated in 2002 were running in races against other incumbents.

Table 1.3 shows the number of House incumbents who have lost in general elections since the 1960s, by decade. In the 1962–70 period, an average of 32 House incumbents lost in each general election. In the 2002 election, only 4 incumbents lost (the smallest number in American history); in 2004 there were only 7 incumbent losses—for an average over the two elections of 5.5, far lower than in previous years (Mann 2005). Political scientists worry about the impact of the decline in competitive seats.

Table 1.2

House Incumbency Trends and Reelections, 1964–2004

Year	Number of Incumbents Running	Percentage Reelected	Percentage Reelected by at Least 60 Percent
1964	397	86.6	58.5
1966	411	88.1	67.7
1968	409	96.8	72.2
1970	401	94.5	77.3
1972	393	93.6	77.8
1974	391	87.7	66.4
1976	384	95.8	71.9
1978	382	93.7	78.0
1980	398	90.7	72.9
1982	393	90.1	68.9
1984	411	95.4	74.6
1986	394	97.7	86.4
1988	409	98.3	88.5
1990	406	96.0	76.4
1992	368	88.3	65.6
1994	387	90.2	64.5
1996	384	94.0	73.6
1998	402	98.3	75.6
2000	403	97.8	77.3
2002	397	96.0	82.7
2004	404	97.8	80.0

Sources: Ornstein, Mann, and Malbin 2002; *CQ Weekly,* Dec. 14, 2002, and Nov. 6, 2004.

Oppenheimer (2005) argues that with the increasing number of safe seats, the opportunity for change in party control becomes more difficult, and an increasing partisanship and growing polarization of parties emerge. With little likelihood of defeat, members of Congress do not need to moderate their positions for electoral purposes—leading them to rely on their ideology and the party for their votes and to ignore district independents and candidates of the other party. Oppenheimer provided as evidence the 1998 vote on impeachment in the House. Although 60 percent of the electorate was opposed to impeachment, nearly all of the Republicans could vote for impeachment because they came from safe districts. Another "enticement" was that party

Table 1.3
House Incumbents Who Lose in General Elections, 1962–2004

Years	Number Defeated	Mean Number per Congress
1962–70	129	32.25
1972–80	116	29
1982–90	78	19.5
1992–2000	91	22.75
2002–4	11	5.5

Source: Oppenheimer 2005, updated with information from Mann 2005.

leaders threatened retribution in the form of lower campaign contributions and strong primary opposition for those who did not vote their way.

Nonetheless, evidence abounds that even incumbents with seemingly healthy electoral situations remain worried about reelection and continue to support their districts' interests. John Dingell (D-MI), who did not face a tough congressional election for nearly three decades, remained vigilant, making no apology for putting forth every effort to support the auto industry in his home state of Michigan. "That's what I'm sent here to do," he said (Duncan 1993, 13).

Members must treat with respect the prospect of being tossed out, because it does happen. The best example was the 1994 election, in which scores of incumbent Democrats (including House Speaker Tom Foley) lost their seats as voter dissatisfaction—largely with the Clinton national health insurance proposal—culminated in a political takeover of both the House and Senate. It was the first time the Republicans had control of the Senate since 1986 and the House since 1954. Similarly, in 2004, Senate majority leader Tom Daschle lost in one of the most expensive Senate races ever, and certainly a record-setting race in tiny South Dakota.

The fear of electoral loss helps keep members accountable and assures that they will carry out the duties associated with reelection: advertising, credit claiming, and position taking. Advertising promotes name recognition and plants an image of personal qualities without the distraction of policy content. Credit claiming paints the member as personally responsible for some desirable policy or program, such as individual casework assistance and bringing specific benefits (pork) to the district. Federal agencies announcing grants phone the good news simultaneously to each member of Congress representing the area, so each can claim credit. Position taking can range from votes on issues, to speeches on the floor or at the Rotary Club, to letters to the editor in the local newspaper. As Mayhew (1987, 23) put it, "The position itself is a political commodity."

Incumbents win in part because they handle constituency issues exceedingly well. They have mastered the art of using the federal bureaucracy to make them look good on pork barreling, casework, and leaning on agencies on their constituents' behalf. Compared with lawmaking, these tasks are a cakewalk. They make constituents happy, and they are rarely controversial. Many legislators have become masters at bringing home the pork. One of the most successful was Sen. Ted Stevens (R-AK), who as chair of the Appropriations Committee in 2005 targeted (or earmarked) $442 million to build two bridges in his home state to connect remote areas serving very few people. But Senator Stevens was not the only senator sending projects to his home state. In the 2005 highway bill, it seemed every senator and member must have gotten something. The $286 billion measure contained a record 6,371 pet projects inserted by members of Congress from both parties (Weisman and VandeHei 2005). The pork seemed so excessive that columnists, reporters, and constituents expressed their dismay, even forcing the Senate to reconsider Senator Stevens's project, which had become known as "the bridge to nowhere." Congress eliminated the earmark for the Alaskan bridges but instead turned the $442 million over to the state to use as it wished (Hulse 2005).

Agency oversight—another task in a member's job description—is even less fun and noticed by very few. Not surprisingly, it often is overlooked, except in dramatic cases or those with photogenic causes. Political scientists call the process "fire alarm" oversight, whereby Congress generally ignores day-to-day oversight until there is a fire, when it brings out the fire trucks: highly televised hearings accompanied by (often) heavily exaggerated accusations about violations of the public trust (McCubbins and Schwartz 1984). Hold an oversight hearing on the evils of smoking, with a teenage movie star talking about her personal convictions on not smoking, and the session has to be moved to the Caucus Room to hold the crowd and network television crews. Similarly, taking an agency head to task for excess spending or an unflattering evaluation often proves appealing—especially to those of the congressional party opposite the party in the White House. Much of this oversight is carried out by staff. When the cameras leave, so do the legislators. Day-to-day oversight is boring and mundane, and not sought out by members, such as the one who described oversight to Segal (1994) as complex and not very "sexy." Partly this reflects the expectations of members of Congress and the enormous demands on their time.

Some members do recognize the importance of oversight. Rep. John

Dingell, long-time chair of the House Energy and Commerce Committee, was one of those who took responsibility for overseeing, sometimes even "bullying," federal agencies. In addition to calling federal bureaucrats to testify before the oversight subcommittee, Dingell also issued hundreds of "Dingell-grams" a year to bureaucrats, asking questions and seeking quick resolutions to issues he found annoying or offensive. During the Clinton presidency, there were numerous House committee investigations on issues ranging from the failed Arkansas land deal called Whitewater to the firing of employees of the White House travel office; from Democratic fundraising to White House efforts to obtain files on former Republican administration officials. However, with the seating of a Republican president and a Republican Congress, oversight of presidential activities was greatly reduced. Even hearings responding to major, highly salient events have been few, and often with little resolution.

Observers from both parties agree that oversight of agencies and programs has waned in recent years. Contributing to this lack of interest are several institutional changes, such as members' shorter workweeks, packed schedules, term-limited chairs, and eroding salaries for the staffers who might conduct investigations (Nather 2004). Good oversight involves long hours of work by well-trained staff. It also requires interest from members of Congress on issues that might not make the network news or Sunday morning talk shows. "Oversight is very tedious work," said Lee Hamilton, former House member from Indiana. "It takes a lot of preparation, and it tends to be very complicated. Members are very busy now and they just don't make oversight that high a priority" (Nather 2004, 1192).

Some observers criticized Congress for failure to adequately address the nation's preparation before the 2001 terrorist attacks, implementation of the Patriot Act, and Iraqi prisoner abuse. The House Government Operations Committee under Democratic leadership and a Democratic president (1992–93) held nearly four times the number of hearings held by the Republicans in 2003–04.

Revealed Preferences and Intensities

Congressional decision making is not easily dissected. The system is complex, including district preferences, interest groups' impact assessments, demands from party leadership, individual members' preferences, the characteristics of the issue on the table, and the distractions of other issues and demands for attention. Some commentators have suggested that how members vote is not as important as where they put their resources and focus their energy. Back in the (what now seem to be) lazy days of the mid-1970s, a political scientist decided that time was "a House member's scarcest and most precious political resource" (Fenno 1978). Today's member of Congress is even more stretched—sandwiching committee introductions, votes, and constituent responses in the few minutes when she is not feeding the persistently yawning jaws of the campaign coffer or questing for 30 more seconds of media coverage.

Deciding How to Vote

Reelection takes top billing in deciding how to vote. Members do a type of personal impact assessment to answer two questions: how will this decision enhance my chances for reelection, and how might it be used against me by opponents? Only those in moderately safe seats enjoy the privilege of frequently pursuing other goals, such as enhancing their influence in Congress or producing good public policy (Arnold 1990).

Sometimes the answer may be to vote yes and no: no to add a provision to a bill, yes to report the bill to committee, no on a rule permitting no amendments, yes to crippling amendments if the member wants to kill the bill, yes to recommit the bill to committee, yes to substitute another bill, no to a motion to cut off a filibuster, yes on a vote to postpone the final vote, no on a voice vote to pass the bill, but yes on a final roll-call vote that may be reported back home. The complicated nature of congressional votes came out in the 2004 presidential campaign when the Democratic candidate, and long-time senator, John Kerry, had to explain his votes for and against the same issue. While congressional scholars might have understood, few others were persuaded that his actions were rational and principled.

Arnold (1990) argued that members will vote in ways that reflect both current and "potential" preferences of constituents. They anticipate what the voters will think, how they will interpret an issue and an action, and respond accordingly. Constituents are not equally informed; only a few can be called "attentives," those who have opinions about a particular policy, know what Congress is doing, and communicate those opinions to their legislator. Interest groups affected by the policy are part of this attentive public. "Inattentives" have no preferences and no knowledge of congressional activity. According to Arnold (1990, 84), to make a decision a legislator needs to

— identify all the attentive and inattentive publics who might care about a policy issue;

— estimate the direction and intensity of their preferences;

— estimate the probability that potential preferences will be transformed into real preferences;

— weight all these preferences according to the size of the attentive and inattentive publics; and

— give special weight to the preferences of consistent supporters.

Conflict can lead to different decision-making strategies. Kingdon (1977) believed that a member will implicitly ask whether there is any controversy in the issue. If no controversy, the legislator votes with the consensus in her "environment" of party members, ideological companions, predispositions, and constituency. But in the face of controversy, Kingdon believed, she subdivides the environment into those actors most critical to her: constituency, party leadership, and fellow members. When these three conflict, she will most likely vote with her constituency. But the reality is that on many issues, the constituency is uninterested or uninformed. This means the choice is between party and policy goals. From that set, the member will most likely choose the policy goal, unless the party makes clear the issue is important and disloyalty will be punished.

The saliency or visibility of the issue in the press and with the public also plays a key role. On highly salient issues, the constituent role is the dominant decision-making criterion. For low-saliency, complex issues of little broad public concern, policy or party considerations are more important. Policy content is also important. Health issues tend to be viewed in an ideological manner, affected by the framing of the problem.

Finally, personalization is important to congressional decision making—what Browne (1993, 22) called the "I Know a Man Theory." Browne's example is a former Senate Budget Committee staffer who said when the time came to make a decision, a member of the committee would say something like: "On the contrary, I know a man from Illinois . . ."; language would then be drafted to avoid that man's problems. A variation of this—the "I Know a Woman Theory"—played out in a turnaround of Sen. Trent Lott's views on drug reimportation. He became an advocate after his 90-year-old mother turned to him one night and asked why she paid so much more for her drugs than did Canadians (Schuler 2004b).

Though legislators prize their own decision-making prowess, they are also affected by the positions of respected colleagues, and, to get their own bills passed, they need to be owed some favors, bargaining and exchanging votes with these colleagues. Bargaining includes more than just vote trading, which also goes on. It can include compromising on a $1.5 billion appropriation rather than the $2 billion the member might have preferred. Bargaining is constrained by the size principle: the bargainer will bargain only as much as necessary to produce a minimum winning coalition, and no more.

While members are generally consistent on votes related to similar issues, sometimes they change their mind. As Meinke (2005) found, members do reverse their positions on important issues, especially when control of the White House shifts, the member's electoral security is high, and the member is subject to cross-pressuring among goals.

Congress at its worst may also be Congress as a collective body. Clearly it seems to suffer from the classic "tragedy of the commons" problem. Individual decision making puts district interests first, as in "that's what I'm here for." But, collectively, that may break the budget and hurt the country. Davidson and Oleszek (1994) referred to this situation as the conflict between the two Congresses: the Congress of individual wills, or guardian of constituent interests, and the Congress of collective decisions. Arnold (1990, 142) argued that legislators will rise above their district's concerns and vote for general benefits over particularized ones under certain circumstances:

— if the general costs or benefits are salient to a large number of citizens;

— if these general effects can be easily traced, permitting credit taking; and

— if the costs to the district are small.

Participation

Members of Congress are buffeted by demands from constituents, special interests, party leaders, committee roles, and their own ideological and personal preferences. The average House member serves on two standing committees and four subcommittees (DeGregorio 1999). Most will serve on at least one informal congressional caucus, and a large number serve in party or other leadership positions. In the 100th Congress, DeGregorio found that 266 members (47 percent) occupied leadership positions, including party leaders, standing committee or subcommittee chairs, or party whips. Members must answer mail and e-mails, spend time in their district, and raise money for the next election. There are well over 1,500 recorded votes per session (Ornstein, Mann, and Malbin 2002). Members simply cannot do everything.

How, then, do they choose where to devote their limited time and energy? Hall's work on participation (1996) deals with individual decisions and the impact those decisions have on the collective body. Members devote what Hall dubbed their "intensity" to measures important to a small number of attentive groups or people in their district, to measures in which the member has a personal interest from experience or background, or to those in which the president has a strong interest. While much of this is played out in sub-committees, even there, the intensity of members varies. On subcommittees, participation is highly selective, with small subsets of members dominating the results. Different subsets dominate on different bills. Few issues elicit involvement by more than a small group of members. Hall concluded that the typical game is played by the few, not by the many. Once again an old saw proves true: the world is run by those who show up.

Caucuses promoting various issues and concerns are also popular and can be used to forge bipartisan relationships. Caucuses range from geographic to ideological, bringing together those of the same gender or race or those who share a concern for a cause. Health causes are very popular as the focus of congressional caucuses, making up around one-fifth of the total in 1998—up from approximately 7 percent in 1987 (Burgin 2003). One of the most effective health caucuses of recent years was the Diabetes Caucus, which was key in passing at least 10 pieces of legislation in the 105th Congress, including expanding Medicare coverage for diabetes, speeding up Food and Drug Administration approval of a noninvasive blood glucose meter, establishing a Diabetes Research Working Group to advise the National Institutes of Health on diabetes, and securing major increases in funding for juvenile diabetes research. The caucus is large (more than 200 members), with powerful members who are leaders of both parties. The caucus used a variety of techniques to focus attention on the problem of diabetes, including organizing diabetes screenings on Capitol Hill for members and staff, press events, and sending group letters to administration officials and congressional leaders. The group also used a carefully crafted message, arguing that diabetes-related spending could help produce budgetary savings by reducing the huge burden the disease places on the nation (Burgin 2003).

Institutional Constraints and Gridlock

Recent political science research has shed light on the role of institutions (including bicameralism, the Senate filibuster, and presidential veto) in voting decisions and in gridlock, the position where no action is taken. Krehbiel (1998) argued that the possibility of a Senate filibuster and possibility of a House override are "pivotal" points in predicting legislative productivity. Chiou and Rothenberg (2003) agree that institutions are important but also found that party unity is key in explaining legislative choices. Martin (2001) documented how the presence of a second chamber and the Supreme Court constrain House and Senate roll-call votes—often leading members to adopt a less-than-optimal policy that will have more likelihood of acceptance in the other chamber or the Supreme Court. Martin did not find that the president constrains behavior—the result, he thinks, of the fact that the presidential effect may appear earlier in the policy process. In an experimental study, Bottom and colleagues (2000) also found the importance of bicameralism—concluding that, much as James Madison hoped, bicameralism helps provide stability, in this case a reduced variance in policy outcomes.

Gridlock or difficulty in enacting legislation is not new in Congress. In fact, some political scientists argue that the Founding Fathers wanted to make law production ponderous and difficult. Others point out that the early leaders also wanted to design a government capable of responding to national crises and problems (Binder 2003). This tension between action and deliberation has been present in the system since its original design. Recent research has tried to better understand why gridlock occurs and its consequences. One influential scholar (Mayhew 1991) found that unlike the common wisdom, there is little evidence that a divided government produces gridlock (or that a unity government produces significantly higher levels of lawmaking). More recent research has countered Mayhew, showing that intrabranch and intraparty conflict (but not interbranch rivalry) are important predictors of deadlock (Binder 2003). Binder also found that while gridlock seems to have a negative effect on the reputation of Congress as an institution, it does not significantly affect members' electoral fortunes, thus limiting legislators' incentive to overcome any gridlock.

THE CONGRESSIONAL ENTERPRISE

Current and former congressional staff and congressional campaign workers who help develop and operate a political policy organization headed by the member of Congress have been called the congressional enterprise (Salisbury and Shepsle 1981). The turnover of congressional staff is so high that an alumni network can be the largest element of the enterprise. Staffers move to executive branch agencies with their bosses, then on to lobbying firms to reap the large financial benefits from their connections. Campaign staffs exist, unnoticed, as ongoing organizations, funded by PAC moneys and other campaign contributions. Yet they may play an important role in defining the policy persona of the member and, especially in the House, provide ongoing political advice. At the center of it all sits the member of Congress—ready to respond to fax machine, phone call, angry letter, or delegation visit, passing on the request to an army of staffers and supporters, tossing a bill in the hopper, or making a speech denouncing an agency ruling or promoting a new program for her district or state.

In recent years, the congressional enterprise has become increasingly active in placing aides in lobbying firms and associations in Washington. Known as the K Street Project, the effort was designed to oust Democrats from trade associations and replace them with Republicans, often those who had worked for House members. House majority leader Tom DeLay placed more than a dozen of his top aides in crucial lobbying and trade association jobs. Confessore (2003) dubbed these placements "graduates of the DeLay school." While these efforts have largely taken place below the radar screen, one effort in 2002 by Rep. Michael Oxley (R-OH) failed when one of his staffers notified a trade group whose legislative interests fell within Representative Oxley's Committee on Financial Services that if it fired its Democratic lobbyist, the chair might go easy on investigating practices in its industry (E. Drew 2005).

Sen. Rick Santorum (R-PA) has held meetings with Republican lobbyists once a week to discuss jobs available in trade associations and lobbying firms and which Republicans might be good for those positions. These efforts were helped by Americans for Tax Relief, which on its Web page (under the heading The K Street Project) identified the political affiliation, employment background, and political donations of Washington's lobbying firms, trade associations, and high-tech companies.

The K Street Project began in 1994 when Republicans won a majority in Congress and warned Washington lobbying and law firms that if they wanted to have appointments with Republican legislators, they should hire more Republicans. Its efforts have stepped up with the dominance of the party in both the executive and legislative branches. According to Elizabeth Drew (2005), a Republican lobbyist explained that "there's a high state of sensitivity to the partisanship of the person you hire for these jobs that did not exist five, six years ago—you hire a Democrat at your peril."

The revolving door of staff from the Hill to lobbying firms, perhaps to the White House or executive branch, provides a close-knit network of like-minded persons that can easily share information and work together. As one Republican lobbyist put it, "It is the hallmark of a very savvy member of Congress to see the departure of staff as an asset and not a detriment. They are building contacts and networks to the good of both sides. Tom [DeLay] has done that as well as anyone" (Justice 2005, A11).

A 2005 scandal involving a Republican lobbyist active in the K Street

Project—Jack Abramoff—turned the endeavor into a liability when former Republican staffers and congressional family members were shown to have benefited financially from their connections.

Congressional Staff

One of the reasons that members of Congress can follow the entrepreneurial path is that they are well staffed. No one would expect the modern Congress to operate without an efficient and capable staff, although until the twentieth century Congress did just that. As Congress began to take on more and more tasks and responsibilities through more committees and subcommittees, it began to hire more staff, especially following World War II and again in the late 1960s and early 1970s as Congress decentralized and worked to free itself from dependence on the executive branch for research and analysis. Overall, more than 22,000 employees work for the legislative branch, a total employment exceeding that of some cabinet departments (Ornstein, Mann, and Malbin 2002, table 5–1). Canada, the next best staffed legislative branch in the world, has around one-eighth of that total—fewer than 3,500 employees.

Figure 1.3 shows the increase in congressional staff since 1965. The biggest growth has been in personal staff—much of it housed in the member's home district, where constituent services are performed. Well over 40 percent of the personal staffs of representatives and nearly one-third of the personal staffs of senators work in district offices. In recent years, the size of staffs in the House and in support agencies such as the Government Accountability Office (GAO; formerly the General Accounting Office) and the Congressional Research Service (CRS) has fallen. In 2001, the House staff was 18 percent smaller than it was in 1979, with most of the decrease occurring in committee staff, which dropped 40 percent over that time period. In contrast, personal staff actually increased slightly. The number of Senate committee staffers also fell substantially over this period, but overall Senate staffing remained fairly stable (Ornstein, Mann, and Malbin 2002).

Personal Staff

Personal staffs are the link between the member of Congress and the district. They keep the legislator in touch and, when the opportunity arises, make the pitch that she is working hard on constituents' behalf. They become

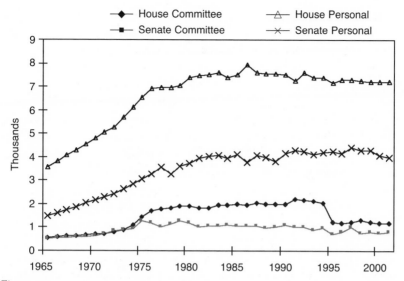

Figure 1.3.

Growth in Congressional Staff, 1965–2001.

Source: Ornstein, Mann, and Malbin 2002.

expert on issues that the member may find boring but that are of concern to constituents. They also offer expert advice on issues in which the member wants to "specialize." Personal staffs work with committee staffs on issues of concern to their bosses in roughly two stages. The first is a monitoring mode, in which personal staffers spend (relatively little) time keeping up with major issues likely to come before the committee. The second is a more active "cramming" mode, gathering information and getting help from committee staff and other sources so they can help the member prepare for deliberations.

As demands on members of Congress have grown, personal staffs have had to assume a greater role in policy making. Staffers consult and engage in initial negotiations with each other, then with their bosses to resolve conflicts. Staffers are expected to come up with new ideas, provide support for desired positions, draft language for proposed laws and press releases, and give advice on political issues. They are also the surveillance crew for legislators on the lookout for issues that will garner media and public attention, whether or not there is a viable solution. Not atypical was the experience of one personal staffer who was given the dates that the member of Congress planned trips home. She was told to come up with a major policy proposal and draft bill for him to unveil at a press conference on each return visit. She did, he did, and one of her ideas—a proposal to remove the requirement for a three-day hospital stay before Medicare home health care eligibility—became law.

Some people worry about these developments. Perhaps congressional staffs play too important a role in policy making, particularly since staffers tend to be young, smart, eager, yet generally inexperienced. "If people only knew how important decisions are really made, with exhausted staffers in their twenties sitting around a table at two in the morning, they would be very upset," confided one health staffer of a U.S. Senator, referring to negotiations in a budget reconciliation package. The story is repeated again and again.

Committee Staff

Committee staffers are, on average, older and more experienced than personal staffers. They also stay longer in their jobs. Compared with personal staffers, they are "the people who really know what's going on" (Whiteman 1987, 223). Whiteman found that on health committees, a small inner core of one committee staffer and perhaps two or three personal staff members who were very knowledgeable on issues dominated things. Staffers outside the core were better informed in the Senate than in the House.

Staffs, of course, tend to reflect the personalities, styles, and political desires of their bosses, although David Price (1971, 325) identified some staffers as policy entrepreneurs who served as independent sources of policy initiation, reflecting "an interest more lively, in some cases, than that of their bosses."

Some observers worry that the staffs are running the place. "There are many senators who felt that all they were doing is running around and responding to the staff . . . It has gotten to the point where the senators never actually sit down and exchange ideas and learn from the experience of others and listen," said Sen. Ernest Hollings (D-SC). "Sometimes when the members do talk, they find that they agree; it was the staff who disagreed" (H. Smith 1988, 282). Staffs are key in translating general congressional desires into legislative mandates. In the hours before the July Fourth weekend of 1994, both the Senate Finance and the House Ways and Means committees passed bills that contained sections with vague directions. Members of Congress fled to their districts or to the beach, leaving it to the staff to fill in the details and produce a coherent legislative product by the time of their return to Washington (Broder 1994a). While the 1995 curbs in committee staffs may help counter this trend toward staff dominance, it is noteworthy that the cuts were not extended to personal staff—the source of major growth. Cynics might point out that it is personal, not committee, staffs that are most closely associated with the reelection of members, clearly an important concern for members of both parties.

Congressional Staff Agencies

Congressional staff agencies—what Martha Derthick (1990) called the congressional generalist staff—have also grown, though not recently. In 1965, the Congressional Research Service, which researches and provides analysis of issues or problems, had 231 employees; by 2001 there were 722 employees—tiny by Washington standards. The CRS is not very visible to the public or even to most policymakers, but it serves an important policy role in congressional decision making. Part of the Library of Congress, the CRS answers questions, provides information, and synthesizes research that is later used in a variety of congressional committee reports and members' speeches.

The Government Accountability Office evaluates the effectiveness of government programs and operations and makes recommendations for improvements. It also alerts policymakers and the public to emerging problems. In the 1970s, the agency changed from a "green eyeshade" agency dominated by accountants to an aggressive policy analysis shop staffed by lawyers, social scientists, and policy analysts. Financial audits are still part of the GAO's mandate—but a small part, making up only about 15 percent of the agency's workload. In 2004, this change in focus was formalized in its change of name from the General Accounting Office to the Government Accountability Office (D. M. Walker 2004).

More than 80 percent of the GAO's work is commissioned by Congress, usually in the form of a request from an individual member. It typically issues well over 1,000 reports and more than 4,000 legal rulings each year, and it claims to save more than $40 billion per year in its advice to Congress. Over the past four years, more than 80 percent of its recommendations have been implemented (Government Accountability Office 2005). Reports on flaws in long-term care insurance oversight by state insurance commissioners, problems with the quality of home health care, and the effects of Medicaid mandates on states are typical of the early, succinct, and provocative reports it issues. In 2004, the GAO sent to the Hill more than 30 reports on Medicare, Medicaid, and preparedness for public health emergencies. It also testifies regularly on the Hill and responds to specific congressional questions with detailed correspondence, also made available to the public.

Nonetheless, the GAO has its critics. A nonprofit research group's study of its performance found that members of Congress increasingly thought it had been giving too many opinions along with its facts. "Some in Congress have expressed concerns . . . that GAO has on occasion moved too far in advocating policy, pushing into policy formulation more appropriate to elected officials," the study found (Pear 1994). But the study noted that Congress was as much at fault as the agency for encouraging findings tailored to the views of the requester. In 1995, a Senate Republican task force recommended cutting the GAO by 25 percent. And the agency has been cut substantially since that time. Between 1995 and 2000, it reduced its staff by 39 percent. In 2005, the GAO had 3,200 employees—down substantially from its heyday in 1988, with 5,204 employees. In 2004, the GAO was given legislative authority to overhaul the agency, including decoupling it from the federal employee pay system.

The Congressional Budget Office is quite small, with only 230 employees in 2005. The CBO was established in 1974 to provide Congress with the institutional capacity to establish and enforce budgetary priorities, coordinate actions on spending and revenue legislation, and develop budgetary and economic information independent of the executive branch. The CBO helps the Budget Committees with the congressional budget resolution and its enforcement, including tracking spending and revenue legislation in a "scorekeeping" system (CBO 2005a). It provides Congress with cost estimates of every single bill reported by a congressional committee, as well as estimates of the costs to state and local governments of federal mandates and laws, and forecasts of economic trends and spending levels. The CBO "mark," or how much money the agency thinks a proposed law will cost, is essential in determining the feasibility of a provision.

Given the importance of health to the budget, the CBO provides major reports on timely health-related issues, and the CBO staff testifies frequently on the Hill. In 2004, CBO health reports dealt with Medicaid's reimbursement to pharmacies for prescription drugs, cost estimates for the Medicare prescription drug benefit (the MMA), financing of long-term care for the elderly, and prescription drug importation.

The CBO's cost estimates were pivotal in the hearings and debates on the 1993–94 health care reform proposal. Although the Clinton White House calculated that its health plan would produce savings in national spending, the CBO concluded that the plan would actually add significantly to the deficit—severely undercutting the political position of the White House and helping to defeat the ambitious plan. Ten years later the CBO played a key role in "scoring" or estimating the costs of the new prescription drug benefit to Medicare. The CBO originally estimated the cost at $400 billion over 10 years—a cost that served as the high-tide mark for many Republicans. In the conference committee hammering out the final version of the bill, CBO staffers were brought in to provide tentative scores on compromises under consideration. They were presented with every new idea or proposal from conferees, in a manner that gave the CBO staff a "sometimes maddening amount of power" (Taylor 2003). The CBO entered another political thicket in 2004 with analysis of the impact of drug importation on U.S. drug spending. It found that permitting importation from Canada would produce a negligible reduction in drug spending, compared with expanding importation to European and other developed nations, which could result in long-term price savings for many consumers (Schuler 2004b).

Another group that advises Congress, the Medicare Payment Advisory Commission (MedPAC) operates below the public's radar screen but is well-known to insiders—particularly to health care providers. MedPAC, established in 1997, provides advice to Congress on issues affecting the Medicare program. In addition to advising Congress on payments to health plans that participate in the Medicare+Choice program and providers in Medicare's traditional fee-for-service program, MedPAC is also charged with analyzing access to care, quality of care, and other issues affecting Medicare. Congress often turns to MedPAC for advice on the legitimacy of provider claims that Medicare payments are too low. Following cuts in hospital payments in 1997, MedPAC urged Congress to hold the course, countering with arguments (and numbers) that hospitals were not suffering from lowered Medicare payments (D. Smith 2002).

MedPAC issues two reports with recommendations to Congress each year. It replaced and consolidated the activities of two previous commissions: the Prospective Payment Assessment Commission (ProPAC) and the Physician Payment Review Commission (PPRC). The success rate of recommendations from these earlier commissions was high. For example, congressional reforms to make the Resource-Based Relative Value Scale (RBRVS) more acceptable to specialists and the decision to include volume performance standards were clearly traceable to PPRC's recommendations. RBRVS is a payment system for physician services intended to increase the payments to primary care physicians.

At a more practical level, MedPAC gives Congress political cover for some of the tough choices it must make if health care costs are to be controlled. Members of Congress simply point to the commission's recommendations and say they had no choice. Drawing outside experts into the inner circle as they do, these agencies also serve that uniquely Washingtonian function of forming informal linkages among experts from the various agencies and institutions of government.

ENTREPRENEURSHIP AND CONGRESS

Although in recent years party leadership has stepped up its grip on members of Congress, and even the minority party leadership is stronger than it was a decade or so ago, it would be wrong not to recognize that individual members are still masters of their own fate on most issues. Members can use modern technology to help assure their reelection, employ staffs who cater to constituents' needs and help the member become expert in desired areas and knowledgeable in many others, and avail themselves of a fairly compliant press corps to get their message across to interest groups, constituents, and colleagues. Several scholars have dubbed modern members of Congress "policy entrepreneurs," who can use staff resources, the media, and technology to promote issues and themselves (Loomis 1988; Parker 1989; Shepsle and Weingast 1984).

Wawro (2000) called activities to achieve a member's policy goals "legislative entrepreneurship" and specifically examined whether legislative entrepreneurship benefits a member in her reelection or in PAC contributions. He found little evidence of this link. However, entrepreneurs are more likely to advance to committee and party leadership positions.

The entrepreneurial member also has her eye on post-congressional status. While moving from legislator to lobbyist is a long-standing political path, few have had a more criticized journey than Rep. Billy Tauzin of Louisiana, chair of the House Energy and Commerce Committee, whose committee's portfolio includes health issues. Tauzin's committee drafted the Medicare prescription drug bill, and he served as a principal negotiator in the conference committee. While serving as a leader in these legislative negotiations, Tauzin was talking with the drug industry lobby group, the Pharmaceutical Research and Manufacturers of America (PhRMA), about taking its top job on his retirement at the end of the 108th Congress. Tauzin eventually stepped down as chair, but nine months later announced his new appointment as PhRMA president. The situation was particularly sticky since one of the most controversial components of the Medicare prescription drug law prohibited the federal government from negotiating lower prices on drugs—a provision strongly supported by the prescription drug industry (Shields 2004).

Congress and the Press

The press plays a crucial role in the packaging of the modern member of Congress. Media representatives are extremely responsive to the actions and reactions of the member and provide her with almost universally positive coverage. Reporters representing local newspapers, particularly those in small or medium-size cities, are generally uncritical and unwilling to examine issues in depth: whatever the legislator says must be true. Local television stations are similarly happy to have video feeds from their district members, even videos produced by the party's own camera crew, often featuring the legislator's press secretary asking the "probing" questions. For members of Congress primarily concerned with reelection, local coverage is more important than national exposure. Kansas Rep. Dan Glickman once said, "I can be on Tom Brokaw but it is not as important to my reelection as being on the NBC affiliate in Wichita" (Benenson 1987, 1552).

The national press, a harder "sell" for many members of Congress, can also be useful if the member is more concerned about influence in Congress or national public policy (or running for national office at a later date). The plethora of talk shows and the advent of C-Span have brought the names and faces of once-unknown legislators into living rooms across the country, and into those of their colleagues. Members can use the media to enhance the importance of and improve public knowledge about favored issues and perhaps persuade viewers to support their position. National media coverage can also serve to inform colleagues, the White House, and top-level bureaucrats and can help build winning coalitions. Rep. Billy Tauzin was a master at generating press coverage for his committee and himself. Before key hearings, he would provide advanced copies of materials that his staff had researched to selected news organizations—to garner headlines and often an appearance on one or more morning talk shows before the hearing (Alpert 2004).

Speaker Newt Gingrich was a popular television guest and was quick with a quote that he knew would be certain to make the network news. He was also a master at intimidating the press. As part of his campaign to pass Medicare reforms in 1995, he wanted to make certain that the press did not describe the Republican bill as "cutting" Medicare. It was not a cut, he and other Republicans emphasized: it was a reduction in the rate of growth. Budget chair John Kasich and Republican National Committee chair Haley Barbour took on the task of calling reporters who described the program as "cutting" Medicare. Barbour called network anchors at NBC and ABC and a correspondent at CBS to complain about the use of the "C" word. He held breakfasts and lunches with reporters to explain the difference between cuts and slowing the rate of growth (Weisskopf and Maraniss 1995).

This media-oriented environment not only has affected the behavior of members of Congress already elected but also has perhaps its greatest effect in attracting a new kind of member—one who is photogenic and fast on her feet. Television personalities, movie stars, and sports heroes have successfully used the media and their experience with it to win primaries and seats in Congress.

Jacobson (1987) concluded that the media, taken together, have not done much to damage members of Congress but have damaged the institution of Congress, at least a little. When an announced Senate candidate appearing on a Sunday television talk show calls the chair of a Senate subcommittee "misinformed" on the president's health care proposal that the subcommittee's staff helped draft, both attacker and attackee are diminished in the process. The confrontational style encouraged by the media may stir the fires of a cynical and dissatisfied public viewing audience.

Public Opinion

It is important to keep in mind that the reason the press is valuable to members of Congress is that it helps link the member with the public. Public opinion clearly matters to individual legislators, party leadership, and other policy participants. Members also use other means to sway public opinion—including personal contacts, grassroots mailings, and orchestrated campaigns. Public opinion is important, particularly as related to the government's role in policy. Kingdon (1995) noted that changes in the public mood or climate have important effects on policy agendas and policy outcomes. DeGregorio (2000) stated flatly that for major policy initiatives, it is essential to have mass public opinion on your side. And Binder's 2003 study of gridlock found empirically that the greater the level of public support for government action, the lower the level of policy gridlock.

Seeking public opinion was a major goal of the early years of Newt Gingrich's reign as Speaker of the House. For example, he developed and implemented an elaborate plan to enact Medicare reform in 1995. A core part of the plan was how to frame the debate. A series of focus groups helped a cadre of political consultants define the "message": to preserve, protect, and improve (*improve* later became *strengthen*) Medicare. Indeed, the name of the Republican House measure, which cut $270 billion from Medicare, was the

Medicare Preservation Act. The Speaker pulled together a group including House members, staff, and press secretaries to sell the plan.

The group met weekly, often with consultants, to ensure that the message was consistent and strong as they met with reporters, wrote legislators' speeches, and issued press releases. One of the tactics was to "flood the faxes" with as much information as possible. When later focus groups responded positively to the idea of long-term consequences of reforming Medicare, the message was honed to include the idea of preserving, protecting, and strengthening Medicare for the next generation. Gingrich personalized the issue as much as possible, highlighting the message that Republicans cared about people (Weisskopf and Maraniss 1995). The measure passed the House with 231 votes.

In recent years, the techniques of framing and packaging issues have become commonplace. For example, in July 2004, House Republicans prepared a "recess kit" for members' dealings with constituents that highlighted the party message. The kit urged members to stress presidential successes in Iraq and improvements in the economy, as well as tax cuts (Dodd and Oppenheimer 2005).

CONGRESS AND THE COURTS

An important balance of power for Congress occupies a lovely building across the park—the U.S. Supreme Court. The Court's relationship with Congress is somewhat cyclical, with some Courts serving to curb congressional actions and others allowing much more leeway. Since the mid-1990s, the Court has resided largely at the curbing end of the cycle—often finding against Congress and for the states. The Rehnquist Court fashioned a federalism agenda that strengthened the notion of state sovereignty and punished Congress if it strayed too much into areas far afield from its enumerated powers (Oleszek 2004, 322). The recent Court has been quite active in nullifying federal laws on federalism and other bases. Between 1994 and 2005, the Supreme Court struck down 64 congressional provisions—almost six per year. Until 1994, the Court struck down an average of one statute every two years (Gewirtz and Golder 2005).

Congress has limited options to change the Supreme Court (except, of course, for approving its members). It has a more direct role in other federal courts and has actively taken on a rather unusual oversight role. One example is a 2003 law limiting federal judges' ability to hand down sentences lighter than those recommended in federal sentencing guidelines for crimes against children and sex crimes. The law requires the Justice Department to inform Congress whenever a judge hands down a sentence more lenient than the federal guidelines, except in cases where the defendant provides substantial assistance to authorities. Another example is the efforts of the House Judiciary Committee to investigate the sentencing habits of specific federal judges viewed as too "soft." Other measures have been introduced to limit the purview of federal courts over such issues as constitutional challenges to the Pledge of Allegiance and the 1996 law against gay marriage. As one scholar put it, "There used to be what we called a reverence for the courts in Congress. Now judges aren't so sure they're safe" (Perine 2004, 2153).

CONCLUSION

In 1965, the executive branch was the primary source of legislation, congressional staffers were few and largely long-time friends of the member they worked for, there were several hundred lobbyists, and a few committee chairs were the dominant players. Today, Congress has no need to wait on the executive branch for ideas or expertise. In a town where power is everything, Congress has the most. The "Imperial Congress" or "King Kong of Washington's political jungle" is how long-time political player and former health advisor Joseph Califano put it (1994, 40). Yet clouds hover over the congressional parade.

Despite the tendency to send incumbents back to the House and Senate, Americans are also willing to express their dissatisfaction with their officials and their government. In 2005, 51 percent of survey respondents said they disapproved of Congress, the highest level of disapproval since May 1994—months before the elections in which Republicans took over the House (NBC News/Wall Street Journal Survey 2005).

President George W. Bush set about to consolidate more power under his presidency and has succeeded (see chapter 2). He has refused to share requested information with Congress and its watchdog agency (the GAO) and has often pursued policy by executive order—allowing him to avoid possible squabbles and to move forward quickly to meet his goals. He set out to strengthen the office of the presidency—and has largely succeeded—with Congress the loser in the power exchange.

But perhaps the biggest cloud on the horizon, and one that worries both political scientists and practitioners alike, is the increasing partisanship that is evident in the halls of Congress. Certainly the long-held Democratic control over Congress promulgated many abuses of power, and the Republicans did not often get their way. But Republicans were not physically excluded from conference committees or given no opportunity to review legislation, much less participate in its drafting. Further, the discourse among members has become increasingly shrill and immoderate—often flowing from a set of talking points produced by party leaders. Even in the Senate, the last bastion of civility and moderation, leaders of the two parties no longer talk regularly, and even personally campaign against each other. With members more and more sure of their seats, there is little reason to seek out colleagues of the other party or to seek a compromise position. And little such consultation and moderation is in play in the modern Congress.

Along with heightened partisanship has come entrenched ideological positions—often with punishment meted to party members who do not toe the ideological line. Although there are examples of moderate Republicans wielding their power, these examples are few, and the number of moderates of both parties elected to office is lessening.

Sometimes ideology becomes so important it seems to trump even constituents' views and long-standing party positions. In 2005, Congress enacted a measure that called for the controversial right-to-die case involving Terri Schiavo to be moved to federal court—in spite of consistent rulings by state courts that the Florida woman be allowed to die. Setting aside both public opinion and the party's support for a strong federal system (with a strong role for states), Congress acted quickly to counter what the majority thought was a moral "wrong."

Ideology has long played a role in congressional action in health, often in positions relating to the role of government versus the market. Conservatives seek a smaller role for government and generally protect the role of the market to solve problems; liberals want government protections. The patients' bill of rights has been stalled in large measure on the issue of the government's role—whether federal law should preempt state laws. Also at issue was the ability of patients to sue insurance plans in court. Similarly, the conflict over prescription benefits was in large part over government versus the free market. Conservatives sought a stronger role for private insurance companies and a small role and lower costs for government. Their position prevailed in the 2003 Medicare Modernization Act.

The Congress emerging in the twenty-first century looks different in crucial ways from earlier ones, but also in important ways looks similar. Partisanship, ideology, strength of party leadership, and public support vary across decades and across Congresses. And because health is a major issue across decades and Congresses, it provides an excellent case for understanding the evolving and ever changing power structure that guides national policy. The willingness of the president to provide policy leadership is a major component in that changing power structure and in health policy. From Lyndon Johnson to George W. Bush, the president has left a mark on health policy—or left a legacy that affected future actions in the health policy arena.

2

The Presidency

A LOOK BACK

1965

ON JULY 27, 1965, President Lyndon B. Johnson and his cabinet, assembled for their twentieth cabinet meeting, congratulated themselves heartily. The Medicare bill had just come out of the House-Senate conference committee and final passage was hours away. The voting rights bill was following close behind it, in conference, with agreement expected within the week. The landmark Elementary and Secondary Education Act had become law in April, and the War on Poverty was a year old. In all, 36 major pieces of legislation had been signed into law by the time of that twentieth cabinet meeting; 26 others were moving through the House or Senate.

Tom Wicker, writing in August 1965, said, "They are rolling the bills out of Congress these days the way Detroit turns super-sleek, souped-up autos off the assembly line" (L. Johnson 1971, 323). The president was an activist, had been elected with 61 percent of the popular vote, and was working with a heavily Democratic Congress (68 percent in both the House and the Senate).

Johnson had strong public support. Although in the fall of 1965 he sensed "a shift in the winds," or a fading of public support for change (reflected in some congressional calls for a slowing down of legislative action), he pushed forward, largely through the work of 10 task forces, each on a critical area of policy.

By the end of the year, major laws had been enacted dealing with issues ranging from higher education to the formation of the Department of Housing and Urban Development (HUD), from law enforcement assistance to workforce training. Of these laws, seven were in health (Medicare; heart, cancer, and stroke program; mental health; health professions; medical libraries; child health; and community health services) and four dealt with the environment (clean air, water pollution control, water resources council, and water desalting). But at the top of the list was Medicare, what Johnson and others considered the premier issue of that year, perhaps of his term.

In 1964, President Johnson was very disappointed when Medicare failed to pass the House after its success in the Senate, and in 1965 he was determined that the Ways and Means Committee should not bottle up the measure again. He worked closely with House leaders, encouraging them to change the composition of the Ways and Means Committee to reflect the Democratic majority in the House, thus adding two crucial seats. He asked the leadership to designate Medicare HR 1 and S 1 (the first bill introduced in both House and Senate), symbolizing its importance. He highlighted the great consequence of Medicare in his state of the union message on January 4 and in a special message on health. When consulted on a compromise proposed by the Ways and Means chair, Johnson (1971, 216) enthusiastically supported any reasonable move "to get this bill now." He met personally with House and Senate leaders following the favorable recommendation of the bill by the House Ways and Means Committee. When the bill passed the Senate, Johnson called it a "great day for America."

1981

The situation facing President Ronald Reagan in his first year after election was not as rosy as that enjoyed by Lyndon Johnson 16 years earlier. Reagan's winning margin was substantial (nearly 10 percentage points over incumbent Jimmy Carter), but he faced a Democratic majority in the House and had only a slim (53–47) Republican majority in the Senate. Nevertheless, Reagan, like Johnson, moved quickly. In his first nine months in office, he helped push through major domestic budget and tax cuts and a massive defense buildup. One of his greatest achievements was passage of the entire administration budget and program reform package in the Omnibus Reconciliation Act of 1981, a legislative coup because it allowed consideration of a large number of important measures in one vote rather than as dozens of bills. Included in this measure was the consolidation of 21 health programs into four block grants: primary care; maternal and child health; preventive health and health services; and alcohol, drug abuse, and mental health. The consolidation included a reduction in federal dollars for the programs—of 21 percent over the previous year's funding (J. Feder et al. 1982).

By the fall of 1981, the congressional tide had turned. Congress was less enthusiastic about the administration's cuts and approved only half of those proposed. By February 1982, even the Republican-dominated Senate Budget Committee rejected the administration's budget, which was defeated 21-0 two months later (Salamon and Abramson 1984). Yet in those early months, some argue, the long-standing principles governing social welfare policy in the United States were questioned, if not revised. The administration thought public welfare should focus only on those unquestionably unable to care for themselves. For those people who were more marginally disabled or less needy, the approach was to reduce or eliminate benefits and encourage them to work or seek help in the private, not the public, sector. In health, President Reagan's philosophy encouraged less government and had the effect of promoting the idea of market competition and the provision of services by the private sector.

1993

The political climate surrounding the newly elected president Bill Clinton was inauspicious. He had been the governor of a small state, with limited Washington experience. Elected with only 43 percent of the vote, he clearly lacked any "mandate." He had what one writer called the "worst first week of any President since William Henry Harrison who caught pneumonia while delivering a long Inaugural speech and died a month later" (Blumenthal 1994, 36). There were problems with nominees for attorney general and enormous opposition to changes in policy on gays in the military. Yet the Congress Clinton faced was seemingly sympathetic, with substantial Democratic majorities in the House and Senate. This president was enthusiastic and diligent in his efforts to court the Democratic members of Congress in his first year of office, making trips to Capitol Hill and inviting members individually and in groups to accompany him jogging, to ride on Air Force One, or to attend meals or movie screenings, to the point that "few on the Hill . . . managed to escape a talk with Clinton" (Blumenthal 1994, 38). Early successes included a difficult budget vote (passing by two votes in the House, one in the Senate), ratification of the North American Free Trade Agreement (NAFTA), legislation on family and medical leave, earned income tax credit, and national service. In his first year, his presidential success rating as measured by Congressional Quarterly was 86 percent—the highest for a president in his first year since Lyndon Johnson's 88 percent in 1964 (Ornstein, Mann, and Malbin 2002). (The score reflects presidential victories on votes on which the president takes a position. It combines major and insignificant bills and reflects the position of the president at the time of the vote.)

Like Lyndon Johnson, Bill Clinton worked Congress to promote his health care agenda, but unlike Johnson, he also used television in what has become known as the town meeting format, in which citizens ask questions of the president in an informal setting. After a highly publicized appearance before a joint session of Congress in September 1993, the real "selling" of the program began. Hillary Rodham Clinton made five televised congressional appearances and had interviews with five network reporters. The president answered questions about his health care proposal for two and a half hours on a popular network news show, conducted a town meeting in California, invited two dozen newspaper reporters to lunch, and allowed 55 radio talk-show hosts to broadcast live from the White House lawn (Kelly 1993).

Clinton, though, faced many more obstacles and had fewer resources than did Johnson. Both were Democratic presidents dealing with a Democratic Congress, but the nature of the relationship was starkly different. The member of Congress of 1994 was largely an independent enterprise and could raise her own money and strike her own "deals." Another "plum" from the Johnson era and before—presidential support and appearances in congressional campaigns—was of little use: Clinton's public support reached a low of 37 percent before the midterm elections and there were relatively few calls for campaign appearances. Party leaders had less power than those of the 1960s and were unable to deliver votes or coerce many votes from party members. With the advent of the Congressional Budget Office, the president's own numbers—on the cost of health care reform, for example—were questioned and discounted in favor of those of the less partisan CBO.

The interest-group world into which President Clinton's health agenda was thrust also varied enormously from that of the mid-1960s. In 1993, numerous interest groups used strategies to mobilize their members and sway public opinion that only one or two powerful groups could have mustered in Johnson's time. Clinton's "bully pulpit" was shared, at least in part, by the fictional characters Harry and Louise, developed by the health insurance industry and wildly successful in framing the public debate on health care reform. Interestingly, Harry and Louise apparently made their biggest initial impact on Washington, D.C., rather than on the people back home. When the Clintons began to refute and parody the ads, they gave the ads more legitimacy and standing (Clymer, Pear, and Toner 1994).

Finally, President Clinton faced budgetary constraints unlike those confronting any other previous modern president. In the summer of his first year in office, Congress imposed strict spending limits, freezing discretionary spending at the previous year's levels with no allowance for inflation. Under the agreement, any new spending had to be accompanied by offsetting spending cuts or revenue increases or both. To make up for inflation and add money for priority initiatives, such as health care, Clinton was forced to cut back on hundreds of programs. It was a far cry from the days of earlier presidential power. Bill Clinton, the president with an activist agenda topped by health care reform as the defining element, was relegated to near-observer status in the spring and summer of 1994, when the legislative drafting set about in earnest.

2005

By 2005, President George W. Bush had been victorious in two very close elections. In 2000 he lost the popular vote and became president with a margin of one electoral vote. In 2004 he fought a highly divisive campaign against Sen. John Kerry (D-MA) and garnered 16 more electoral votes than the 270 he needed to win (with a popular margin of 50.7 percent). In both terms, however, he governed without apology or a middle ground. Further, he worked to strengthen the institution of the presidency, which may have been tarnished by the personal activities of the previous president, Bill Clinton, and weakened by the diligence of special prosecutors probing the alleged unethical conduct of presidents, their aides, and cabinet secretaries. The law authorizing the independent counsel, first enacted in 1978, expired in 1999.

The 43rd president's primary concerns in the beginning of his term were tax-related—specifically, fulfilling a campaign promise to lower taxes. Indeed, over the first term, he spearheaded an effort that led to adoption of two of the three biggest tax cuts in American history (Cochran 2004). His presidency was indelibly changed on September 11, 2001, when terrorist attacks on New York and Washington led to a national fixation on both safety and retribution. Military efforts in Afghanistan and later Iraq dominated the presidency, the Congress, the media, and the public throughout the months following 9/11 and the invasion of Iraq. President Bush was not engaged in health policy issues in the first years of his administration, an absence reflected in the fact that a listing of the top 100 players in health policy in 2002 did not include the president of the United States.

With the coming of the presidential elections of 2004, domestic issues began to come to the fore for both the president and Congress. And Medicare was at the top of their concerns. In his state of the union address in 2003, President Bush called for reform and strengthening of Medicare, including providing access to prescription drugs and a greater choice in plans that offer those drugs. In an incredibly short period of time for major legislation, Congress followed the president's advice and enacted the Medicare Modernization Act, signed by President Bush in December 2003. The law for the first time included prescription drugs in Medicare coverage, expanded the appeal of managed care plans for seniors, and contained a host of other benefits for providers, insurance companies, and health interests (Heaney 2003). Bush not only put the item on the agenda in January 2003, but he also served as "cheerleader in chief," highlighting the need for reform in speeches, public sessions, and private discussions as Congress worked out the details (A. Goldstein and Dewar 2003).

Medicare was part of a broader Bush agenda promoting the idea of an "ownership society," in which the people, not the government, make major decisions on programs affecting their lives (Cochran 2004). In health care, this means a society in which more people "own" their health plans and (with physicians) make their own health decisions, instead of "bureaucrats in Washington, D.C." (Bush 2004). By 2003, Bush was number one in a list of the most influential people in health care (Romano 2003)—clear evidence of a president's dominance when he decides to enter the policy fray.

President Bush seemed personally committed to increasing the power of the office of the president. Unlike his immediate predecessor, who was relatively forthcoming in providing information to Congress and the special prosecutor, George W. Bush fought for his right to withhold information—and won. Federal courts upheld the White House assertion that it did not have to turn over to the General Accountability Office, Congress's primary investigative agency, the names of lobbyists and company officials who helped craft the president's energy plan. President Bush also fought to protect the ability of his office to block Congress from calling on White House aides to testify and imposed new restrictions on public access to presidential papers (Stevenson 2005). Bush took on the power to set policy on the detention and interrogation of individuals involved in terrorism. When Congress was not forthcoming on legislation he desired, he often pursued his goals through executive orders or regulations.

One long-time presidential observer, Abner Mikva, described Bush's use of power in terms of body building: "The separation of powers works because of who makes the biggest muscle. When the president makes a big muscle, as George Bush is currently doing, he has a lot of power. He's willing to take on the courts and Congress and exercise power in a big way" (Stevenson 2005).

PRESIDENTIAL POWER, SYMBOLS, AND ROLES

The presidency is the institution of executive power in the United States; the president is the person who exercises that power for a limited period of time. Many young boys and girls (and their parents) may aspire to be president, but few will achieve it, and those few will be closely watched, examined, and analyzed. Yet, as Charles Jones (1994, 281) pointed out, the U.S. presidency "carries a burden of lofty expectations that are simply not warranted by the political or constitutional basis of the office." The president, analysts say, is one institutional player among many in the crafting of national public policy.

One of the primary policy-making roles of the president is to put items on the agenda. When a measure is introduced in Congress, his role shifts to one of monitoring and encouragement. The president's margin of victory, his popularity with the public, and the dominance of his party in Congress make up what is known as political capital, an important factor in the president's ability to persuade Congress to adopt his programs. Presidents like to "go public," or take their case to the American people, in the hope that constituents will then pressure their members of Congress to support the president's policy. In 1994, going public was not a successful route for President Clinton and his health care reform initiative, since strong interest groups also invested in advertising to inform the public on issues not to the president's liking. Like Congress, the presidency is much affected by public opinion and the press. The press coverage of presidents is massive; it can be helpful or harmful. The president is responsible for overseeing the executive branch, a task that many presidents do not like but some try to use to their advantage. Finally, presidents appoint members of the Supreme Court and other judicial posts, subject to Senate advice and consent. The president's most significant role in health policy has traditionally been in putting health issues on the national agenda and urging public support for their adoption by Congress.

Presidential Power

The Founding Fathers were leery of giving presidents too much control; their experience with kings and their henchmen had convinced the founders that control vested in one individual was a bad idea. Yet they were also fearful of the "impetuous vortex" of the legislative branch and wanted to prevent "legislative usurpations" as well (Publius [1787–88] 1961, 309). So they set up a system of balanced powers, with three branches of government, each providing a check to any overzealousness of the others. Since ratification of the Constitution, the struggle between Congress and the president over control has waged almost continually, with some presidents exercising strong leadership and others acquiescing to a more dominant Congress.

The president personally embodies most of the power of the executive branch (unlike Congress and the judiciary, where power is highly decentralized and dispersed). This gives the president power because he can act more quickly than other branches and can be the center of press coverage, thus focusing the attention of the entire nation on a particular matter. The president is the only person (except for the vice president) elected to represent the nation as a whole, and thus he has a national constituency. The president represents all the people and is the personification of the national interest. In the development of policy, presidential concerns for the broad national interest can conflict with more specialized congressional concerns focused on the costs and benefits of policies to members' local constituencies.

Another way to look at the president is as the representative of the 200 million or so Americans who are not directly represented by lobbies of some sort. This was the role President Lyndon Johnson described when he explained to a group of Southern senators why, as president, he was proposing major civil rights and other "liberal" issues that he had not supported as a senator. He said, "I'm president now—president of all the people" (Thomas 1999, 37). President Clinton seemed to be appealing to all the people when he said in August 1994 that his White House was really "the home office of the American Association for Ordinary Citizens" (Wines 1994, A9). Later, looking back at his presidency, he had the same view: "I've tried to make my government the government of the people of Watts as well as the people of Beverly Hills," he told a predominantly African American crowd of enthusiastic Democratic supporters in Watts, California, as he stumped for candidate Al Gore in the final days before the 2000 presidential election. "Four more years," his listeners responded, indicating that in their view he had succeeded and, if they had their way, the Constitution would be changed to let him keep up the good work (National Public Radio 2000).

Presidents are a symbol for the country as a whole, and people sleep better when a president they trust is watching over the country (Kernell, Spelich, and Wildavsky 1975). Journalists focus Washington coverage on the White House, and scholars highlight the power and leadership of the office of the president. Presidents themselves encourage their identification with the nation and the national interest in their speeches and addresses (Hinckley 1990). In his emotional speech on resigning from the presidency, Richard Nixon drew on this bond, which he called "a personal sense of kinship with each and every American" (R. Price 1977, 348). President George W. Bush frequently talks about "the people's business." Yet a president soon learns that promoting unity in the face of the pluralism of the U.S. political system is extremely difficult. Much is expected—often too much. Brownlow (1949) noted that whatever else a president newly arrived in the White House might look forward to, he would be wise to realize from the first moment that he is certain to disappoint many of his constituents, who collectively compose the nation. As George W. Bush (2004, 2072) put it in his speech accepting the Republican nomination in 2004, "One thing I have learned about the presidency is that whatever shortcomings you have, people are going to notice them; and whatever strengths you have, you're going to need them."

Presidential Roles

The president is clearly the most visible government official in the land. Television seems to cover his every move—even stops at fast-food restaurants while jogging, helicopter trips to a forest getaway, and attendance at church worship, parents' funerals, and parent-teacher meetings. The formal speeches, press conferences, and state dinners are well covered by the press and closely followed by many others. Yet the presidency is more than a photo opportunity or dress-up dinner. The president must lead. But how? And in what direction?

Cronin and Genovese (1998) described seven functions of the presidency:

recruitment of leadership, crisis management, symbolic and morale-building leadership, priority setting and program design, legislative and political coalition building, program implementation and evaluation, and oversight of government routines and establishment of an early-warning system for future problem areas. The first function facing presidents is selection of leadership. President George W. Bush launched his administration flanked by many old hands brought back to Washington from the days of the first Bush administration or the Gerald Ford administration. His cabinet did not have to spend the first days and months figuring out where to park and how to run their office, as is typical for newcomers to the capital. The experience of these officials was helpful when the president confronted crisis management early in his presidency with the events surrounding 9/11 and when the press and Congress made demands on the new administration. President Bush, like his predecessors, was least interested in oversight and early-warning systems for future problem areas. Presidents are, of course, politicians interested in promoting their policies, building their party, and leaving a legacy.

While presidents are viewed by the public as the epitome of power in the United States, political scientists have debated whether the president is in fact a leader or a clerk (Neustadt 1960). Those who subscribe to the clerk mode argue that understanding the presidency is a matter of understanding the institution of the presidency, in which presidential behavior is fully (or mostly) subsumed under the institutional setting, dimensions, and constraints. The president has little individual leeway under this model—rather, any president in the same institutional setting would do pretty much the same thing. The counterargument, the president-centered approach (Gilmour 2002), is that the president is a leader and imposes his own will on those institutional constraints and opportunities. As in many such debates, the truth may lie between the two models or have a few components of each. The president has institutional constraints but can choose to push those constraints to the limit or live with them. George W. Bush tends to push and generally has succeeded in protecting private documents, initiating policies through executive orders, and limiting congressional inquiries.

A president has to deal with two distinct policy domains: domestic affairs and foreign and defense policy (Wildavsky 1966). Of the two, the president has more control over (and perhaps more success with) the second. He must deal extensively with Congress on domestic issues, and convincing legislators can be tough indeed. Presidential time and attention are often devoted to mustering congressional support rather than determining the desired policy. In foreign and defense policy, the reverse is often true: "selling" the plan is not the hard part; coming up with the best policy choice seems to be much tougher. The public knows little about foreign policy or defense and tends to trust the president on his proposals. Voters generally like a president to be decisive in foreign affairs; support for the president, as measured by polls, often rises after presidential action to deal with a difficult foreign issue. Also, the interest groups opposing presidential actions in foreign policy are relatively weak.

In domestic policy, especially economic issues, the public is more informed and is more likely to object to presidential preferences when interest groups are active. And the preferences of the president and Congress may differ more markedly on domestic than on foreign policy issues (Rohde 1990). Indeed, for many years, members of both congressional parties frequently announced that they honored the principle that "politics stops at the water's edge." Although the growth of free trade has eroded this bipartisanship principle by mixing foreign and domestic issues concerning exported jobs and imported workers, human rights concerns, and other matters, when the nation is engaged in a foreign policy crisis, there is still a tendency to rally behind the president and save the second-guessing till the dust settles. The country's bipartisan response to the 9/11 terrorism attacks is a case in point, with initially very little second-guessing from Congress, the press, or the citizenry. The benefit of the doubt is less likely to be given in domestic policy, where frequently the opposition party deliberately tries to differentiate itself from the president's policy choices, and members of his own party may feel pulled away from their leadership by constituents, policy, or interest-group pressures.

Our focus here is on the domestic presidency, the one in which the president has major roles in setting the policy agenda, persuading Congress and the public to support the proposed policies, and overseeing the implementation of the policies once enacted.

Setting the Agenda

For the president, unlike members of Congress, reelection is not viewed as the raison d'être of decision making. Presidents also want their policies to be adopted, they want the policies they put in place to last, and they want to feel they helped solve the problems facing the country (Ceaser 1988). But for the first-term president, reelection is an ever present concern. In *The Agenda*, Woodward (1994) reported that reelection concerns came up in the first term of the Clinton presidency over issues such as NAFTA and a freeze on Social Security cost-of-living increases and their likely effects on key states such as Florida and California in the 1996 election. The closer to an election, the more likely the president is to be concerned with reelection. Other presidential goals are historical achievement, power, and the ability to solve the country's problems. George W. Bush recognized the importance of agenda in his 2000 campaign biography: "The first challenge of leadership . . . is to outline a clear vision and agenda" (F. Greenstein 2004, 197).

When a president decides an issue is a national concern, whether health care reform, drug abuse, energy conservation, or Social Security, that issue is propelled to the top of the nation's policy agenda. Typically, presidents use the prestige and prominence of their office to focus national attention on the desired policies. As Davidson (1984, 371) noted, "Framing agendas is what the presidency is all about." Presidents communicate their agendas through state of the union addresses and other major speeches, television addresses and televised news conferences, and the release of special reports and analyses. They use highly visible cabinet members to spread the word and highlight key issues across the country. To effect policy they must convince Congress, and the president has little trouble getting members' attention. Kingdon (1995, 23) quoted a lobbyist as saying that "when a president sends up a bill [to Congress], it takes first place in the queue. All other bills take second place."

President Clinton was committed to health care reform in the early years of his presidency and used the state of the union and a special address to Congress to make his case. President George W. Bush was less concerned with health, but nonetheless did speak about his concerns about access and costs of health care and offer some proposals for Congress during his first term. In his state of the union address in 2003, President Bush called for Medicare reform, including improved access for seniors to preventive medicine and new drugs. He also called for more choice in the Medicare program. He got all of one and much of the other in the 2003 MMA. However, it is noteworthy that he did not succeed with other health issues he placed on the agenda, including a patients' bill of rights (2002), tax credits for uninsured/lower-income Americans (2002, 2004, 2005), association plans in which small businesses could work together to negotiate for lower insurance rates (2004, 2005), malpractice reform (2003, 2004, 2004), expanded health savings accounts (2004, 2005), and technological improvements (2004, 2005) (Government Printing Office 2005).

According to Light (1991), presidents choose issues to minimize political costs and maximize political benefits. One way to do this is to alternate the promotion of broad policy redirection and noncontroversial incremental change. Indeed, not all presidential agenda items are bold steps. Mark Peterson (1990) found that of the presidential initiatives he examined, only 12 percent involved large new programs. Most of the proposals (58 percent) were best categorized as small changes to existing programs.

Presidents can choose certain issues for strategic, political gain. For example, Torres-Gil (1989) argued that part of the rationale behind President Reagan's decision to put catastrophic health insurance on the agenda was a careful determination that the Republicans needed an issue that would demonstrate their compassion and family orientation. Torres-Gil noted that the "compassion agenda" came on the heels of the Iran-Contra hearings and a loss of party control in the Senate, at a time when the president needed to regain public support. Similarly, the push for Medicare prescription drugs in 2003 was seen as a way to undercut the Democrats' domestic policy positions in the 2004 congressional and presidential campaigns.

Although the president cannot introduce legislation, he can and does provide draft legislation or legislative guidance for translating his agenda into legislative language. A leader of the president's party or another prominent party member usually introduces the president's proposal. The president is also responsible for the presidential budget proposal, submitted to Congress in January before the fiscal year begins, which often sets the baseline for further discussions. Congressional budget reforms adopted in the mid-1970s dramatically affected the president's budget-making power, providing Congress with the staff and procedures to formulate its own budgets and allowing it to declare that the president's proposed budgets were DOA—dead on arrival. However, the president can use the budget process to his advantage as well. President George W. Bush urged Congress to set caps on domestic spending, and President Clinton worked closely with Congress on the 1997 reconciliation measure.

In 1995–96, Congress learned the power of the presidency in the budget process the hard way. Republican leaders refused to compromise with President Clinton over their plan to balance the budget in seven years through major cuts in virtually every area of government spending while also providing a sizable tax cut. Clinton twice vetoed the temporary spending authority for the federal government, and federal offices were shut down. The shutdown was a public relations nightmare for the Republicans, whom the public blamed by a margin of two to one (Quirk and Cunion 2000). The impasse was resolved, of course, but with considerable loss of face by the Republicans. As Sen. John McCain (R-AZ) said of the experience, "I have to give President Clinton credit. He played us like a violin" (Congressional Quarterly 1997).

The president must make three decisions concerning his agenda: the problems to be addressed, the solutions that seem most appropriate, and the relative priorities (Light 1991). The decision calculus for the three differs markedly. Light argued that the evaluation of which problems to address is based on which are most likely to be politically beneficial to the president—generally chosen from problems that have been around for a long time rather than newly identified problems. The evaluation of solution options relies on costs; solutions that involve high costs—either budgetary or political—will likely not be proposed. (An exception here is the 2003 MMA, which was costly to the budget; see chapter 7 for more on the politics of the MMA.) The search for alternatives is important yet very difficult, particularly with the budgetary and political constraints of recent years.

Light (1991) advised presidents to adopt a "satisficing" approach, choosing the first alternative that meets the policy needs rather than continuing the search for a "better" solution. The Clinton administration sought to change the U.S. health care system dramatically—after extensive study by some 500 experts for nearly six months. A year later, the task force process and the product were roundly criticized and were credited, at least in part, with the failure of the Clinton health care plan. Clearly he would have been better advised to follow the recommendation of Light (1991) and others to adopt and amend proposals already before Congress rather than embarking on a new policy path.

We need to clarify that although the agenda-setting role for presidents is important, the agenda is full of nonpresidential initiatives as well. Studying the sources of agenda topics in speeches, hearings, and media—measured in inches of type and minutes of talk—between 1986 and 1994, Edwards and Wood (1997) found that presidents mostly react to events and are generally unable to overcome inertia, world events, and an already full congressional agenda of leftover issues. Only in the area of health did President Clinton seem to be the dominant agenda setter, and even that dominance disappeared if the weeks following introduction of the Clinton national health insurance proposal are omitted from the study sample.

Presidential priorities are crucial. The president often chooses to put his prestige behind one or two issues prominent in the campaign and those ideologically important to him. As Sullivan (1991) expressed it, the lesson is one of "concentrate or lose." Edwards and Wood (1997, 342) expanded on this: "Under special circumstances, presidents may concentrate their resources and move issues onto the agendas of other institutions and focus issue attention, especially when the issue is a major administration initiative. Under these circumstances, presidents operate as issue entrepreneurs, essentially creating attention where little existed before."

The targeting of priorities is necessary because resources, especially time and energy for both the president and Congress, are scarce and need to be directed to those programs with highest support—usually only one or two key issues. President Carter discovered the value of prioritized issues in 1978, when he began sending to Congress a variety of programs with little guidance on the relative standing of each—with minimal success. President Reagan learned from the Carter experience and was clear about his priorities: cutting government spending, reducing taxes, and increasing defense spending. President Clinton came in with two top priorities: health care and economic stimulus. He had difficulties with both, but especially health care reform. He promised he would introduce his plan in the first 100 days, but it was actually nine months into his term before he gave a major speech to Congress outlining the goals of his plan. And it was another two months before the legislative proposal itself was presented. In the meantime, he dealt with a number of issues not high on his priority list, including gays in the military and Haitian immigration policy, which used up valuable time and effort. But putting items on the agenda and getting them passed are very different; the second is much harder.

Monitoring and Encouragement

Once the president has put the item on the agenda and offered a preferred solution, it is up to Congress to act. At that point, presidents operate "at the margin" of coalition building in Congress: they must rely on congressional party leadership for support, and their legislative skills are essentially limited to exploiting rather than creating opportunities for leadership (Bond and Fleisher 1990; Edwards 1989). Presidential skills have less to do with changing votes than with getting the right issues on the floor (Schull 1989), and presidents prefer to influence the design of legislation rather than the votes on it.

The president's proposals can be dismissed, ignored, substituted for those more acceptable to Congress, compromised, or (sometimes) adopted in full. Most presidents recognize that the probability of success is improved with their active monitoring and encouragement. Presidents can help mobilize public support and assist in the coalition formation necessary to guide the bill successfully through both houses of Congress. They can use their office to encourage legislators "leaning" in their direction and to provide encouragement to friends. They can use their prestige and visibility to counter strong interest groups by alerting the public to their tactics.

Personal appeals, on the telephone or in person, can be persuasive, although not conclusive. Harry Truman summed up his role as sitting all day "trying to persuade people to do things they ought to have sense enough to do without my persuading them . . . That's all the powers of the president amount to" (quoted in Neustadt 1960, 10). Such persuasion includes inducing people "to believe that what he wants of them is what their own appraisal of their own responsibilities requires them to do in their own self interest, not his" (Neustadt 1960, 10).

In the 1994 congressional consideration of health care reform, President Clinton was asked by congressional leaders to stay out of the first round of decisions and refrain from public comment on what was going on. The White House activity directed at Congress in the spring and summer of 1994 was confined largely to providing expertise when asked and inviting pivotal members of Congress to the White House for special attention and persuasion (Kosterlitz 1994). Yet by summer, the president was more visibly concerned about the slow congressional pace and began meeting with key congressional leaders and stepping up his public appearances and those of the first lady and prominent cabinet members.

Hands-On Negotiations

Sometimes presidents become much more than monitors and cheerleaders. They can be intensely involved in the day-to-day negotiations in major legislation. These bargaining sessions, sometimes called summits, include chairs of the Budget, Ways and Means, and Finance committees, party leaders, and the president. A case in point was the Balanced Budget Act of 1997, a measure that made major changes in Medicare and Medicaid policies. From the release of his budget in February of that year, President Clinton played an active role, informing Republican leaders of his budget in advance and calling for two reconciliation bills—one to balance the budget and one with tax amendments. When congressional action was stalled, the president would invite congressional leaders to meet with him at the White House to reach agreement. President Clinton was also actively involved in the conference committee, sending letters and statements, calling strategy meetings, and providing staff for day-to-day drafting tasks. Negotiations were not the usual House versus Senate, but rather the Republican Congress versus the president, and the final solution reflected these actors—with both sides giving and taking until they found common ground (D. Smith 2002).

THE PRESIDENT'S RELATIONSHIP WITH CONGRESS

In the early days of his presidency, George W. Bush was asked how he would deal with Congress. "A dictatorship would be a heck of a lot easier, there's no question about it," he joked (Crawford 2005). On a more serious note, Lyndon Johnson once said, "There is only one way to deal with Congress, and that is continuously, incessantly, and without interruption" (Kearns 1976, 226). Indeed, Johnson understood the workings of Congress and was able to work with it very successfully. His successors had a more difficult time.

Woodward's 1994 chronicle of the first year of Clinton's presidency frequently illustrates the presidential preoccupation and frustration with Congress—a Congress where both houses were controlled by his party. On the budget deficit and economic stimulus package of 1993, the president was involved daily, counting voters, making calls to key members, sitting in on strategy sessions with congressional leaders. At one point, Hillary Clinton claimed her husband had become "mechanic-in-chief"—put in a position of "tinkering" with policy rather than leading the charge to a higher vision (Woodward 1994, 255). Yet President Clinton managed to squeeze out success with the closest of votes on several issues important to him, including his economic plan and NAFTA. Clinton expressed his frustration by using the analogy of the nation as a ship: "I can steer it but a storm can still come up and sink it. And the people that are supposed to be rowing can refuse to row" (Woodward 1994, 330).

Clinton learned early that sometimes capitulation to members of Congress is necessary to move legislation. When the votes are close, the president even has to persuade members of his own party. Sometimes the price he must pay is fairly low: a round of golf, mention of an issue in the state of the union address, fund-raising help, or a job for a long-time aide. Sometimes it is higher, such as arranging an appointment to chair a high-profile commission or acceding to a demand on a preferred policy. In one case, in 1994, Sen. Herbert Kohl (D-WI), a crucial vote on the gas tax, set the ceiling on a gas tax increase as the price for his vote. He got it.

Some researchers believe there are swings in dominance between the White House and Congress such that in some years the president is more powerful, in other years Congress. Others see the system as much more stable and cooperative, what Mark Peterson (1990) described as tandem institutions both contributing to national decision making. Indeed, as Davidson (1984) noted, cooperation between Congress and the president is at least as common as conflict, although we hear more about the latter. The president's relationship with Congress is far from static, varying with the president's political capital, outside influences, and the nature of the policy proposed. One thing that can affect the relationship is scandal or low popularity, making it easier for members to vote against the president. As one presidential aide put it, "When the president's popularity is low it's advantageous and even fun to kick him around" (quoted in Collier 1995, 6).

The president's influence is greatest when some recent event shows that current policy is no longer acceptable and presidential leadership can help forge the alliances in Congress necessary to come up with a new solution (Miller 1993). The president plays a much less important role in issues that are not salient and on which Congress has already reached agreement.

Presidential styles in working with Congress vary greatly. While Bill Clinton was often accused of "policy wonkism," or involvement in details of policy, his successor, George W. Bush, prefers a different style: setting forth broad parameters of his vision and leaving much of the detail work to Congress. And blessed with a Republican Congress and leadership closely attuned to his views, Bush has been extremely successful. When he has failed to achieve the desired vote in one house, he has often been able to recover in conference committees closely controlled by Republican leaders (J. Schatz 2004). One example of Bush's policy leadership style was his approach to the signature health law passed during his first term: the MMA. Bush's overall goals for the program were outlined in the document "Framework to Modernize and Improve Medicare," released in March 2003. The framework included some specific suggestions, including allowing private health plans to provide additional prescription drug benefits, but had few details about how the overall program would work. It stuck by the $400 billion price tag first mentioned in the state of the union address a few months earlier, but it did not include detail on how that money would be allocated.

This hands-off style is one that many members of Congress prefer. For example, veteran senator Charles Grassley said, "Those of us who have been working on Medicare and prescription drugs for the last two or three years, we feel like we know how to do it. So what we finally talked the president into back in probably February or March, was, 'We ain't going to wait for a bill, we're going to go ahead'" (Krane 2003, 22). This more general approach contrasts sharply with the effort of the Clinton administration to produce a 1,342-page proposal to Congress on reforming the health care system—an approach, it might be noted, that did not result in a bill that passed any committee in either house.

Yet, even with a Republican majority in Congress, in summer 2003 some intraparty opposition arose over the MMA, particularly from rural-state senators, including the chair of the Finance Committee. Some conservatives were concerned about the costs of creating a new entitlement program without adequate changes in the program itself. By June, the president was meeting with conservatives and rural solons about their concerns (Toner and Pear 2003). In an effort to influence a close House floor vote, Vice President Cheney visited the House to meet with members and sent a signal that the White House strongly wanted a bill. President Bush strongly supported the measure, even though it did not contain his preferred provision relating to better drug benefits for Medicare patients willing to join private plans (A. Goldstein and Dewar 2003). Importantly, the bill did pass—and the president took full credit. Late in his first term, some Republicans complained that they were not included in discussions on key policy, but the dissent was muted in part by the importance of the upcoming presidential and congressional elections.

Political Capital and Midterm Elections

Political capital is the strength of a president's popularity and of his party in Congress, and his electoral margin. Political capital is important because it affects Congress's receptivity to the president's proposals. Presidential popularity, reflected in public approval polls, is a crucial component of political capital, given that presidents who can arouse and mobilize the public are apt to "greatly lessen" their problems in Congress (Sullivan 1987, 300). Rivers and Rose (1985) estimated that a 1 percent increase in the president's popularity leads to a 1 percent increase in his legislative approval rate. Even legislative sponsors can be persuaded by public opinion influenced by the president (MacKuen and Mouw 1992). Similarly, potential opponents may think twice about voting against a measure supported by a particularly popular president. The president's popularity is especially important when he is of the party of the congressional majority. The components that make up the political capital of presidents since Lyndon Johnson are shown in table 2.1.

The strength of the president's party in Congress is an important component in political capital. Thomas Jefferson is purported to have said that "great innovations should not be forced on slender majorities" (Light 1991, 106). Indeed, Lyndon Johnson's successes of 1965, including the passage of Medicare, must be attributed mainly to the election of a large number of liberal Northern Democrats in November 1964. There were 295 Democrats

Table 2.1

Presidential Political Capital, 1965–2005

President	Year	Senate Seats Held by President's Party	House Seats Held by President's Party	Public Approval (percent)	Percentage of Popular Vote in Presidential Election
Johnson	1965	68	295	80	61.1
	1967	64	248	46	—
Nixon	1969	42	192	59	43.4
	1971	44	180	51	—
	1973	42	192	65	60.7
Ford	1975	37	144	39	—
Carter	1977	61	292	66	50.1
	1979	58	277	43	—
Reagan	1981	53	192	60	50.7
	1983	54	167	38	—
	1985	53	182	62	58.8
	1987	45	177	48	—
Bush, G. H. W.	1989	45	175	51	53.4
	1991	44	167	58	—
Clinton	1993	57	258	58	43.0
	1995	47	204	47	—
	1997	45	207	58	49.2
	1999	45	211	63	—
Bush, G. W.	2001	49	220	57	49.8
	2003	51	228	63	—
	2005	55	232	52	51.3

Sources: Light 1991, table 1, p. 32; updated with information from Ornstein, Mann, and Malbin 2002; *CQ Weekly,* Nov. 6, 2004; and information from the House Clerk's Office.

Note: First approval rating of the year from the Gallup Opinion Index.

in the House in 1965—a level not met in the decades since. The amount by which presidents lead or trail congressional candidates of their party can be important as well. If individual members drew more votes in their district than did the president, the perceived political value of the president to that member is reduced. Mark Peterson (1990) found that when the opposition controlled Congress, the proposals of presidents who had smaller winning margins than did their party's House candidates had difficulty finding a consensus, and public fights over the proposals were common. Although Bill Clinton did not face a House controlled by the opposition party in his first two years, he was in the unenviable position of having trailed every member of the House and one-third of the Senate at the polls in November 1992. And in the fight over health care, consensus was slow in coming, and public fights, even among members of his own party, were frequent.

A second important component is a public approval that is often extremely volatile. Lyndon Johnson enjoyed strong public approval in the first year following his election but saw it nearly halved by his last year. Presidents Reagan, George H. W. Bush, and Clinton saw major changes in their approval as well. Figure 2.1 shows the volatility in public support during the first term of George W. Bush. His approval ratings spiked shortly after the 9/11 attacks in 2001, had a small spike in May 2003, shortly after he declared the end of major combat operations in the Iraq War, and a smaller spike shortly before the 2004 election, after which they began to fall again. Generally, however, the pattern is one of declining popularity. Ironically, as Light (1991) noted, the cycle of decreasing presidential influence coincides with a cycle of increasing effectiveness as the president learns about the office, makes mistakes, and learns from those mistakes.

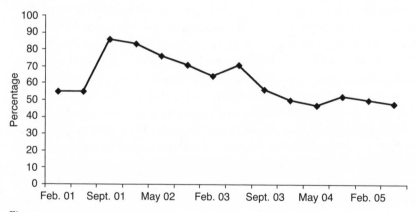

Figure 2.1.

Approval Ratings of George W. Bush, February 2001–May 2005. From ABC News / Washington Post poll of 1,000 likely voters (margin of error ±3.0). Question: "Do you approve or disapprove of the way George W. Bush is handling his job as president?"

Source: PollingReport 2005.

Interestingly, President Clinton maintained relatively high popularity throughout the years of investigation for his alleged sexual harassment and lying under oath. Even during his removal trial in the Senate in January 1999, his approval ratings were no lower than 60 percent (in contrast, Ronald Reagan in his last year had only 48 percent approval). In Clinton's case, the public disliked the person of the president but liked his policies—or the booming economy they enjoyed during his terms of office. In polls taken over 1998 and 1999, two-thirds of respondents repeatedly said they did not like Clinton as a person but more than 60 percent consistently said they liked his policies (Sonner and Wilcox 1999).

The third measure of the president's popularity in a new term, the size of his electoral victory, is also a factor in political capital, to the extent that it provides a president with a mandate to act. Lyndon Johnson, Richard Nixon in 1972, and Ronald Reagan in 1984 could (and did) claim a mandate for change that Congress recognized. Members of Congress are sometimes reluctant to face the wrath of an electorate by opposing the implementation of such a mandate.

But some presidents don't have much of an electoral mandate. John Kennedy squeaked by in 1960; a change in one state, or even a large city like Chicago, could have changed the outcome of the election. Similarly, Bill Clinton was elected by a scant 43 percent of voters in 1992; the margin was only slightly improved in 1996, at 49 percent (table 2.1). George W. Bush became president without a plurality of the popular vote in 2000 and with a small majority in 2004. Yet his administration has expressly ignored this lack of mandate.

Political scientists have examined the linkage between approval and policy success. The assumption is that high approval leads to more success with Congress, since high approval levels either (1) affect/alter citizen approval or (2) reflect public preferences about the president's agenda. There is some evidence that high presidential approval is a significant determinant of policy success in Congress, especially when the issue is complex and salient (characteristics that define many health policy issues) (Canes-Wrone and de Marchi 2002).

Presidents tend to think of themselves as being strongest politically in the earliest months of their tenure and act accordingly. Lyndon Johnson (1971, 323) was especially concerned in the early days following his election that he should "use his strength while it still existed," pointing out that the popularity of other presidents had diminished and their problems with Congress increased very quickly. Edwin Meese, a key Reagan aide, told a reporter that the White House knew that if it wanted to get the radical changes it proposed through Congress, it had to do so in the early months of the administration. "We're fighting the clock," he said. "We think about that all the time" (Kernell 1984, 256). Indeed, by the fall of the first year of the Reagan administration, the presidential victories declined abruptly, and the following spring even the Senate Republicans on the Budget Committee voted against the president's budget (Salamon and Abramson 1984). However, some political scientists believe the value of "hitting the ground running" has been overestimated. Sullivan (1991), for example, argued that quick action is secondary to the value of a focused presidential agenda.

As if to follow Sullivan's advice, George W. Bush was very focused during his first term. "The president doesn't like to lose," said one observer. White House officials are "very attuned to which bills and legislation they should let Congress write and which ones they should write" (J. Schatz 2004, 2900). The president was very active on the issues he cared most deeply about, such as tax cuts and education policy, while "staying on the edges of many debates, even some of the ones on which he eventually takes a decisive position" (2903).

The midterm elections, the end of the president's second year when one-third of the Senate and all seats in the House are up for election, are an important outside influence affecting the relations between the president and Congress. As election day nears, members may shy away from controversial issues and may prefer to provide visible programs to their districts. After the election, the president may be worse off, because midterm elections generally go against the incumbent's party, regardless of his efforts or popularity. In the 1994 health care reform debates in Congress, the approach of midterm elections was a crucial outside influence. The Republicans wanted to delay a vote until the new Congress was seated in January 1995, hoping they would have greater numbers, perhaps even a majority, in one or both houses. (They were right: they took over both houses in 1995.) The Democrats wanted to make health care a campaign issue, ideally taking credit for the passage of a laudatory bill or, alternatively, taking the opportunity to blame the Republicans for any failure to do so. Yet health was markedly absent from most campaign debates. And, most significantly, Sen. Harris Wofford (D-PA), whose election to an abbreviated term in 1991 was credited with alerting politicians to the public's concern about health care and catapulting health care to the top of the national agenda, lost in November 1994. Some thought his defeat symbolized the coming dormancy of comprehensive health care reform in Washington.

Presidential Persuasion

The "power to persuade" is one of the most important aspects of the presidency. One foremost presidential scholar, Richard Neustadt (1990), argued that presidents get what they want through persuasion, not through command or institutional authority. Kernell (1991, 90) called the president "doubtless the Washington community's most prominent and active dealmaker" who can provide the "much-needed coordination in assembling coalitions across a broad institutional landscape."

Consultation with Congress is important. The likelihood of meaningful consultation between the president and Congress is greatly enhanced when the issues involved are salient and when the president wants a solution, the White House cannot solve the problem alone, and prominent figures on the Hill want to reach an agreement or the president wants to work with Congress on a solution (M. Peterson 1990).

Bargaining, whereby a legislator agrees to vote with the president in exchange for presidential support for her pet issue, is extremely common and an important weapon in the presidential arsenal. The president must bargain even with those who agree with him, because most members have interests of their own beyond policy objectives and their votes cannot be guaranteed (Edwards 1980). Bill Clinton was accused of "giving away the store" for crucial votes on the 1993 budget bill and NAFTA. Other presidents have been similarly accused. Ronald Reagan, for example, angered party leaders when he offered not to campaign personally against Southern Democrats who supported him and gave them policy concessions beneficial to their constituents (Salamon and Abramson 1984). Coercion, or arm-twisting, is generally the last resort, and then only on particularly important votes (Edwards 1980).

Compromise is obviously an important factor in the relations between the president and Congress, but compromise can be difficult for a president whose every move makes national news. In the spring of 1994, for example, Bill Clinton was criticized for compromising too much to make his health care reform plan pleasing to a variety of people. When he seemed to be wavering in his support for universal coverage—or at least its definition—he was criticized for retreating or backsliding and was forced to reiterate his full support for coverage of all Americans. Interestingly, Ronald Reagan was criticized for the opposite behavior—not compromising enough, what Salamon and Abramson (1984, 59) called "ideological intransigence." Senate majority leader George Mitchell (D-ME) described the situation in 1994 as one in which Clinton would be criticized for whatever he did. If he took an inflexible position or refused to compromise, he would be attacked for not knowing the ways of Capitol Hill or not having the experience to win. If he participated and made the necessary compromises to get the plan approved, he would be attacked for being willing to give in. "You can't escape criticism in the process," Mitchell said (Woodward 1994, 183).

The personality component of the presidency can be of great importance on some issues but may be overstated. Some presidents (Clinton and Johnson) seemed to enjoy meeting with and attempting to persuade members of Congress; others (Nixon and Carter) preferred a hands-off approach, with minimal personal interaction. President Reagan was widely viewed as an excellent communicator whose informal, friendly style was disarming and charming to members of both parties. Barber (1985) characterized presidential personalities into four types based on the level of energy and enthusiasm the president brought to the job and his positive or negative views about himself in relation to that activity. Reagan would be classified as passive positive, Clinton and George W. Bush as active positive, Eisenhower as passive negative, and Nixon as active negative.

Vetoes and Threatened Vetoes

Another presidential "tool" is the veto, a disapproval that requires a two-thirds vote in both houses to overturn. Unlike 43 state governors, the president of the United States does not have a line-item veto but is forced to veto an entire law rather than just offensive parts of it. In 1996, Congress enacted a law allowing the president a type of line-item veto in which he could cancel specific items of spending or specific tax breaks (but only when the budget was in a deficit). Two years later the Supreme Court overturned the law, saying it was incompatible with Article 1 of the Constitution. Within that short period, Clinton vetoed 82 items, including 38 in a military construction appropriations bill (Aberbach 2000).

While presidential vetoes are most likely when Congress passes legislation that is objectionable to the president, some presidents are more likely than others to veto bills. Gerald Ford, the only unelected president who assumed office without serving as an elected vice president (having been appointed as vice president when Spiro Agnew resigned), had no electoral margin of any kind and faced a heavily Democratic Congress. He used the veto more than any other modern president, vetoing 37 bills in the 94th Congress (1975–76), compared with Reagan's 15 vetoes in the 97th Congress (1981–82) and Carter's 12 in the 96th Congress (1979–80).

Typically, the presidential veto has served more as a threat than a reality, although presidents facing a Congress controlled by the opposite party and those with declining public popularity are particularly likely to use the veto (Rohde and Simon 1985). A veto override is relatively difficult to achieve. For example, George H. W. Bush vetoed 46 bills in four years and was overridden only once (Ornstein, Mann, and Malbin 2002). His son, George W. Bush, did not veto any bills in his entire first term—the first president to avoid the veto over a four-year period since John Quincy Adams (Cochran 2004).

The president's threat of a veto, particularly one issued early in the policy process, greatly increases his stake in the policy outcome and clearly articulates his priorities. Such a threat means that the president has thrown down the gauntlet (especially to the opposition party), that certain policies must be enacted (or omitted) or he is willing to sacrifice the entire policy package. It also provides "comfort and cover" to members of Congress inclined to follow the president but wanting assurances that he will back them up (Priest and Broder 1994). President Reagan "drew the line in the dirt" on tax cuts in 1981. President George H. W. Bush uttered a "no new taxes" pledge. President Clinton, in his speech to a joint session of Congress introducing his health care reform proposal, used the threat of a veto to attempt to prove his intractability on universal coverage. Although he offered to compromise on other aspects of the proposal—managed competition, health care networks, and global budgets, to name a few—he continued to demand that universal coverage be in the legislative package or the package would be vetoed. The use of the veto reminds Congress that the president can be a powerful constraint, especially since successful override votes are difficult to muster. Franklin Roosevelt was known to ask his supporters for something he could veto as a reminder to Congress that this form of policy enforcement could and would be applied (Spitzer 1983).

Executive Orders

Presidents have one way to make policy without congressional approval: they can issue executive orders, which have the force of law and establish requirements for the agencies and departments under the president's direct authority and supervision. Presidents have great leeway in executive orders;

the only constraint is that they must have the statutory or constitutional authority to support their actions. Since the late 1970s, presidents have relied less on statutory authority and more on their constitutional powers when justifying their executive orders. Executive orders can be especially attractive to presidents facing a Congress controlled by the opposite party. For example, in his first year in office (with a Democratic Congress), President Clinton issued 27 executive orders; in the first few months of 1998, with a Republican Congress, he issued 102 (Aberbach 2000). But another analysis of executive orders between 1936 and 1999 found little evidence that the party of Congress was a significant factor in the number of executive orders issued. Only twice has Congress overruled an executive order—most recently in 1998 when Congress prohibited expenditure of federal funds to carry out implementation of an executive order on federalism (Mayer 2001).

The assumption is that what presidents cannot get through Congress they implement through executive orders. President Clinton was straightforward about this when he said in a July 2000 radio address that if Congress did not act, he would use his own authority to create a home heating oil reserve to help avoid shortages in the Northeast (Lacy 2000). He issued several orders in his last days in office, including one requiring Medicare to cover the costs of clinical trials for testing the value of new drugs and procedures intended for use by beneficiaries who are elderly and disabled (Pear 2000a)—a change long sought by beneficiaries, many of whom have chronic illnesses. Before this order, Medicare did not cover experimental drugs and procedures. Another order required plans offering health insurance to the federal government's nine million employees to provide mental health parity—equally generous coverage of mental health services and physical health services. Supporters hoped the order would inspire private employers to adopt similar standards (Goode 2001). Though Congress passed the mental health parity act in 1996, the act's many loopholes allowed plans to continue to limit mental health coverage. President George W. Bush has used executive orders frequently, many associated with homeland security and the war in Iraq. His first executive order established a White House Office of Faith-Based and Community Initiatives. As with other presidents, health has not been a major focus for executive orders in the George W. Bush White House.

In one count, domestic policy (not including civil service, public lands, and labor policy) accounted for less than 4 percent of executive orders between 1936 and 1999 (Mayer 2001). Nevertheless, it is important to recognize the importance of executive orders as a policy tool available to the president. With the stroke of a pen, the president can issue a directive that has the force of law (although, if it conflicts with a statute, the statute will prevail). Presidents have used the executive order to establish or abolish executive branch agencies, determine how legislation is implemented, launch dramatic civil rights policies, determine how national security information will be handled, and set up dozens, if not hundreds, of commissions and advisory bodies.

Possibly the most interesting saga of executive orders has concerned abortion. In January 2001, the newly elected president used an executive order to ban federal aid to international organizations that promote or perform abortion as a way to implement family planning, reversing an executive order that President Bill Clinton issued in his first month of his presidency, January 1993. Clinton's executive order reversed the ban imposed by the Reagan administration and maintained by the administration of President George H. W. Bush (Pal and Weaver 2003).

Institutional Constraints

Historically, among the institutional constraints on presidential action are the decentralized nature of congressional policy making, the expansion of interest groups and policy networks, and the reduced importance of political parties in the past 30 years. A modern president cannot work with a few key committee chairs and party leaders and a few dominant interest groups; rather, he must deal with a spate of individuals and groups, all of whom have their own particular interests. As Jimmy Carter (1982, 80) put it, "Each member had to be wooed and won individually. It was every member for himself, and the devil take the hindmost!" Further, the underlying consensus animating the national majority politically and philosophically is different from that which animates the majority party of the legislature (Marini 1992). In a time of weak party discipline, ideology, not partisanship, is key.

In Light's view (1984), presidents must now "pay more for domestic programs." And the cost is high. Joseph Califano (1994, 41), White House staffer and secretary of Health, Education, and Welfare (HEW) in the Carter administration, noted that President Clinton's willingness to compromise on most things in his health care package reflected the dominance of Congress and the recognition that he would have to sign whatever it sent to him and "declare victory." In Lyndon Johnson's time, wrote Califano, the president had some leverage over Congress with campaign contributions, patronage jobs, and assistance in writing bills. Today, Congress needs little help in those areas. In fact, as Light (1984, 207) noted, the president often does not get "star billing" for his domestic agenda; the presidential aura has lessened because of increased competition among the other policy initiators, more resources for such initiation, and less reverence for the wisdom of presidential planning.

President George W. Bush has benefited not only from Republican majorities in both houses but also from strong party leadership. While the Republican Party in Congress is far from homogeneous, it nevertheless understands the importance of staying in the majority and working with the White House to do so. President Bush trusts the House and Senate party leaders to hold their party members in line and deliver the vote on important legislation. They have been able to do so by taking advantage of rule changes and curtailing the independence of committee chairs (see chapter 1). In return, the congressional party has benefited from a popular president who campaigns enthusiastically for members, helps raise money for the party, and articulates a strong ideological position shared by many in the party.

Presidential Successes

The president generally has an easier time when Congress is controlled by members of his own party: his legislative success scores do not drop below 75 percent (Ornstein, Mann, and Malbin 2002, 198). Ronald Reagan was successful an average of 62 percent of the time over his eight years in office. Richard Nixon's average success rate in office was 67 percent; Gerald Ford's, 58 percent. Lyndon Johnson's, in contrast, was 83 percent. When Bill Clinton had a Democratic House and Senate to work with, his success rate was 86 percent; when the Republicans took over both houses in 1995, it dropped to a low of 36 percent. Over the four years of his first term, George W. Bush had an average success rate of 82 percent—the highest of any president since Lyndon Johnson (J. Schatz 2004).

The success rates shown in table 2.2, compiled by Congressional Quarterly, are used frequently by presidential researchers and the press. However, these ratings probably overstate presidents' successes, for several reasons. First, the scores are based on issues on which the president took a clear-cut position, and they treat seminal legislation and more trivial pursuits equally. Second, the Congressional Quarterly score considers the president's position at the time of the vote, not his position much earlier when the item was first placed on the agenda. Finally, roll-call measures such as this understate the

Table 2.2
Presidential Victories in Congress

President	Year Elected (or assumed office)	Percentage of Bills Supported by the President That Were Enacted		
		Highest	Lowest	Mean
Johnson	1963	93.1 (1965)	74.5 (1968)	82.6
Nixon	1968	76.9 (1970)	50.6 (1973)	67.2
Ford	1974	61.0 (1975)	53.8 (1976)	57.6
Carter	1976	78.3 (1978)	75.1 (1980)	76.4
Reagan	1980	82.3 (1981)	43.5 (1987)	61.9
Bush, G. H. W.	1988	62.6 (1989)	43.0 (1992)	51.6
Clinton	1992	86.4 (1993; 1994)	36.2 (1995)	61.4
Bush, G. W.	2000	87.8 (2002)	72.6 (2004)	81.5

Sources: Data from Ornstein, Mann, and Malbin 2002; Congressional Quarterly Almanac 2001–4.

complexity of the policy process, in which the president is only one of many actors, and making "victories" attributable to the efforts of one player can be somewhat suspect.

In a more in-depth look at a sample of some 300 presidential proposals of five presidents (Eisenhower through Reagan), Mark Peterson (1990) found that about 54 percent of the proposals between 1953 and 1984 were passed, in some form, with more than one-third passed exactly as introduced. However, presidential success varied with the nature and scope of the proposal. Presidential proposals involving new and costly comprehensive policy initiatives often engendered opposition and were defeated outright 40 percent of the time. An analysis of 20 health policies in the final two years of the Carter administration and first two years of the Reagan administration found that half were initiated by the White House, but only 12.5 percent of those proposals were enacted (Heinz et al. 1993).

Divided Government

A president facing at least one house controlled by the opposite party has to use a different strategy from the president blessed with a Congress led by his own party. Traditionally, presidents facing a unified Congress often rely on informal party mechanisms to achieve their goals. When facing a divided

Congress or one controlled by members of the other party, the president must resort to the veto (or threat of the veto) and support from the public. Yet both strategies are somewhat risky. Clearly the president cannot veto every bill he does not like but must pick those that arouse public interest or strong public opinion. Similarly, the president cannot take every issue to the public.

One reason that relations between the president and Congress are especially dicey when government is divided is that opposition politicians often gain electoral advantage in frustrating the president. According to Kernell (1991), the main business of an opposition Congress is to prepare for the next election. Members of the minority party will tend not to bargain in good faith—it is not in their best interest.

Interestingly, President Clinton had a Democratic Congress in his first year yet encountered difficulties (from his own party and the opposition) not unlike those of a president in divided government. The Republican leadership talked about "sitting at the table" but spent more time carping at the Democrats' health care plan and forming coalitions with conservative Democrats to defeat key portions of the proposal. In the remaining years of his two terms, Clinton faced an opposition Congress, and his tactics changed as expected. He had fewer meetings with members, was less visible to the public, and offered little in the way of legislative initiatives.

In his second term, Clinton played obstructionist politics, reverting to fighting Republican initiatives rather than launching his own. He also compromised with the Republican leadership, often to the point of alienating some members of his own party. In fact the president tried to distance himself from both congressional Democrats and Republicans in his second election campaign, adopting a centrist strategy between traditional Democrats and Republicans.

GOING PUBLIC

Closely tied to presidential success in Congress is the desire of the public at large. Lincoln once commented on the strength of public approval: "Public sentiment is everything. With public sentiment, nothing can fail; without it nothing can succeed" (Collier 1995, 1). Presidents often make direct appeals to the public, urging constituents to put pressure on their elected officials, in a manner Collier called "merchandising." Ronald Reagan often tried "to go over the heads" of members of Congress to mobilize public opinion behind a desired policy. Though this tactic is not new—Woodrow Wilson used it in an attempt to engender public support for the League of Nations—it has been used increasingly in the past two decades, thanks to advances in technology that allow interactive communications from a variety of sources and direct, targeted satellite feeds to television stations across the country. From Franklin Roosevelt's fireside chats to Bill Clinton's town meetings, the purpose is the same: to mobilize public support and build coalitions. As Miller (1993, 314) put it, "The president's most powerful weapon . . . is a public aroused on a specific issue." Public support can be important in building coalitions. It can help convince members of Congress that it is safe to support the president. This is especially important for members of the opposition party.

Presidents and their advisors fully understand the role of strong public support. Kernell (1984) recounted the desires of Reagan and his staff to take advantage of the president's popularity after the assassination attempt in 1981. They decided to push the president's desired budget cuts in a televised joint session of Congress, the first major appearance of President Reagan since the shooting. The broad public support helped; the budget passed, nearly intact. The problem with such an appeal is that the public is typically fickle and can often provide only fleeting support. It is also susceptible to messages from other interested parties and can easily grow bored with a subject. Jeffrey Cohen (1994) found that presidential attention to economic, foreign, and civil rights policy led to increased public concern with these policies. But presidential leadership effects decay within a year (except in the area of foreign policy). To keep the item on the public agenda, presidents must repeatedly rally the public.

Presidents also use sympathetic interest groups to help arouse public support. Since Gerald Ford, presidents have established an Office of Public Liaison that mobilizes interest-group allies. In Clinton's health care reform strategy, core natural allies included senior citizens' associations, consumer groups, unions, liberal health care provider organizations, religious associations, and several organizations representing women, children, and minorities. As it turned out, Clinton did not get this base of support. Only a quarter of the Democratic target group was in favor of the plan (M. Peterson 2000). President Nixon also fully understood the importance of developing a message and making certain it got out. According to speech writer David Gergen, Nixon would repeatedly say that "about the time you are writing a line that you have written so often that you want to throw up, that is the first time the American people will hear it" (Gergen quoted in Kelly 1993, 68).

Presidents can help define public opinion by framing issues in appealing ways. One example from the presidency of George W. Bush concerns his opposition in 2005 to a measure that would permit the importation of prescription drugs from Canada and allow the government to negotiate drug prices. While Democrats viewed the measure as giving seniors more access, the president saw the measure as a threat to the 2003 Medicare law and said, "Any attempt to limit the choices of our seniors and to take away their prescription-drug coverage under Medicare will meet my veto." His press secretary reiterated the "straw man" approach: "He's not going to let anybody take away what we have provided to you" (quoted in Loven 2005).

A president's access to the media and strong allegiance to the national interest make the public approach appealing. A crucial challenge to the president comes in seeking to shape opinion. The Clinton administration recognized the importance of public opinion and established a "war room" that served to put the best "spin" on information such as the CBO's cost estimates for the Clinton plan and congressional pronouncements such as New York Sen. Daniel Patrick Moynihan's questioning of the seriousness of the "health care crisis." But the Republican opposition and interest groups opposing the plan were better at shaping the message than was the White House. An early and successful spin on the president's plan was that it would lead to more bureaucracy, lower standards of care, decreased choice of provider, and increased costs. Public support for the plan began to drop in the spring of 1994, when, for the first time, more Americans opposed Clinton's plan than favored it—although, ironically, they continued to like many aspects of it (Kosterlitz 1994). As the vote on health care reform neared, the White House stepped up its efforts, scheduling a Health Security Express bus tour and offering nightly short addresses on cable television in which the president highlighted health issues of public concern. But the public's support continued to dwindle. In its "selling of the health care reform plan," the Clinton administration tried to promote broad principles and goals, such as health security, and to avoid details on such matters as health alliances and employer mandates. This policy backfired when interest-group commercials took the opportunity to inform and persuade the public that such aspects of the plan were harmful and unwise. President Carter had also found the public difficult to persuade on rising health costs, since most people were insulated from the problem by insurance and could not get worked up over the need for change (M. Peterson 1990).

Probably the best example of public misunderstanding involved the passage, then repeal, of catastrophic health insurance for elderly people in 1988. Passed by substantial margins in both the House and the Senate and strongly supported by the president, the law was not well explained by elected officials and the public was easily led astray by opponents' scare tactics. Although the bill adversely affected primarily the well-to-do and helped the poor, many poor elderly people thought they would have to pay high premiums for services they valued little. The final blow came when the initial cost estimates of the program turned out to be much too low; the new figures predicted costs of six times the first estimates (Broder 1994b).

Sometimes the president uses the public as a sounding board for possible solutions—solutions quickly forgotten if the cues are wrong. For example, the Clinton administration abandoned consideration of a new value-added tax (VAT) to finance its health program, because a poll conducted by the White House indicated no support for it (C. Peters 1994). However, recent research on the politics of polling indicates that polling is used more for finding the catch phrases and arguments to shape issues that will win public support than for figuring out what the public wants and how to respond. Jacobs and Shapiro (2000) found that since the 1970s, the policy decisions of presidents and members of Congress have become less responsive to the substantive policy preferences of Americans.

THE PRESIDENT AND THE PRESS

The days when a small close-knit press corps crowded around Franklin Roosevelt's desk to hear the latest presidential pronouncements are long gone. Today's White House press corps numbers in the hundreds, and it covers the president's every move, and failure to move, in seemingly excruciating detail. The first modern media president was John F. Kennedy, who used television to project the image of an energetic, talented, and handsome leader. Richard Nixon, "burned" by television in his campaign against Kennedy in 1960, learned to use it to his advantage in his effort to remake his political career in the mid-1960s. Nixon institutionalized the process of communications and put in place a series of innovations designed to control the news and put the best spin on it.

Nixon established an Office of Communications and Office of Public Liaison, which worked to "orchestrate" the news and organize grassroots efforts supportive of the president. The Office of Communications focused in large part on local media, using them to reach the people without filtering through the larger, more cynical (and perhaps unsupportive) Washington and East Coast media. This office understood the importance of symbols to presidential activities and worked to provide short, meaningful messages that could be captured in brief "sound bites." The Nixon staff developed the notion of a "line of the day," highlighted on a given day by the president and other spokespersons. The communications staff tried to control the media's agenda and access, rewarding reporters who wrote good stories and attacking those who were critical. The communications staff met weekly with public relations staff from federal agencies to make certain the message was clear and unified.

President Reagan, using some of the staff members trained in the Nixon White House, followed the same highly coordinated, well-developed plan to control the media and reach the public. James Baker, while chief of staff, spent 35 hours a week talking to journalists. He gave an hour a day to three networks and four major newspapers (Kelly 1993). The Reagan team was also good at "leaking" information to reporters in exchange for information from the press, such as what members of the White House press corps were working on and what they were hearing from other people.

President Clinton had a tough time getting his message across in the first two years of his term. Such missteps as troublesome nominees for attorney general, expensive haircuts, and aides using helicopters to travel to golf courses were emblazoned across newspapers with headlines such as the *New York Daily News*'s "Bumblin' Bill" and *Time* magazine's "Incredible Shrinking President." More serious issues involving allegations of influence peddling and sexual harassment during his gubernatorial tenure followed Clinton into his second year. He seemed to suffer from what political scientist Larry Sabato (1991) called a "boom-and-bust cycle—where things are either perfect and beautiful and wonderful or they're terrible and awful" with little in between. In Sabato's view, the press tends to follow public opinion rather than help shape it, but others think media coverage helps define the presidency and form the perceptions essential to public opinion (H. Kurtz 1994b).

POLICY IMPLEMENTATION

The president may spend enormous amounts of time setting the policy agenda and trying to get desired policies put into place, but the office also brings with it another important policy function: carrying out, or executing, those laws. The president is charged with overseeing the executive branch of government—some 2.8 million strong, with about 300,000 employees working in the Washington, D.C., metropolitan area.

One important way the president exercises such oversight is through appointing cabinet positions, commissions, and subcabinet posts, offices with leadership responsibility for federal programmatic functions. There are 15 cabinet posts and around 200 important subcabinet posts, all subject to Senate confirmation. The "inner cabinet" is made up of the secretaries of Defense, State, Justice, and Treasury. "Outer cabinet" members—secretaries of the Interior, Agriculture, Commerce, Labor, Education, Housing and Urban Development, Transportation, Health and Human Services, Energy, Veterans Affairs, and Homeland Security—do not generally have the access and influence of inner cabinet members. They deal with groups whose political resources are few (welfare recipients, Native Americans) and those whose well-established influence presidents could not change substantially even if they wanted to (large manufacturers, corporate farmers, organized labor). However, some outer cabinet members can exercise more power if they are particularly close to the president, such as Robert Reich, President Clinton's first-term labor secretary, or if the issue is extremely timely and salient, such as homeland security. George W. Bush also recognizes four additional staff as having cabinet rank: the administrator of the Environmental Protection Agency, the director of the Office of Management and Budget, the director of the National Drug Control Policy, and the U.S. Trade Representative.

Cabinet members are appointed by the president and serve at his pleasure. The popular Joseph Califano, secretary of HEW in the Carter years, discovered the tenuous nature of his position when he was rather ignominiously fired for reasons quite apart from his role as cabinet secretary (he got too cozy with potential presidential primary challenger Sen. Edward Kennedy). Or, as Abraham Lincoln said following a cabinet vote over a heated issue, "One aye, seven nays. The Ayes have it" (Light 1984, 436). The presidentially appointed cabinet serves important functions linking the president and his plan for government with a huge body of civil servants who do the day-to-day work of implementing federal programs. Cabinet members also advise the president on issues and represent him in hearings before Congress. They chair commissions and other efforts to seek information and reach consensus. For example, in 1999 President Clinton directed the treasury secretary and the attorney general to develop a strategy on gun violence.

There is usually a fairly high turnover of presidentially appointed heads of agencies. Only 4 of the 15 cabinet secretaries in George W. Bush's first term retained those positions in his second term. Interestingly, Clinton administration appointees were longer lasting than most. For example, Donna Shalala was HHS secretary during the entire eight years of his presidency. There were three HHS heads in the eight-year Reagan administration. Former Wisconsin governor Tommy Thompson served as HHS secretary through the first term of the George W. Bush presidency but left that position at the start of the second term.

The Bureaucracy

Presidents are important to federal agency employees. In addition to appointing the agency leadership, presidents and the OMB recommend agencies' budgets to Congress and oversee the promulgation of agency recommendations.

The bureaucracy is important to the president. It can provide useful expertise and an institutional and policy memory that can mean the difference between the success and failure of a treasured policy or program. Ironically, though the president often understands the importance of "getting the bureaucracy under control," he is usually relatively uninterested in administration, and presidents of both parties tend to distrust the federal bureaucracy. Some presidents try to control federal agencies with careful selection of agency heads who share the president's ideological and policy vision. Others prefer to "work around" agencies by locating policy expertise and control in the White House rather than relying on the agencies. President Nixon tried both. He carefully selected cabinet members and other high officials to ensure that the bureaucracy would be helpful, not harmful, in his policy goals, and he also centralized control of policy making in the White House, using agencies as little as possible.

Presidents can also reorganize the executive branch to best fit their goals and to improve overall efficiency—to some extent. For example, in 1971 President Nixon sent to Congress a reorganization plan that would have abolished the departments of Agriculture, Labor, Commerce, HUD, Interior, HEW, and Transportation and consolidated their functions into four new "superagencies": departments of Human Resources, Natural Resources, Community Development, and Economic Affairs. His plan went nowhere in a Congress that was lobbied by groups wanting to keep the existing agencies and in which such a shakeup would change congressional committee responsibilities—meaning that some committee chairs and members could lose authority and standing. Nixon later accomplished some of his changes with a functional reorganization corresponding roughly to the proposed superagencies, with staffers responsible for coordinating policy in those areas. Recent presidents have not attempted major reorganization—with the notable exception of the George W. Bush administration, which formed a new cabinet agency for homeland security and incorporated a number of existing offices from different departments within the new agency. Not surprisingly, the implementation of this effort was difficult and slow-moving. The reorganization proved controversial following Hurricane Katrina in 2005, which devastated New Orleans and the Gulf Coast. Some observers thought that inclusion of the Federal Emergency Management Agency (FEMA) in Homeland Security diluted the agency's ability to respond quickly and effectively.

President George W. Bush is an active user of signed statements that outline how his administration plans to implement the law. Signed with the law, these orders can send the message to Congress that the president has his own ideas about how the law should be implemented, and as such they can be viewed as the last word on the law before its implementation (Cochran 2004).

The White House Staff

The White House staff typically consists of about 1,000 people. Like the congressional staff, the White House staff is an important source of expertise and political guidance—often more of the latter than the former. While most presidents fill these positions with trusted and loyal assistants and aides, sometimes the persons who are most trusted are not the best staffers. Bill Clinton's first chief of staff, long-time friend Thomas McLarty, was loyal but not best suited to the tough job of gatekeeper, and he left after 18 months. Many of the Clinton White House aides were young (in their twenties) and inexperienced in Washington norms. Not a few "old hands" were offended by what they felt was brusque or inappropriate treatment by the "youngsters." Having such young and inexperienced staffs has been a recurring problem for presidents. George W. Bush has been the exception. His staffers tend to be middle-aged or older and highly experienced—several having served with his father.

Problems can arise if aides isolate the president and tell him only what he wants to hear (Presidents Nixon and Johnson are possible examples) or are not well informed on political relationships and mores in Washington (President Carter comes to mind here). President Clinton was criticized for "government by inner circle" and for relying for advice on an "adhocracy," or ad hoc groups, rather than established experts in the bureaucracy and elsewhere (Haass 1994). Traditionally, Democratic presidents have preferred what is known as a spokes-of-the-wheel organization, whereby the president works with a few cabinet-level persons who report directly to him. Republicans tend to use a chief-of-staff model, with one person serving as gatekeeper to the presidential office. In reality, however, these organizational models oversimplify the differences in presidential interaction with staffs (C. Jones 1994).

In recent years, the White House staff has grown considerably as the president wants to have more of his "own people" in central policy-making roles. For example, the Domestic Policy Council often serves as a president's window on domestic policy and the mechanism for presidential coordination of agencies. The Office of Communications in the White House is a very important vehicle for presidential links with people—especially important since Nixon. The Council of Economic Advisers is responsible for the annual economic report and provides advice to the president on economic issues. The National Security Council provides advice on defense issues. The staffs of these agencies are usually small. "The number of [White House] staff directly involved in policy choice is quite restricted," Light (1991, 55) noted. "The bulk of the staff is usually engaged in firefighting while the rest are forced to tackle one or two problems at a time."

The Office of Management and Budget

Of the agencies within the executive office of the president, the OMB is particularly pivotal to domestic policy making. Established in 1921 as the Bureau of the Budget, its formation is viewed by some as the beginning of the institutional presidency (Moe 1985). In 1970, it added *management* to its name and function and became the "eyes and ears" of the president (Benda and Levine 1986). The OMB has increasingly taken on broad domestic policy coordination issues, in addition to its traditional budgetary role. Its primary function is the preparation of the president's budget; it reviews agency requests and coordinates them with presidential priorities and desires.

The OMB has long played the role of budgetary "heavy," arguing for reductions in spending or the elimination or scaling back of programs. Although most of the OMB's actions in drafting the president's budget occur behind closed doors, sometimes actions and rationales become known. Clinton's HHS secretary Donna Shalala typically requested major funding for the nation's community health centers, only to have the requests slashed drastically by the OMB. For example, in 1997 she requested $100 million in appropriations and the OMB reduced it to $8 million. When questioned about the severe cuts in a program that provides care to many of the nation's poorest residents, an OMB official replied that the agency has to operate under budget caps and that "we have a holistic approach to public health. The system is under strain and we are being innovative. We have given increases to the Centers for Disease Control, which also serves minorities and the poor" (quoted in McGrory 1999). In an equally telling remark, the official also noted that the Republicans in Congress could always restore the funds.

In the 1980s and early 1990s, the OMB took on a stronger regulatory role. Agencies were required to submit "major rules" (those involving an estimated economic impact of more than $100 million a year) to the OMB 60 days before publication of notice in the *Federal Register* and again 30 days before publication. The OMB could delay or recommend the withdrawal of regulations. The agency promulgating (or writing) the regulations was also required to submit a cost-benefit analysis of the regulations' expected impact. In 1994, the OMB was reorganized to recognize some similar administrative roles of the National Performance Review, a nonstatutory ad hoc organization tied to the vice president's office. The OMB's management capabilities were diminished, but do remain in some statutes. For example, the agency must make yearly estimates of the overall cost of regulation in the United States ($190 billion in 1999) and approve agency requests to collect information.

The OMB's budgetary role remains strong and powerful. Its officials work closely with Congress in drafting appropriations and authorization bills, monitor spending and surpluses, work with agencies to make congressional cuts, and sometimes play politics in speaking for the president on budgetary issues. The OMB director Franklin Raines, for example, fought hard against the inclusion of health savings accounts in the 1996 Health Insurance Portability and Accountability Act (HIPAA), arguing that these would "provide a tax break for the healthiest and wealthiest individuals . . . and attract them out of the general insurance market, potentially raising premiums for all other people" (Congressional Quarterly 1997). Raines's successor, Jacob Lew, was even more visible and outspoken in efforts to influence Congress. He described one Republican budget plan as being "as phony as a three-dollar bill" (J. Harris 1999) and called another a "bankrupt approach" (OMB Director Lew 2000). Lew threatened Congress in May 2000 with several presidential vetoes of appropriations and other important bills unless it made "significant improvements" by increasing funding or altering priorities. In conference committees, the OMB director is often an active participant in deliberations, representing the president.

When HHS secretary Tommy Thompson stepped down in 2005, he was highly critical of the OMB's role in policy making. He asserted that the OMB acted as "super God." "They turn you down nine times out 10 just to show you they are the boss," he told reporters in a candid interview expressing his frustrations with Washington's bureaucracy. He also complained about the White House staff, who "do not believe that anything smart or original can come from a secretary or a department" (Pugh 2005, 4A).

THE PRESIDENCY AND HEALTH POLICY

Since Harry Truman, every president, Democrat or Republican, has proposed major health legislation, much of it involving national health insurance. Most presidents wanted to expand the federal role in health; the Reagan and Bush administrations of the 1980s proposed the addition of protection against catastrophic losses under Medicare and several additional Medicare benefits, in an effort to make public coverage more efficient and better targeted. Presidents vary in their efforts to inform the public and influence Congress, and in their success at doing so. President Ford offered a major plan and (largely because of economic considerations) never pursued it with Congress. President Clinton pulled out all the stops in drafting a comprehensive plan and encouraging its adoption. Yet no comprehensive national health insurance reform plan has been enacted, although some president-supported cost controls and efforts to revamp the delivery system have been put in place.

One reason for the notable lack of success of presidential proposals in health care reform may be the different constituencies. For the president, concerned with a national and broad constituency, national health insurance is easily understood and explained as making broad policy changes that will improve the efficiency and effectiveness of health care for all Americans. For a member of Congress, national health care reform comes down to the effect on her local hospital, medical school, or small businesses. Each legislator sees the issue in terms of pharmacists and optometrists and nurses and drug companies and dry cleaners—many of the health care sector's components—rather than the entire issue. When the national program for the public good is thus deconstructed into its 535 component parts, problems arise, and these have so far stymied the enactment of a comprehensive, universal health policy for the country.

Other major sticking points for presidents have concerned the cost of a broad, comprehensive health care program—and how to pay for it. Increased taxation is something no president relishes, yet any major change must be accompanied by the resources to pay for it. Issues of unemployment also arise, although not as closely or personally at the presidential level as in congressional districts. And all modern presidents have promoted cost controls. Going back to the Nixon—and indeed even the Johnson—administration, there was a great deal of concern about rising health care costs and how to get a handle on them. So far, answers have been elusive to presidents and Congresses alike. Finally, as Steinmo and Watts (1995) noted, there are institutional constraints against passage of comprehensive health care reforms: the fragmented political power in the United States, congressional rules allowing a minority to block legislation, fragmented power in the entrepreneurial Congress, and the increasing importance of the media.

Although many earlier modern presidents proposed major health care reforms, none did so with the fervor and dedication of President Bill Clinton. He dubbed health care reform the "defining issue" of his presidency. With the first lady as the point person, a major effort involving more than 500 experts in a dozen or more task forces was launched to write a health care reform plan in 100 days. The effort was largely conducted in secret, without the involvement of key interest groups that would be directly affected by the reforms, and it was highly decentralized, with task forces working independently and generally without concern for potential costs and likely political support (or opposition). The result—the American Health Security Act—was sweeping in scope. It called for universal health care coverage by 1998 for all Americans. It would have made changes in the way health care is structured by setting up regional insurance purchasing alliances, mandating that employers pay a substantial amount of health insurance for employees, and creating a national health board to establish national and regional spending limits. The plan would have meant major changes for employers, insurance companies, health care providers, and consumers.

In a speech before Congress in September 1993, President Clinton challenged the members to ignore scare tactics by groups that may benefit from the waste in the current system and produce a program that would provide universal, comprehensive health care for American citizens. But it was too late. A plethora of interest groups were lying in wait to attack the parts of the proposal they did not like (while remaining largely silent on those parts they did approve of), with millions of dollars at their disposal. Several weeks later, some 280 days after the process began, a 1,342-page bill was unveiled to Congress, the public, and the affected interests. The timing, the process, and the product were problematic. Criticism was rampant and shrill, and questions designed to shake public support were being asked in television commercials and emblazoned across full-page newspaper ads.

The timing—nine months into the presidency—was well past the "honeymoon" period, the time when Presidents Reagan and Johnson had been most successful with their sweeping new proposals. In those nine months, Clinton had been engaged in other high-visibility issues such as NAFTA and an economic stimulus program. These issues were hard-fought, even with the Democratic Congress, and involved presidential persuasion and arm-twisting that used up valuable good will and support. Meanwhile, the process used to draft the health plan enraged those who were not a part of it. The press railed against the secrecy and complained about the waste of money. It was a "policy wonk's" dream—months of high-level policy deliberation. But the political realities were sorely misjudged. The product, a reflection of the rarified air of a protected policy analytical discussion, was simply too complex and too academic, containing something to offend everyone. As noted by Light a decade earlier (1984), a president can often succeed by adopting and amending proposals already before Congress. But the Clintons chose not to take this path. Rather, they forged an ambitious, comprehensive proposal for making massive changes in the current system, with limited congressional involvement.

The public, which initially seemed supportive of the proposal, began to question the need for and complexity of national health care reform. In public polls conducted in February 1994, those against the plan and those supportive of the plan garnered the same percentages. After that time, the nays began to pull ahead. Even those in favor of reforms may have had a rather modest adjustment in mind. Focus groups and some polls found that many people were interested mainly in the forms of insurance rather than the problems of the uninsured, and in whether they could obtain insurance if they left their jobs, an issue of portability, rather than whether the entire system needed a major overhaul (Clymer, Pear, and Toner 1994).

The reasons for the demise of the Clinton health care reform are many. They include budgetary constraints and an antigovernment mood that doomed any comprehensive plan from the beginning (Skocpol 1996); the White House's inability to define the issue and frame the debate, and its lack of sustained effort (Edwards 2000); the plan's complexity, liberal approach, and cost (Quirk and Cunion 2000); the inability of the experts to agree on the reform (White 1995); the lack of support from the business community (Morone 1995); a deeply divided public, which wanted reform but balked at the actual policies (Brodie and Blendon 1995); and low levels of support from elites (Jacobs and Shapiro 1995).

President Clinton, given an opportunity to choose early in his term between a more targeted program to cover only large, catastrophic costs and a more comprehensive, universal approach chose the latter (Woodward 1994). He was simply unwilling to compromise his vision of major reform. To do so, he felt, would be to violate the trust of the people and his office. As he said later, when the prospects for success of any plan were bleak, "We didn't say, 'vote for me, in a representative form of government and I will make all the necessary decisions to solve the problems of the country, except those that are difficult, controversial and make the people mad.' That was not the deal" (Wines 1994, A9). But it was a deal, at least in health care, that was not to be. President Clinton joined his predecessors in his inability to fashion a successful health care reform package.

Though comprehensive health care reform never again was a major policy theme of his administration, Clinton did not give up. Rather, he adopted an incremental approach, and if he did not succeed in the first year, he came back year after year seeking Medicare buy-in for those aged 55 to 64, prescription drug coverage for Medicare beneficiaries, and a tax credit to assist people caring for relatives with chronic illnesses or disabilities. In his final state of the union address, he put it this way: "The lesson of our history, and the lesson of the last seven years, is that great goals are reached step-by-step, always building on our progress, always gaining ground" (Pear 2000c).

President George W. Bush has not attempted a national health insurance initiative, but he was successful at the most significant reform of the Medicare program since its founding in 1965. The politics and policies surrounding the president's role in that initiative are analyzed extensively in chapter 7. It is interesting to note here that Bush's success in health and other areas flies in the face of some conventional wisdom and political research on the presidency. He had no electoral mandate yet acted decisively; in his health proposal, he shunned incremental approaches and proposed a program with huge costs; and he turned serious attention to Medicare reform in the middle of his first presidential term, not in the earliest days. The importance to his success of having a strong, united party in the presidency and both houses of Congress should not be underestimated. The Republican leadership was focused and determined to give the president a Medicare package—and they succeeded.

CONCLUSION

In Number 70 of the *Federalist Papers*—the collection of political tracts arguing for support of the U.S. Constitution—Alexander Hamilton argued that "energy in the executive is a leading character in the definition of good government" (Publius [1787–88] 1961, 423). While other Founding Fathers were less enthusiastic about a strong executive, they agreed that their desired system of checks and balances required roughly equivalent components—strong executive and legislative branches.

There is variance in the perception of strength in the presidency. Some presidents, including Abraham Lincoln, Franklin Roosevelt, Harry Truman, and George W. Bush, have been willing to push the limits of presidential power and, in the process, have expanded that power—at least for the short term. Other presidents have had a harder time dealing with Congress. Certainly Bill Clinton's presidential clout was weakened by the dozens of congressional and special investigator probes, one of which led to his impeachment by the House in 1998.

The president can command the public's attention and garner massive press attention, but the public is also hearing contrary messages from other interests, and the press attention is often critical and downright negative. In health, the presidential role has long been as an initiator of change in health care access and delivery. But the president is stymied at many points and has been generally unsuccessful in achieving major health legislation since the passage of Medicare in 1965. (The adoption of the Medicare Modernization Act in 2003 serves as the sole exception here.) Republican and Democratic presidents have offered surprisingly similar proposals for national health insurance, which have met similar, unsuccessful fates in Congress.

Supreme Court Justice Robert H. Jackson noted in a 1952 decision that power migrates between the branches of government, and quoted Napoleon as saying, "The tools belong to the man who can use them" (Stevenson 2005). President George W. Bush has used those tools. The question remains whether the next president will build on this foundation or whether the power will migrate back to Congress.

3

Interest Groups

1965

CHARLS WALKER, a top Washington lobbyist, described lobbying Congress in the days of Sam Rayburn (D-TX; Speaker for the 10 sessions between 1940 and 1961) as highly personal, direct, and easy. In a fifty-minute meeting with Speaker Rayburn, "for forty-eight minutes we would talk about Texas, family and friends. In the remaining two, we would settle what I had come to talk about. He always knew what I was there for, and would say, 'It's taken care of, Charlie,' or 'I just can't do that for you'" (Colamosca 1979, 16). John McCormack (D-MA), who took over when Rayburn died, was similarly low-keyed and circumspect.

   In 1965, the American Medical Association (AMA) was the strongest health lobby and probably the most powerful lobby of any kind in the country. A spokesperson for the AMA could say that "medicine" opposed a bill and be correct. According to a *Yale Law Journal* article of 1954, the *New York Times* had recently claimed that the AMA was the "only organization in the country that could marshal 140 votes in Congress between sundown Friday night and noon on Monday" (quoted in Morone 1990, 256). Yet in 1965, the powerful AMA met its first major defeat with the passage of Medicare, after spending $1.2 million to fight it.

The 1965 Medicare fight was unusual, a blip on the otherwise relatively blank screen of national health insurance. By 1966 things had settled down, and the physicians' group spent $49,000 on lobbying in Washington, D.C.—a small amount even in today's dollars. That same year, the American Dental Association (ADA) spent $18,000 on lobbying; the American Hospital Association (AHA), $41,000; and the American Nurses Association (ANA), $45,000.

Political action committees were few and not very noticeable in 1965. Those that did exist were mostly associated with labor unions, PACs set up to fight federal prohibitions on labor contributions to federal candidates. The American Medical Association's PAC (AMPAC), formed in 1961, was one of the very few nonlabor PACs.

1981

The pace of politics and interest-group competition had picked up by the early 1980s. A plethora of health-related interest groups had opened offices in the capital, along K Street, N.W. More and more of the lunches consumed at the Rotunda, the Monocle, and other long-time power-lunch eateries huddled at the foot of Capitol Hill were being bought by professional lobbyists whose clients wore white coats to work, or worked closely with those who did. President Jimmy Carter's demand for spending controls on hospitals had aroused the powerful Chicago-based AHA, which stepped up its lobbying and built up its campaign contribution base. Business lobbyists, too, had health care on their menus. Costs had caught the eye of business executives as the fringe-benefit line in their annual reports began to show a higher rate of growth than wages, sales, or profits.

Chatty lunches were only a small part of the story on what was influencing health care policy. Reelection campaign costs had mushroomed as expensive television ads became the weapon of choice in the battle for votes. Campaign costs had risen tenfold in less than two decades. With so many digits in their reelection budgets, those who were elected might not even notice the generosity of moderately sized individual contributions. Enter the PAC, bundling the campaign contributions of interest groups, corporations, labor unions, and others to represent a single set of interests (Sabato 1985). By 1981, PACs had become a major factor in helping to fund (and speed the growth of) the campaign vortex.

Though the AMA and a few other organizations had PACs in the 1970s, PACs became a noticeable feature of the political landscape only in the 1980s, thanks in part to the reforms of the 1970s. In an attempt to shrink the influence of a few well-heeled givers, those who wanted more citizen-financed campaigns had pressured Congress to cap contributions from individuals and interest groups and to set up a public financing mechanism for major party candidates for president. The authorization of PACs in the 1974 law led to an extraordinary increase in their number and influence.

Health care associations took notice. Clearly there were many whose interests were not being represented by the AMA, the AHA, or the insurance companies. With their own PACs, optometrists, chiropractors, dentists, nurses, nursing homes, group practice associations, family doctors, pharmacists, drug companies, occupational therapists, and others could mount lobbying efforts or make campaign contributions to ensure that when the body politic wrote national health insurance legislation, it did not neglect the part of the human body in which they had a particular interest. Well-placed contributions could ensure that the giver's services—optometry or dentistry or whatever—were included in insurance coverage proposals and that the giver's scope of practice was protected from would-be poachers.

Cash became a p.r.n. (physician notation for "take as needed") prescription for the whole health care industry. The 1978 spending totals for federal elections alone reached huge proportions for a wide range of groups: the AMA, nearly $2 million; the dental PAC, $573,000; nurses, $100,000; for-profit hospitals, $144,000; and optometrists, $112,000.

Political action committees seemed to be taking on a life of their own. Groups without them needed them; those with them needed bigger ones; and those in a PAC representing interests that might be a bit too broad for their particular concerns splintered off, forming their own PACs. But there never seemed to be enough. More money chasing the same number of candidates inflated the cost of campaigns, intensifying the need for larger and larger PAC contributions and more and more fundraising efforts by the candidates. More PACs would have to raise more money.

1993

At the start of the Clinton administration, Washington seemed to be over-run with lobbyists—many with health care reform on their minds. Groups had proliferated, mutated, multiplied, spread, bred, and fed on one another: specialized physicians' groups, specialty hospitals, insurers, businesses, labor, corporate interests, pharmaceutical firms, home care companies, prepaid health plans, walk-in clinics, and groups representing people who are poor, elderly, or disabled, and children. Nursing homes in one Southern state could not afford their own lobbyist, so they retained a Washington professional who lobbied for a variety of health care groups; enterprisingly, he then contacted the nursing home association in a contiguous state and picked up another client. The story was being repeated all over town. When White House staffers began to count noses as they sized up the potential opposition to the president's reform plan, the numbers took their breath away. They identified more than 1,100 interest groups with substantial stakes in the health care battle (Broder 1994c). No one wanted to be left out. Every interest group in the land seemed "to have something to say on health care restructuring—from dentists to the Christian Coalition. It has created a daily, unrelenting round of Health Care Events" (Toner 1994, 1). "This is the biggest-scale lobbying effort that has ever been mounted on any single piece of legislation—both in terms of dollars spent and people engaged," said Ellen Miller of the Center for Responsive Politics, a watchdog group that keeps an eye on lobby activities and spending (Seelye 1994, A10).

The *New York Times* described a "typical day" in the capital—March 8, 1994—in the "Year of Health Care Events":

> [Eight hundred] doctors were massed at the American Medical Association conference; 210 restaurateurs were tromping to Capitol Hill, ventilating their opposition to the idea of requiring businesses to pay for health insurance; President Clinton was making the case for health care overhaul to the American Society of Association Executives (a kind of trade group for trade groups); Ralph Nader was denouncing the AMA at a news conference; former First Ladies Rosalyn Carter and Betty Ford were arguing for mental health coverage before the Senate Labor and Human Resources Committee, and the line of interested parties stretched down a very long hall when the House Ways and Means Subcommittee on Health began considering a health care bill. And this was all before noon. (Toner 1994, 1)

Health care lobbying had become a team sport. The AMA was just a player. No longer could its president boldly declare that "medicine is opposed to this measure as a total package" (Campion 1984, 275). There were no "genuine peak associations" in the health domain, concluded Salisbury and his fellow researchers (1987, 1227); they found that the AMA was best described as only one among several sets of interest-group participants, though a highly significant set.

Style changed too. "It's not about going up and tugging on Rosty's sleeve [Dan Rostenkowski of Illinois, chair of the House Ways and Means Committee] and saying 'I need something,'" a former Clinton administration functionary told the *Washington Post.* "That gets you absolutely nowhere. It's knowing how to mobilize, having access to information, making the right moves at the right time" (Boodman 1994, 6).

2005

There were 35,000 registered lobbyists by 2005, double the number in 2000; this works out to 65 lobbyists for every member of Congress (Jump 2005). By 2005, the AMA had been deposed as the dominant player in the world of health-related interest groups by a group known only by its initials: the AARP. Long an important voice in health policy, the AARP was a pivotal player in the 2003 Medicare Modernization Act. By strongly endorsing the measure in late 2003, the AARP put Democrats in the unfortunate situation of having to explain to constituents why they voted against an AARP-supported prescription drug bill—not an impossible task but certainly a difficult one, given the complicated nature of the measure.

The AARP, formerly known as the American Association of Retired Persons, often takes positions on health issues, and its endorsement of proposals is sought after by both Democrats and Republicans. Its 35 million members make the AARP a formidable proponent—or opponent. Once a bit stodgy and politically cautious, the AARP remade itself in the early twenty-first century to appeal to the 78 million baby boomers entering or soon to enter their fifties. The AARP launched a series of ads featuring vigorous 50-plus athletes and business leaders and put out a new magazine geared to 50- to 55-year-olds. The AARP also expanded its scope in state capitals—opening offices in all 50 (up from 22) states to lobby and stay in touch with local groups (Kondracke 2001). But it was the association's decision in 2003 to support the Republican Medicare prescription drug bill that indicated a major political shift.

The AARP had long supported a drug benefit but preferred a comprehensive benefit and was skeptical of the use of private plans in Medicare—preferring the traditional fee-for-service approach. But in November 2003 the AARP strongly endorsed the Republicans' prescription drug bill, in part because, in its judgment, given the federal government's weak fiscal outlook over the next few years, taking a deal on the table was imperative. The organization backed up its position with a grassroots campaign designed to convince wavering legislators to support the package. The AARP endorsement was seen as a turning point for the legislation (Pear and Hulse 2003). At the time, one reporter noted that "while other organizations like the American Medical Association and the American Hospital Association have backed the Medicare deal, none has the cache of AARP" (Bresnahan and Billings 2003).

The other dominant health interest group in 2005 was one that had operated quietly, out of the limelight, until recent years: the Pharmaceutical Research and Manufacturers of America (PhRMA), which represents the nation's drug manufacturers. Unlike the AARP, which spends only 15 percent of its budget on lobbying and advocacy, PhRMA and the companies it represents are generous contributors to elected officials and to nonprofit conservative groups. In 2004, the pharmaceutical and health products industries contributed more than $17 million to federal candidates and parties, with two-thirds going to Republicans (Center for Responsive Politics 2005). The money was well spent. Although PhRMA had strongly opposed previous congressional efforts to include a prescription drug benefit in Medicare, in 2003—with Republicans in control of Congress and the White House—the group urged quick action. It was rewarded for its support with at least three provisions in the MMA: prohibiting the Centers for Medicare and Medicaid Services (CMS) from negotiating drug prices for the voluminous Medicare market, encumbering drug reimportation with impossible-to-meet conditions, and taking the states out of the drug purchasing picture so they could no longer demand discounts.

However successful with Congress, the pharmaceutical industry has suffered bad press related to popular drugs with unexpected adverse reactions, and it typically has been the lightning rod for criticism about rising health care costs. The industry's vehement opposition to importing drugs from Canada flies in the face of strong public support for this, especially from the elderly. A 2005 survey found that 70 percent of respondents said drug companies put profits ahead of people, and that people are more likely to cite drug company profits as the major cause of rising health care costs than any other cause (Kaiser Family Foundation 2005a). PhRMA is working to polish its image and provide an alternative to legislation that would allow drug importation: a new project providing national call centers to hook up low-income patients with state and local drug-assistance programs (National Journal 2005).

One of the biggest changes in the lobbying world in 2005 may have been in the political realm. While in the early 1990s, political scientists were still arguing that interest groups generally avoided becoming too beholden to a particular party, by 2005 such disdain for partisanship had largely disappeared. Between 1995 and 2005, the K Street Project, directed in large part by House Republican leader Tom DeLay (R-TX), had succeeded in populating major interest groups and associations with Republican lobbyists and then ensuring that those lobbyists directed funding to Republican candidates. While some Democrats complained and some formal allegations were made against DeLay, his former staff, and favored lobbyists, the K Street network was powerful and successful at "growing the Republican majority in Congress, passing business-friendly legislation, and collecting more than $25 million since 1994" (Justice 2005).

The law that eliminated soft money contributions to political parties, the Bipartisan Campaign Reform Act of 2002 (BCRA), also spawned a new, and in many ways more fearsome, political entity—Section 527 groups. With few controls and great partisanship, these entities became a major force in political discourse in the 2004 presidential election and in issue-related advertisements on Social Security and Medicare.

OVERVIEW

The body of theory that describes interest groups and their actions reflects the changes these groups have undergone. Key elements of this theory include how and why interest groups form and why they persist. Interest groups have evolved rapidly from close-knit alliances into diverse, large, and powerful players in federal (and state) policy making. Many groups occupy somewhat narrow "niches" in policy, but they also participate in coalitions that allow them to pool their efforts to effect or deflect broad policy change. Interest groups provide information and campaign support to elected officials and use several strategies to influence policy, including direct lobbying, grassroots organizing, campaign contributions through PACs, and participation in coalitions. Though interest groups spend most of their time attempting to influence Congress, they also recognize the importance of lobbying the executive branch. Interest groups also use the courts, often as a final avenue for action when other means fall short. Interest groups play an important role in both electing members of Congress favorable to their cause and working with these members to enact the policies the groups desire (and stop the policies they oppose). In sum, the role of interest groups in defining and shaping health care policy is pivotal. Next to Congress, interest groups may well be the most important actors in health policy.

HOW AND WHY INTERESTS ORGANIZE

Interest groups consist of individuals who have organized themselves around a shared interest and seek to influence public policy. Interest groups include organizations as diverse as the Federation of Behavioral, Psychological, and Cognitive Sciences and the Association of State and Territorial Health Officials, as broad as the American Public Health Association and as narrow as the American Society of Gastrointestinal Endoscopy. They also include corporations and institutional interests such as hospitals, medical schools, HMOs, and schools of public health.

Table 3.1 lists some of the 171 organizations and groups that were most active on health care advocacy (including registered lobbying and testimony before committees) between 1997 and 2002, as identified by Heaney (2004a). It includes well-known groups such as the AARP and the American Hospital Association and little-known groups such as the Renal Physicians Association and the Society for Investigative Dermatology. It includes broad health groups (Families USA), narrow health groups (Autism Society of America), nonhealth groups that lobby on health issues (American Society of Association Executives), advocacy groups (NARAL Pro-Choice America), and citizen groups (Public Citizen). What table 3.1 illustrates is the enormous scope and range of health issues across interest groups—and why understanding interest groups is crucial to understanding health policy.

Interest Groups and Policy Making

Lindblom (1980, 85) described interest groups' role in policy making as "indispensable." These groups clarify and articulate citizens' preferences, warn policymakers of problems with their proposals, and suggest ways to make proposals more palatable or point out why they will damage and enrage a group's membership. Simply put, groups represent the interests of their members and supporters, whether the American Social Health Association or the Association of American Medical Colleges or the nation's Catholic hospitals.

Interest groups also serve to educate their members and others on issues and to help form a feasible public agenda. They monitor activity, public and

Table 3.1

Some Health Interest Groups Lobbying Congress between 1997 and 2002

AARP

Advanced Medical Technology Association

American Academy of Child and Adolescent Psychiatry

American Association of Dental Research

American College of Cardiology

American Hospital Association

American Public Health Association

American Social Health Association

American Society of Association Executives

Arthritis Foundation

Association for American Medical Colleges

Association for Schools of Public Health

Autism Society of America

Citizens for Public Action on High Blood Pressure and Cholesterol

Coalition for Health Funding

Crohn's and Colitis Foundation of America

Families USA

Federation of American Hospitals

Greater New York Hospital Association

International Council of Cruise Lines

Joint Commission on Accreditation of Healthcare Organizations

Medical Library Association

NARAL Pro-Choice America

National Association of Chain Drug Stores

National Breast Cancer Coalition

National Governors Association

National League for Nursing

National Union of Hospital and Health Care Employees, Local 1199

Planned Parenthood Federation of America

Public Citizen

Renal Physicians Association

Seniors Coalition

Society for Investigative Dermatology

Vietnam Veterans of America

Washington Business Group on Health

Source: Heaney 2004a.

private, and can blow the whistle on a bad idea when it is proposed. Their job is to make the case for their constituents before government, plying the halls of Congress, the executive branch, the courts, and the offices of other interest groups to provide a linkage between citizens and government. For many decades in the United States, it was political parties that provided this linkage. But in recent years, surveys show that people prefer to have more clearly kindred spirits minding the store for them. The more well-heeled the group, the more likely it is to make its own way rather than turn the job over to a broader group such as a political party.

Interest groups are as American as talk shows, and much older. James Madison, in Number 10 of the *Federalist Papers,* bemoaned the mischiefs of "factions," which he defined as "a number of citizens . . . who are united and actuated by some common impulse of passion or of interest" (Publius [1787–88] 1961, 78). Though Madison put a negative "spin" on the factions by suggesting their interests might be adverse to the rights of other citizens and to the interests of the community, the right to associate is one of the first defended in the Bill of Rights. A century later, Alexis de Tocqueville, the French visitor to the United States whose uncannily accurate observations still resonate today, observed that "in no country in the world has the principle of association been more successfully used or applied to a greater multitude of objects than in America." He continued, "Wherever, at the head of some new undertaking, you see the government in France, or a man of rank in England, in the United States you will be sure to find an association" (de Tocqueville [1835] 1956, 95, 198).

Interest-group representation has long been a fact of life in Washington, D.C.—much to the chagrin of many in government. Woodrow Wilson said in 1913 that "Washington was so full of lobbyists that 'a brick couldn't be thrown without hitting one.'" Eighty years later, President Bill Clinton, outlining his economic plan to Congress, noted that "within minutes of the time I conclude my address to Congress . . . the special interests will be out in force . . . Many have already lined the corridors of power with high-priced lobbyists" (both quoted in Brinkley 1993, A14). Some presidents have been less disparaging of lobbyists. For instance, when Harry Truman was asked about men twisting arms on his behalf, he argued that "we wouldn't call those people lobbyists. We would call them citizens appearing in the public interest" (Cotterell 2004).

Groups are essential to the American notion of pluralism—groups competing to put items on, or keep them off, the agenda and to achieve their members' goals in public policies. Ideally, as Madison speculated, groups check one another and come to agree only on the common interest. Madison's ideal has not emerged, however. Groups are not equally endowed, and they fail to provide representation for all. As Schattschneider (1960, 35) put it, the pluralists' "heavenly chorus sings with a strong upper class accent." Poor people, immigrants, and ethnic minorities are often not as well represented as are middle-class business interests. And all middle-class interests are not equal. The National Rifle Association (NRA) is a very strong national lobby whose success is only partly checked by anti-handgun groups and police associations. Powerful interests such as the AMA have a greater potential to be heard than do organizations of nurse-midwives or health care consumers.

Nor do groups always act in the public interest. Frequently, their contribution to public policy making is to exercise a veto power over policy changes and innovation. Kingdon (1995) found that interest groups' power lies less in moving subjects onto the agenda than in keeping other subjects off. A common goal is to block new initiatives from gaining widespread support, and the groups tend to be very good at this. A minority, represented by a strong interest group, can stop or delay legislation or a proposed rule. The system of government is set up that way, to make it hard to change policy: lose one round, live to fight another; move from subcommittee to full committee to house floor; repeat the process in the second house; move to the more informal setting of the conference committee; and, if you still have not succeeded, seek a presidential veto, or try to influence the agency writing the regulations, or sue the agency in federal court for violating the due process clause of the Constitution. "A lot of the best lobbyists are like paid assassins," a spokesperson for the Center for Responsive Politics told the *New York Times* (Abramson 1998). And Ellen Miller, of the same center, commented that PAC money "buys silence, hearings are not held or amendments not introduced" (Matlack, Barnes, and Cohen 1990, 1479). Lowi (1964) termed this ability of a strong interest-group minority to ride roughshod over majority interests "interest group liberalism." President Jimmy Carter tried to sound the alarm that it was not good for the republic. Making the growth of special interest organizations the topic of his farewell address, he said that "the national interest is not always the sum of all our single or special interests" (Carter 1981). He called the growth of these groups a "disturbing factor in American political life."

Those who run these lobby groups do not see it that way. Karen Ignagni, chief executive officer of the American Association of Health Plans and one of the most important lobbyists in Washington, described her organization's efforts as simply doing its job of professional, hard-hitting work on behalf of its membership—people with an important stake in the policy process. "Most people think of trade associations making backroom deals and buttonholing legislators," she told *Washingtonian Magazine.* "That is not the way it is anymore. You run an association with all the vehicles of a political campaign with polling, grassroots organizing, and all the earned media attention you can get. The tired view of associations from the outside is that it is lowest-common-denominator advocacy. The fact is, we are not your father's Oldsmobile anymore" (Eisler 1999).

Lobbyists are also paid as skilled professionals, commanding annual salaries of up to a million dollars, and those with the right backgrounds face a seller's market. A Washington headhunter said she could not believe what a hot property a former senior aide at the Health Care Financing Administration (HCFA; now the CMS) turned out to be when he sought a lobbying job: "I felt like I was representing Michael Jordan," the headhunter said. "The demand for knowledgeable people who can track what is going on on Capitol Hill and [in] the government and can figure out the pressure points that companies should be touching in Washington has greatly increased," said another placement-firm spokesperson (both quoted in Abramson 1998).

How Interest Groups Form and Persist

Analogies help scholars make sense out of complexities. Madison wrote Number 10 of the *Federalist Papers* at a time when educated people thought of the universe as a collection of forces pressing against one another. The point at which these forces were equal, the equilibrium, seemed somehow natural or right. Applied to politics, scholars concluded, this point of equilibrium was the public interest. Political scientist David B. Truman (1951) used the term *equilibrium* in one of the first efforts to describe why interest groups form. Some disruption or disturbance upsets the equilibrium; people then band together to restore equilibrium by exerting countervailing force. Sometimes the formation of one group might lead to a disturbance that upsets another group, which might in turn cause another group to form, until a new social equilibrium is reached. Group formation might stabilize for a while, only to start up again with another disturbance. Though this explanation goes a long way toward explaining the formation of most groups, it does not explain why groups stay together once the threat or event causing the group to form has disappeared or attenuated. It also assumes that during a disturbance, anyone can easily organize those who share their interests into a group.

A second explanation for group formation highlights selective benefits. Olson (1968) offered what can be viewed as a "rational choice" argument: people join groups because they will directly benefit from membership through material rewards such as the ability to serve on the staff of a hospital, to bid on certain construction jobs, or even just to receive discounted travel services or an informative magazine. Selective benefits also help overcome another problem for groups seeking public policy change: the free rider. Why join the Sierra Club when anybody can enjoy the clean water and unspoiled wilderness that the club's policy advocacy has helped produce? One answer is selective benefits: to receive maps, camping tips, and other benefits of membership. Nobody does this better than the AARP, the group that claims 35 million members, roughly one-fourth of the registered voters in the United States. With a low membership fee, anyone 50 years of age or older qualifies for rental car and hotel discounts, cut-rate prices on drugs, group health insurance, investment programs, and reduced-price car and mobile home insurance.

Other explanations have also been put forward. Clark and Wilson (1961) built on the selective benefits notion, describing three types of benefits that attract group membership: material benefits (magazines, discounts, tips, etc.); purposive benefits (those associated with ideological or issue-oriented goals without tangible benefits to members); and solidarity or social benefits, which can also include benefits from achieving worthwhile policy goals. Salisbury (1969) offered a market-oriented view. He believed that interest groups are formed by entrepreneurs who invest capital to create benefits that they offer, at a price, to a market of potential customers. In effect, an "exchange" takes place between leaders who provide the incentives and members who provide their support. Exchange theory is useful because it explains not only how groups begin but also how they retain their membership and survive. According to Jack Walker (1991), 80 percent of U.S. interest groups have emerged from preexisting occupational or professional communities. He could have been looking at health groups, where the link to jobs is clear: groups representing health professionals, health providers, and the health industry dominate the field.

Today's interest groups have moved beyond membership fees as the sole source of support. The AARP gets substantial resources from insurance and mutual fund companies. The AMA secures about two-thirds of its resources from real estate and business transactions (Ainsworth 2002). In a well-publicized but embarrassing bid for money, the AMA agreed to let the Sunbeam Corporation use the AMA logo on its home health care products, in exchange for a reputed cash settlement and an agreement to promote AMA health care information (Ainsworth 2002; Carney 1998). When AMA members complained, the group reneged and Sunbeam sued. The case was settled out of court for a substantial AMA payment to Sunbeam.

Interest groups can be launched directly or indirectly by government action. More government equals more groups. Jack Walker (1991) noted that groups are created more as a consequence of legislation than as an impetus for it. Government policies provide new benefits or jobs to people who form groups to protect (and expand) those benefits or jobs. The American Farm Bureau Federation and the U.S. Chamber of Commerce are the two best-known examples of groups started by government agencies. An example in the health sector is the genesis of the National Association of Community Health Centers. Federal grant dollars helped establish neighborhood health centers across the country, and the centers then formed an association to lobby Congress for more funding. The federal funding agency facilitated the survival of the fledgling group by giving it additional grant money. Groups are also formed in anticipation of federal action; for example, hospitals that wanted reclassification from rural to urban (to qualify for higher reimbursement) formed a lobby-oriented association (Kosterlitz 1992). Other groups start up to prevent federal action: the Tobacco Institute was formed to fight the regulation of cigarettes (J. Walker 1991); the American Association of Blood Banks organized to fight a proposal for a national blood system (Tierney 1987).

Economic interests play a big role in interest-group formation. Health economist Paul Feldstein (1977) noted that health associations pursue policies that allow a monopoly position for their members. This applies whether the group consists of professional members or nonprofit organizations. Feldstein argued that health interest groups will likely support policies that increase the demand for their services, enable them to be reimbursed as price-discriminating monopolists, lower the price of complementary inputs, increase the price of substitutes, or restrict additions to their supply. Simply put, economic interests support policies to help health care providers get more patients, set their own prices, reduce their costs, make their product the best deal, and freeze out the competition. Clearly, the battle in the 1990s over the patients' bill of rights legislation supports this notion that groups vigorously oppose government policies that will increase their costs, including transaction costs or legal liability. In 2004 and 2005, the gun industry successfully fought to enact legislation that gives them legal immunity from cases in which guns are used to maim and kill people. While pursuing these policies of self-interest, the groups say they are acting in the best interests of the public.

Nonoccupational Interest Groups

Most interest groups represent occupations and companies, but others are brought together by ideology or a common purpose, such as Mothers Against Drunk Driving (MADD). Though many such groups are small in both numbers and resources, they often garner considerable public and media support for their public interest lobbying. In the past 25 years, more and more of these citizens' groups have sprung up in Washington and the states.

When pitted against the organized and well-funded groups of health providers, citizens' groups in the health area can be overshadowed, if not ignored. A few well-known citizens' groups target health issues, such as Planned Parenthood, the Health Research Group, the National Women's Health Network, and the National Citizens' Coalition for Nursing Home Reform. The AARP is the largest—and best-known—of the citizens' groups. It is so large that its headquarters in Washington, D.C., has its own zip code (D. West and Loomis 1998). Unlike most citizens' groups, the AARP is well funded and highly visible. When asked to name the citizens' groups active in the 1994 health care discussions, one well-placed participant named only the AARP. Though the AARP fits Jack Walker's definition of a citizens' group, its role of protecting current and expanding future benefits under Medicare seems to fit the spirit of an occupational or professional group protecting its concentrated interest in regulation (or, in this case, reimbursement) and in imposing costs over a broad population base.

A subset of citizens' groups is those that Foreman (1995) called grassroots victims' organizations, made up of persons who are directly and often suddenly and tragically affected by a health hazard or disease. Such groups, such as the Love Canal Homeowners Association and the AIDS Coalition to Unleash Power (ACT-UP), can achieve limited, targeted policy success. People with cancer, in particular, have from time to time successfully drawn thousands of their peers to march and rally on the Washington Mall and descend on Congress. MADD is another type of grassroots victims' organization.

One of the most successful grassroots groups is the National Breast Cancer Coalition, which over the past 15 years has grown from small groups of women meeting in living rooms across the country to a well-financed, highly organized group with considerable visibility and legislative effectiveness. Casamayou (2001) credits its success to a mixture of strong leadership and extraordinary passion for action—notably, more funding for breast cancer research.

Anecdotal evidence suggests that single-issue citizens' groups can eventually succeed in health policy—largely by persistence. The federal requirement that states enact a 0.08 percent blood alcohol level as the standard for drunk driving was passed in 2000, after 16 years of aggressive lobbying by MADD and many earlier defeats under pressure from the restaurant and alcoholic beverage industries. Likewise, citizens' groups succeeded in getting Medicare coverage expanded to include preventive services—again after a very long and persistent effort.

Surprisingly, perhaps, citizens' groups are often politically hampered by their focus on local rather than national issues. Browne (1993) concluded that environmental public interest groups are often disadvantaged in their interactions with Congress, since members of Congress, when they go home to their districts, rarely hear from constituents who are also representatives of these groups. Local activists often are more concerned with local issues than with national ones and have only general views about better national environmental conditions.

FRAGMENTATION, COALITIONS, AND CHANGES IN AFFILIATION

For many years the interest-group world was dominated by "peak associations," umbrella organizations representing large groups of farmers, businesses, or labor unions. In the 1990s, the landscape became much more varied, with the larger organizations still in existence but sharing space with smaller, more focused groups, often splintered off from peak associations. For example, complementing the AMA at the time of the Clinton administration's health care proposal efforts were at least 80 medical specialty groups representing surgeons, pediatricians, emergency room physicians, ophthalmologists, plastic surgeons, and others. Similar diversification occurred in the hospital industry, where the interests of small community hospitals, large nonprofit hospitals, teaching hospitals, and inner-city hospitals differed so substantially that a single organization (the AHA) could not fully represent them all. What frequently happens is that the larger umbrella organizations must take less specific, more general positions that minimize conflict, while the more specialized, smaller groups are free to adopt more specific positions targeted at their members. As Rep. Pete Stark (D-CA), long-time health advocate, described it, "I think that the specialty [physician] groups are often more effective because their issues are more focused. The AMA suffers from the same problem the American Hospital Association does. When you try and represent everyone, you basically can't represent anyone" (Carney 1998).

Indeed, the AHA has had great difficulty in keeping its hospitals happy.

Teaching hospitals, rural hospitals, Catholic hospitals, and inner-city hospitals—to name a few—have varied interests and often pursue policies that benefit themselves to the exclusion of other hospitals. For example, in 2002, the Catholic Health Association (CHA), which represents Roman Catholic hospitals, released a report arguing that Catholic hospitals play a special role in the health care safety net and should be reimbursed for that role (Reilly 2002).

Interest-Group Coalitions

The proliferation and fragmentation of interest groups and the rising stakes have made the formation of coalitions especially important. In these coalitions, interest groups can maximize their resources and their lobby strength. They can work to influence a wider array of policies than groups working alone. They can also help with a group's visibility and image. One interest group lobbyist put it this way: "Coalitions show that we are in good company. They allow other groups to see us as a contributor to the community. Smart people on Capitol Hill frequently think of us as the 'go to' group" (quoted in Heaney 2004b, 1).

Some coalitions are long-standing, with groups working together over many years and numerous policy battles. Such groups can be considered "policy communities," networks of interest groups active in a particular domain or representing similar constituencies. Sometimes these coalitions are well funded and staffed. An example is the 100-plus-member National Health Council, founded in 1920 to improve the health of the nation. With a budget of about a million dollars, the National Health Council encompasses voluntary and professional health societies, federal agencies, national organizations, and business groups with strong health interests.

More typical are temporary coalitions, formed to work together on one issue or policy, then disbanding when the issue dies or becomes law. Several such coalitions formed during the lobbying for the MMA in 2003. Opponents of competitive bidding for medical equipment and services, such as home health providers, formed the Coalition for Access to Medical Services, Equipment and Technology (M. Carey 2003). Twenty-five state medical societies and a group of rural physicians formed the Geographic Equity in Medicare Coalition to encourage higher payments to rural hospitals (A. Goldstein 2003). Coalitions are so important that several congressional leaders have designated staff to assemble and keep in touch with coalitions, and some lobby firms specialize in a brokering service to help assemble coalitions (Birnbaum 2004). One of the benefits of such a service may be in helping the coalition to select a name—often a name that has little to do with its purpose or its sponsors. The Consumer Foundation is dominated by large retailers such as Sears and large drugstore chains; the Coalition for Health Care Choices is primarily financed by the Health Insurance Association of America (HIAA) (Wilcox 1999).

Sometimes coalitions bring together unusual collaborators. For example, to fight the 2003 drug reimportation bill, PhRMA joined with abortion opponents in a direct-mail campaign that focused on conservative House members. The jointly sponsored material warned that the drug reimportation measure would make the RU-486 abortion pill as "easy to get as aspirin" (Stolberg 2003a).

Groups are free to join multiple coalitions, and many do. The U.S. Chamber of Commerce is a member of at least 300 coalitions on issues ranging from highway construction to expansion of the nation's visa program (Birnbaum 2004). Heaney (2004b) identified 231 health coalitions, many of them small. His work focused on 80 coalitions made up of six or more groups. The coalitions ranged from Citizens for Better Medicare and the Coalition for Fair Medicare Payment to the Coalition for Genetic Fairness and the Friends of Indian Health (table 3.2). Heaney found that patient advocacy groups and groups representing medical service providers were most likely to participate in coalitions, and business groups least likely. But coalition membership is widespread. More than 90 percent of the interest-group representatives interviewed by Heaney reported membership in one of the coalitions in the study.

Sometimes coalitions are useful for helping highly visible groups get support for their preferences from other, more "legitimate" groups. For example, in 1993 the Pharmaceutical Manufacturers' Association (PMA) formed a coalition of citizens' groups and public health advocates that opposed limits on Medicaid spending for prescription drugs. A PMA spokesperson acknowledged that the coalition was formed to give the association more credibility with Congress than if the PMA itself made the apparently self-serving arguments (Pear 1993). Later the association added *research* to its name to add to its status, becoming PhRMA.

Coalitions allow groups to pool their resources to fund media campaigns and research papers. They may be funded primarily by larger lobbying groups with a common interest in a major bill, with important grassroots support provided by advocacy or membership groups. Interest groups see coalitions

Table 3.2

Some Health Coalitions Lobbying Congress between 1997 and 2002

Ad Hoc Group for Medical Research Funding

Alliance to Improve Medicare

Americans for Long Term Care Security

Association Health Plan Coalition

Campaign for Quality Care

Campaign for Tobacco Free Kids

Citizens for Better Medicare

Coalition for Affordable Health Coverage

Coalition for Fair Medicare Payment

Coalition for Genetic Fairness

Coalition on Human Needs

FamilyCare Act Coalition

Friends of Indian Health

Genetic Alliance

GINE Coalition

Health Professions and Nursing Education Coalition

Independence Through Enhancement of Medicare and Medicaid Coalition (ITEM)

Independent Budget

Long Term Care Campaign

Mental Health Liaison Group

National Council on Folic Acid

National Health Council

One Voice Against Cancer (OVAC)

Partnership for Prevention

Patient Access Coalition

Research!America

Women's Health Research Coalition

Source: Heaney 2004b.

as a way to maximize their likelihood of success with a minimum of staff effort, by devising joint strategies with like-minded groups. They can also use a variety of resources to achieve a common goal. For example, in one coalition designed to promote regulatory relief, the members targeted legislators who had district ties to their businesses. The Johnson and Johnson lobbyists concentrated on members of Congress from districts where the company's plants were situated; Federal Express lobbyists targeted Memphis (home of

FedEx headquarters) legislators; a retail farm supplier group took responsibility for rural legislators (Weisskopf and Maraniss 1995).

Coalitions sometimes exaggerate their size, hoping to parlay the perception of a vast nationwide membership into political influence. The Christian Coalition, a dominant voice in several national elections, was revealed in 1999 to have deliberately misled the press and others about its size. Discontented leaders who abandoned the group after it fell into financial trouble disclosed how it had routinely employed deceptive techniques to give the appearance of a large office staff, a huge national membership, and active chapters in 48 states. Techniques included maintaining membership rolls with wrong addresses, duplicates, and the names of dead people; hiring temporary staff to look busy in the mail room when reporters or camera crews showed up; and using their few actual staff to run ahead of reporters to occupy empty offices, "leapfrogging" the reporters as they moved from office to office (Goodstein 1999). Printing millions of voter guides that would never be mailed to non-existent members was also part of the ruse. The group's actual size, clearly much smaller than the 2.8 million members it once claimed, continued to be a point of contention, but its ability to organize a campaign effort of significant size seemed to be limited to just seven states in 1999. "We never distributed 40 million guides," a former director told the *New York Times*. "State affiliates took stacks of them to recycling centers after the election. A lot of churches just put a pile of them on the back table. I never considered effective distribution anything short of inserting them into church bulletins, but in very few churches did that actually happen" (Goodstein 1999).

Coalitions are sometimes difficult to form, especially for groups fearful of surrendering some of their "turf." Wood (1999) found that disease-related associations did not work together effectively, even when there was good reason to do so. He described a situation in which five associations concerned with Parkinson's disease could not work together even when an Arizona legislator had a bill calling for additional funding for research ready for action.

Niche Theory

In contrast to the pluralistic notion of interest groups competing against one another to reach some type of accommodation, in some interest areas the groups tend to stake out policy domains that are theirs and are recognized as such and accommodated by other groups. A group does this by finding a recognizable identity, defining a highly specific issue niche for itself, and fixing its political assets (that is, recognition and other resources) within that niche. Groups with special expertise can establish a niche, unthreatened by other interests. Clearly, such a staking out of territory has a practical appeal, since one interest group cannot influence everything. Another important reason for finding a niche is the instability of the policy world. Without the security of friends in Congress and the bureaucracy, and with forces such as citizens' groups, the president, the press, and the decentralization of Congress all exerting their influence, interest groups can attain some sense of security by staking out a policy niche and devoting their resources there (Browne 1991). For example, the Association of American Medical Colleges (AAMC) focuses on policies affecting the nation's 125 medical schools. This association has not often ventured into broader health care issues, but it has been perceived as the dominant force in issues related to medical education. Similarly, many patients' organizations focus only on the disease or condition at hand, refusing to participate in larger battles such as the 1993–94 health care reform debate.

Niche politics prevail when the issues are narrow and involve few interests. Cigler and Loomis (1991, 392) thought the "bulk of group politics" takes place within these policy niches, or policy communities. As long as discrete policies do not cross niche boundaries, these accommodations can continue, even as more and more groups are added. A study of lobbyists and the issues they deal with confirmed this idea. Baumgartner and Leech (2000) found a highly skewed pattern of lobbying when they examined the 1996 Lobbying Disclosure Reports. A few issues involved a very large number of lobbyists (an obvious one was health care reform), but most issues were much lower key. The top 5 percent of issues accounted for more than 30 percent of the lobbying; in contrast, the bottom 50 percent accounted for only 3.5 percent. In other words, most issues involved few lobbyists. Not surprisingly, business was overrepresented in issues that drew few or no competing interests.

Niche politics can benefit both the interest group and the member of Congress. Both enjoy the benefits of low transaction costs. Interest groups with well-defined niches do not have to explain to legislators which groups they represent and what they stand for—thus they are able to use time with a legislator to pursue policy objectives. Members of Congress benefit for the same reason: they do not have to listen to explanations and descriptions of the group. These saved transaction costs are especially important given that the competition for legislators' time is becoming more and more limited as groups increase in number but members of Congress, of course, do not (Heaney 2004a).

Expertise is key to understanding niche politics. One example noted by

Heaney (2004a) was when, during the 2003 revision of Medicare, congressional sponsors of a provision to create an outpatient prescription drug benefit needed to learn more about the role of pharmacy benefit managers (PBMs). Two interest groups were happy to help out: the Academy of Managed Care Pharmacy and the Pharmaceutical Care Management Association. Both Congress and the groups benefited from the interaction.

Comprehensive proposals for change can disrupt interest-group niches. When reforms affect financing, education, quality, cost, and a host of details, the scope of the conflict is widened. Choices have to be made about what to fight for and against. Old alliances and the dominance of a particular issue can break down, opening opportunities for new patterns of dominance (Baumgartner and Jones 1993). Niche groups often participate in coalitions when comprehensive change is proposed. This gives them a way to ensure that the change will encompass issues of concern to them, or at least that damage will be minimal.

Health policy is sometimes characterized as niche politics, with highly specialized groups dealing with focused, even arcane, issues. The issues are often resolved without much outside attention. But not all issues are niche issues and not all groups are niche groups. Health politics and policy are not quite so easily explained.

From Iron Triangles to Issue Networks

The dominant political model of interest-group influence for many years was the iron triangle: congressional committees, interest groups, and bureaucrats—the three vertices of the triangle—did all the decision making. This triumvirate was so strong that it tended to prevail over all other actors, including the president. Sometimes called subgovernments, or policy subsystems, or policy monopolies, these relationships were considered impermeable and lasting. Major decisions, so it was said, were made by a few experts who benefited from working closely together. The interest group benefited from close access to decision makers and implementers. The bureaucracy benefited by ensuring adequate appropriations and public support. Congressional staffers benefited by garnering the substantive and political resources of these key actors—making members of Congress look good to other members and to constituents.

Though intuitively persuasive, the notion of iron triangles proved to be simplistic and wrong as U.S. policy making moved into a world of competing interests, complexity, and tough choices. With the decentralization of congressional power, interest groups could not simply work with leaders or with a few committee chairs and a handful of legislators to maximize the likelihood that their positions would prevail. Today's interest-group world is much more complex and less easily defined. In what are called issue networks (Heclo 1978) or policy subsystems (Stein and Bickers 1995), policy is shaped by loosely connected interest groups and experts within and outside government, working together on some aspect of public policy. The definition of these entities is somewhat nebulous, because members of issue networks or policy subsystems can have varying degrees of expertise and commitment to the policy and can move in and out of the policy domain. Issue networks are sloppy and unpredictable and very difficult to describe, much less predict or explain. Another aspect of the shift to networks relates to the complexity of such issues as health care policy. Because jurisdiction for health care is widely shared among many congressional committees rather than focused in one or two committees, most interest groups now tend to work with four or five separate committees or agencies and, on some issues, with committees not generally in their purview.

Empirical studies of interest groups have increased our understanding of these entities by charting the acquaintance networks of groups identified as influential in several key policy domains, including health (Heinz et al. 1990; Salisbury et al. 1987). The researchers looked for interest groups that were influential in more than one of several different fields: health, labor, agriculture, and energy. They found none. Had the research been done 30 years earlier, they would have found that the American Federation of Labor–Congress of Industrial Organizations (AFL-CIO) was influential in multiple issue areas such as health, income, poverty, aging, and housing policies and labor relations. Likewise, for each issue, the researchers found few examples of mediators or facilitators who worked closely with a variety of colleagues concerned with the same issues. Instead, influential people talked with people who agreed with them, based largely on their organizational or client interests. The researchers dubbed this phenomenon a network of interest groups with a "hollow core," or empty center, sans actors who could bridge various aspects of policy. Again, 30 years earlier, they might have found such mediators or coordinators in the form of the Farm Bureau in agriculture and the AMA in health care policy.

In short, the interest-group world has changed. It seems to have swung from a tightly knit, closely coordinated, impervious, and closed world to an atomistic, uncoordinated, and highly permeable one. Nevertheless, it would be misleading to say the iron triangle has completely gone from the scene. For some complex, nonsalient issues or those with little opposition, the iron triangle may still prevail. Veterans' policy is heavily dominated by the associations for veterans with disabilities and a few other veterans' groups, a small number of House and Senate committees, and the Department of Veterans Affairs. Few others concern themselves with policy decisions affecting veterans. When veterans' groups decided that Clinton's Veterans Affairs secretary, Togo D. West Jr., had not fought vigorously enough for the agency's budget, their attacks led West to write a memo to the president indicating that he would resign before the end of his term. Meanwhile, he promised the groups he would seek additional funding, sent a plea to the OMB, and braced himself to battle for more money in the coming budget cycle (Becker 1999). Similarly, at the state level, groups representing people with mental retardation or developmental disabilities often work closely with legislative supporters and agency staff to achieve policy goals, rarely questioned by other policymakers.

HOW INTEREST GROUPS INFLUENCE DECISION MAKING

Lobbying today looks much like a political campaign. Issues are defined through research and polling; public support is garnered through media campaigns, often targeted to constituents of key members of Congress; and organization is paramount at the local or grassroots level where the voters reside. Simply knowing the committee chair is not enough (Andres 2004). It all starts with information.

Information

Salisbury (1992) found that lobbyists report spending most of their time monitoring issues and providing information, much of it to other groups. This makes sense, given the rapid expansion of new groups and the growing list of activities into which government now injects itself. Information provided by lobbyists may help legislators make (and defend) public policy *and* get reelected. The information may include data on the problem, on the impact of the proposed new policy, and, importantly, on the effects of the new policy on the legislator's constituents. Wright (1996) argues that the NRA's success over the years has flowed from a large membership that presents compelling information to members of Congress about the electoral consequences of their stands on gun control. Wright (1996, 199) says of legislators that "to stay apprised of the political situations at home and in Washington, they must frequently turn to others for information and advice. Among those they turn to are organized interests." Lobbyists can provide procedural information on which other members of Congress are supporting the legislation and what procedural strategies might be used in markup. Lobbyists can help frame the issue in ways that legislators can use to support their own positions and to engender constituent support.

More and more interest groups are commissioning research to support their positions. As one lobbyist put it, "Commissioning studies gives us a more persuasive position to argue from" (P. Stone 1994, 2842). When interest groups were active in calling for provider "givebacks" following the 1997 Balanced Budget Act (BBA), home care and hospital lobbies released "research" showing how their industries had been undermined by the law. To buttress their case that Catholic hospitals were "special," the CHA funded research quantifying their uncompensated care and medical education and research. The information was used, said a CHA spokesperson, to provide "credibility when we get into a public discussion" (Reilly 2002). Sometimes the research is proactive. For example, anticipating criticism about rising drug costs, PhRMA produced research in 2004 showing that in recent years health plan co-payments had increased at a faster rate than drug costs (PhRMA 2004a).

Interest groups have also found the Internet extremely useful in providing information to policymakers, journalists, and the public. The Internet has dramatically lowered the per-unit distribution costs and has proved a great boon for less wealthy groups, especially those with large constituencies. Groups use the Internet for getting out their message, mobilizing supporters, fundraising, and fostering grassroots activism (Bosso and Collins 2002).

The AMA has been extremely engaged in providing information on an issue near and dear to physicians' hearts: malpractice reform. The association has not shied away from strong language, saying that 20 states are in a "full-blown medical liability crisis." In fact, the GAO found mixed evidence in five states that were identified as in crisis. Other observers have pointed out that malpractice claims and awards have declined, rather than increased, in several "crisis" states identified by the AMA (Herbert 2004).

Information is most useful in the early stages of consideration of a bill, when members of Congress must get up to speed on the issue and its likely impact on their district. Later in the process things change. "We've long passed informational lobbying; now we're at the break-your-arm lobbying," said Sen. John Breaux (D-LA) late in the 1994 health care reform debate (Seelye 1994, A10).

Gaining Access

To make use of what they see and learn, lobbyists must meet the most important proximate goal of their profession: gaining access. A chance to tell their story is essential to most lobbying strategies. To the interest group, access may mean telephone calls and regular meetings with members of Congress and their staff. Sabato (1985, 127) quoted one PAC official as saying, "Frequently all it takes is the opportunity to talk to a legislator 10 or 15 minutes to make your case. He may not have 10 or 1 minute to hear the other side." Wright (1990) found that the number of lobbying contacts was a better predictor of legislators' votes than the amount of campaign contributions.

Access alone is not always enough, of course. Lobbyists must be able to present a case so persuasive that the legislator will support their position. They do this in part with good, timely information on complex issues. The form and content of this information are crucial. Baumgartner and Jones (1993) referred to this as the "policy image," or definition of an issue. Ellen Merlo, a Philip Morris executive, described how this is done: "Once you have the access, you have to be able to deliver a message that makes sense. If it's a tax that we're against, then we have to be able to prove that there are going to be job losses, that it's not going to produce the revenue that is being projected, that if a state raises its taxes so high and it's next to another state with low taxes, there are going to be cross-border sales and those sales will not only be a loss in tobacco revenue, but once someone goes over a border to buy their tobacco or their liquor or something else, they're probably making a lot of other purchases" (Roger Rosenblatt 1994, 55).

Framing Issues

There are many examples of health groups "framing" an issue so that support of the issue is seemingly in the public interest. In a typical example, a PhRMA-funded group called Citizens for the Right to Know argued that the high price of drugs was due to drug stores overcharging clients rather than any actions the pharmaceutical industry might have undertaken (Ainsworth 2002). In another case, in a 2001 press conference featuring a congressional sponsor, one interest group accidentally handed out a memo on its strategy for how to pitch a national energy package, instead of the press release describing that package. The memo included talking points on key provisions of the bill and provided suggested answers to likely media questions (McCutcheon 2001).

The framing usually skirts the issue of self-interest and the ways in which groups will benefit from or be harmed by any changes. A 1998–2001 (and continuing) battle in Congress over the roles of nurse-anesthetists highlighted the not-so-hidden role of self-interest. Congress was considering legislation to give states discretion to decide whether nurse-anesthetists should be allowed to work without being supervised by anesthesiologists during surgery paid for by Medicare or Medicaid. The nurse-anesthetists argued that passage of this law would return power to the states. The anesthesiologists made the case that patients' health would be endangered without the presence of a physician during surgery. Neither side noted that the law could have a substantial, positive effect on the incomes of nurse-anesthetists and a countervailing negative effect on those of anesthesiologists (Salant 1998).

A final example of rather sophisticated framing—targeting different audiences—is provided by the case of a tobacco company that wanted to prevent the Food and Drug Administration (FDA) from regulating cigarette manufacturing and sales. It organized three groups. Smokers were organized around the theme that the government should stay out of their lives. Small stores were mobilized around the notion that FDA involvement would lead to more taxes and more regulation. Finally, and more originally, gay rights groups were organized with the message that the FDA's preoccupation with tobacco might distract the agency from approving new drugs for HIV/AIDS (K. Goldstein 1999).

The increase in the numbers of interest groups and lobbyists has made it harder for lobbyists to get noticed and have their way. The addition of grassroots strategies, research, and polling, however, has greatly enhanced their job and led to specialization within lobby firms. Some firms specialize in such approaches as polling or grassroots organization; others specialize in the target of lobbying—for example, specializing in a certain committee or even committee member.

Finally, lobbying can be about raw power. A case in point was the effort in 1999 to include anti-alcohol messages in a national advertising campaign against illicit drug use. The proposal, supported by MADD, was defeated in large measure by the efforts of the National Beer Wholesalers Association and its lobbyist, who was a member of the small group that met each week with House majority whip Tom DeLay. The lobbyist became an issue in the MADD campaign, which highlighted his comment to a newspaper reporter that each lawmaker should look in the mirror and say, "It's not worth messing with the beer wholesalers" (Eilperin 1999). The lobbyist-led effort against the proposal was focused on how a change in the meaning of *illicit drug* might weaken the message of antidrug efforts. This view was legitimized when reiterated by

Barry McCaffrey, President Clinton's national drug policy director. The beer wholesalers won when the measure was rejected in committee.

While lobbyists' power is usually out of the spotlight, sometimes their importance literally stops congressional action. In 2003, a compromise version of a bill sponsored by Sen. Bill Frist (R-TN) on vaccine liability was expected to quickly pass the Senate Health, Education, Labor, and Pensions Committee, since it had agreement from all sides. But just before the vote, lobbyists for several vaccine manufacturers talked hurriedly with Sen. Judd Gregg (R-NH), chair of the committee, who then announced that action on the bill would be postponed. His explanation? "My staff told me we didn't have an agreement. In this business, things move back and forth pretty often" (Stolberg 2003c).

Media, Message, and Polling

In 1998–2000, a national association of health provider groups developed major media efforts to inform constituents (and, importantly, their elected officials) of the adverse effects of cuts in health services in the BBA. The ads were generally targeted to the media markets of key members of the subcommittees and committees considering "giveback" legislation. The AHA, the Federation of American Hospitals, and the Coalition to Protect America's Health Care ran newspaper ads protesting the 1997 cuts in six GOP districts and composed a television ad to run in other districts. The ad featured an emergency room and argued that "one-third of hospitals are losing money . . . yet some in Washington want to cut payments by billions." Interestingly, the television ads were never aired in the targeted districts, but they were played several times on Capitol Hill (Kondracke 2002).

In the 1993–94 health care battle for the public's support, television was the weapon of choice for grassroots campaigns. An estimated $60 million was spent on television time alone—$10 million more than the total spending on advertising in the 1992 presidential campaign (Seelye 1994, A10). The most highly visible ad campaigns launched in 1993 were those of the insurance industry, featuring a fictitious Harry and Louise, sitting at the kitchen table, questioning the Clinton health care plan. Several coalitions and the Clintons themselves tried to counter, and later parody, the ads, but the commercials were widely viewed and remembered and set a questioning or dubious tone for the public debate. The sponsor of the ads, the HIAA, spent more than $12 million on this and related advertising. Evidence of the success of the Harry and Louise campaign was its potent role in the HIAA's negotiations with a key health committee. The HIAA agreed to muzzle Harry and Louise in particular states while the House Ways and Means Committee considered health care reform legislation. In return, the committee made some concessions in insurance reform that were being sought by the insurance industry (D. West and Francis 1996).

The success of the Harry and Louise campaign spawned further broadcast and print issue-advocacy pieces during the 107th Congress. Some $20 million was expended on health care advertising over that two-year period. The largest spenders were industry groups, including pharmaceutical manufacturers and insurance companies, which spent more than $7 million. Health care providers spent nearly $5 million. Consumer groups, such as the AARP, spent about $3 million (Falk 2003).

Sometimes media ads are targeted primarily to policymakers and other elites, including journalists. One way to do this is through "advertorials," or sponsored messages placed in the media by organized interests to create a favorable environment for their group or their issue. Brown and Waltzer (2002) classified advertorials into three types: image advertorials, designed to create a favorable view; advocacy advertorials, which explain the group's views on controversial issues; and journalism advertorials, which target the press. Journalists are important to interest groups, not only to help "frame" an issue in the way desired by the group but also for "priming," or helping to put the issue on the public agenda. In advertorials targeted to journalists, the group may also hope to get on the journalists' list of sources to call on for comment in stories relating to the group's interests.

Also part of this new lobbying approach are polling and focus groups. In the 2002 campaign to persuade Congress to "give back" provider payment cuts, hospital groups circulated a survey conducted by a GOP pollster showing that more than 70 percent of potential voters opposed cuts to hospitals (Kondracke 2002). In 2003, the AARP used polls and focus groups of Americans aged 45 and older to help determine that the organization should support the Republican legislation to reform Medicare and provide for prescription drugs. The support was highly controversial, however, and some 85 House Democrats announced they would either resign from or refuse to join the AARP (Stolberg 2003b).

The Party–Interest Group Connection

A good example of the connection between interest groups and congressional parties was the development and implementation of the 1995 Contract with America by the newly elected Republican House leadership. Even before they assumed the majority, the House Republicans, led by Newt Gingrich, had developed a list of 10 issues that Republicans would address when they took over Congress. The issues ranged from "loser pays" laws that discouraged litigation to denial of increased welfare payments to mothers receiving Aid to Families with Dependent Children (AFDC) if they had additional children. The list was carefully designed and honed over a seven-month planning period, with a careful eye toward public support. To make it onto the list, an item had to have the support of at least 60 percent of the public, as measured by polls and focus groups. The framers of this contract avoided issues that might divide constituents (such as environmental issues). They also avoided issues on health care, which were still under active debate while the contract was being developed. The contract items had carefully scripted names such as the Personal Responsibility and Work Opportunity Reconciliation Act (PRWORA) for welfare reform and the American Dream Restoration Act for tax relief (D. West and Francis 1995). For each of the 10 contract positions, a working group was formed, composed of legislators, staff, and interest groups. The working groups were closely screened to include only those interests that shared the contract framers' ideology—mostly conservative interest groups and think tanks. These were also groups that the Republican House leadership would work with on policy issues and in the election campaign.

The process of writing the contract may have been more important than its role in the 1994 campaign. Polls after the election found that 60 percent of those who had voted in the election had not even heard of the Contract with America (D. West and Francis 1995). However, once in the majority, the Republican leadership could use the contract to set the agenda of the House—and it had a ready-made, well-informed group of interest-group supporters. The working groups, now designated to promote the contract, were composed largely of lobbyists who met weekly with members of Congress and their staffs. Lobbyists often sat on the committee platform with the legislators during hearings. They helped develop the strategy and funded it. They sponsored broadcasting ads, ran phone banks, sent direct mail, and contributed money for research (D. West and Francis 1995). A contract information center helped coordinate the efforts among the groups.

Another important conduit for interest groups was the Thursday Group of lobbyists who met with House and Senate leaders each week to develop strategy. The role of interest groups was so central that reporters described the situation as a "triumph for business interests," which now found themselves "a full partner of the Republican leadership in shaping congressional priorities" (Weisskopf and Maraniss 1995). Interestingly, one potential lobbying ally was largely ignored in this effort: big business. The Republicans focused on small businesses, which they considered more ideologically compatible. The House majority leader Dick Armey (R-TX) told the *New York Times* that "small businesses tend to be more ideological and principled in what they expect from the Government." In contrast, big business executives were "prags"—pragmatics—who "go where the wind blows" (Berke 1995).

In the Contract with America, the scope of issues was pointedly narrow and most issues remained highly focused, reflecting strategists' understanding that to broaden the contract would invite controversy—which would slow the policy process and reduce prospects for enactment (a lesson learned from the failure of the Clinton health care reform, which touched so many areas that every interest had a stake in changing or defeating it).

The bottom line is that many interest groups are using sophisticated communications tools to present their positions (framed in the most positive manner) to members of Congress and their constituents. Yet the campaigns are not cheap and are waged by the wealthiest groups—or coalitions—perhaps leaving out other worthy groups and their positions (D. West and Loomis 1998).

Direct Lobbying

The old adage "it's whom you know" has traditionally been very important in the lobbying business. Lobbyists rely heavily on legislative "friends" or advocates and spend much of their time trying to retain or increase the intensity of legislators' commitment to an established, favored position. Groups also target committee and subcommittee members, chairs, and party leaders, because they set the agenda, and provide policy cues to other members (Hojnacki and Kimball 1998). The point is to convert these supporters of a group's interests into advocates who will then convince other members of Congress of the value of the group's position. However, lobbyists often must cast their legislative nets wider than the already converted and spend at least some of their time on uncommitted members, or fence sitters. Neither side can ignore the uncommitted, since in a close vote they can make the difference.

Both supporters and opponents of the Clinton plan targeted the same 100 House members and 15 to 20 senators, mostly moderate Democrats, for special attention during the 1994 health care reform debate (Boodman 1994). Similarly, lobbyists seeking deregulation in 1995 recognized that they needed some Democratic votes and closely examined the list of 72 Democrats who had voted for the Republicans' balanced budget. They then divided the list into "tier one" for gettable and "tier two" for questionable. They focused on tier one legislators, especially those with large business interests in their districts (Weisskopf and Maraniss 1995). The Health Benefits Coalition targeted 10 wavering Republican senators in its effort to win passage in the Senate of a much weaker version of the patients' bill of rights than the one promoted by Democrats and liberal Republicans. Of the 10 senators, 9 wound up supporting the bill favored by the coalition: "We found that when we argued the big numbers . . . people were kind of unimpressed," the director of communications for the Business Roundtable told the *Los Angeles Times*. "But when we started breaking things down into the impact on individual states and individual districts, we had much more impact" (Rubin 1999).

Research by Hall (1996) found that this attention to the uncommitted is largely confined to close votes—particularly floor votes. Of course, most policy conflicts do not become close floor votes. Instead they are resolved in subcommittee or committee markup sessions or informally. In these settings, legislators friendly to the interest groups garner most of the lobbyists' attention as they mutually support one another's efforts in pressing an issue important to them.

Groups without paying members seem to prefer to hire external lobbyists, in part because lobbying may be backed by corporate or union treasuries rather than personal contributions to PACs. Spending on lobbying is less regulated than campaign or other PAC contributions. The 1995 Lobbying Registration Act required groups that spend more than $20,000 on lobbying to report their expenditures. But there is no limit on the amount a group can spend.

In 2003, lobbying for the MMA pulled out all the stops in direct, personal lobbying that involved most, if not all, the major health interests—health providers, insurance companies, the pharmaceutical industry and retailers, and consumer groups. Unlike the experience during work on the Clinton health care plan, there was a sense that something was going to happen and that groups needed to act, not stonewall. Indeed, at the end, many of the groups got what they wanted. In addition to making major changes in Medicare, the MMA also provided dozens, if not hundreds, of provisions desired by various groups—ranging from the funding of diabetes diagnosis and cardiovascular screening (supported by the American Diabetes Association and the American Heart Association) to increased reimbursement for chiropractic services (supported by the American Chiropractic Association) (Heaney 2003).

Sealing the Deal

Lobbyists can and do participate in the legislative process at all levels: in encouraging introduction of a bill and in helping to shape the language of that bill through committee and house votes. But even if a lobbyist is unsuccessful in one or both houses, the effort continues in conference committee and finally in lobbying the White House and executive branch during the writing of rules or other implementation-related issues.

Lobbyists are frequently present at strategy sessions with House and Senate party leaders, determining the best way to achieve mutually desired goals as the bill proceeds through the legislative process. While this generally benefits both legislators and interest groups, sometimes it can backfire. Heaney (2004a) reported one such instance when, in 2003, the American Society of Clinical Oncology (ASCO) was allowed to negotiate directly with members of a conference committee in negotiations over reform of average wholesale prices for oral cancer drugs. During the negotiations, the ASCO sent out a grassroots e-mail alert urging opposition to the direction in which the conference committee was headed (a direction not known to others outside the conference room). When a congressional staffer received the group's e-mail, he alerted Rep. Nancy Johnson (R-CT), who terminated the negotiation with the group.

Members of Congress must balance the desires of interest groups with those of their own constituents. After all, they want to keep their seats, to continue being reelected. Some political scientists have examined how members of Congress can maintain their popularity with constituents while at the same time keeping interest groups happy—often with policies that are not in the broad public interest. Lohmann (1998) argued that legislators can benefit more from catering to a well-informed minority (interest groups) than to an ill-informed majority (including their own constituents). They benefit because their constituents are generally not well informed about the policy choices of members of Congress, whereas interest groups are better equipped to monitor an incumbent's activities. Lohmann thus concluded that public policy is biased toward special interests because of an information asymmetry between the general public and those interests.

Good lobbyists work with key officials in the executive branch as well as Congress, but they focus more of their attention—and often rack up more successes—on Capitol Hill than elsewhere in Washington. Former AHA president John McMahon put it this way: "Congress has a greater understanding and more sympathy with our problems" (Iglehart 1977, 1527). The understanding stems, in no small measure, from the important role of hospitals in the economies of local communities; the standing of hospital administrators, boards, and staffs in the legislator's district; and the likely campaign support derived from hospitals and their employees. Probably the most effective lobbyists are hometown folks directly lobbying their representatives in person. A senator from Utah, say, may not make time to meet with a lobbyist from a large conglomerate or interest group but will agree to see the manager of a company branch located in Utah or a delegation of local physicians. As frequent AMA critic Rep. Pete Stark (D-CA) noted, "My colleagues listen to folks from home and that's the AMA's strength" (B. Feder 1993).

Sometimes lobbying means cutting deals. The 1997 Balanced Budget Act cut $115 billion in Medicare provider payments over five years. Unlike other health care providers, physicians suffered few major cuts. It soon emerged that in the early 1997 debates, an AMA official sent Speaker Newt Gingrich a letter asking that physicians be spared from disproportionate cuts. The day the letter was written, the AMA announced it would support the Partial-Birth Abortion Ban Act, a bill banning late-term abortions that was strongly supported by many Republicans. While AMA officials denied any "deal," many physicians, Democrats, and fellow lobbyists were not convinced, particularly since the AMA did not discuss its pending position with the leading specialty group of obstetricians and gynecologists, and the position seemed to run counter to the AMA's own policy that lawmakers should not dictate specific medical procedures (Carney 1998).

Lobbyists also buttonhole congressional staffers. It gives them someone to work on when the legislator is too busy, but they also recognize the reality that staffers make many of the decisions on specific issues of concern to interest groups. Groups often sponsor staff seminars in exclusive resorts, where lobbyists have a chance to fully discuss issues of common interest.

THE ELECTORAL LINK

Interest groups attempt to influence public policy choices (legislative influence) and to help determine who is elected (electoral influence). The two roles are closely linked. One key linkage is interest groups' ratings of members of Congress on a selected range of issues. Many groups determine their electoral endorsements—and campaign support—based on legislators' support of issues of concern to the group. For example, the National Federation of Independent Business (NFIB) polls its members to determine their top priorities before each session of Congress and sends the results to congressional offices. Just before a vote on one of these issues, the group sends a special green-edged postcard to legislators warning them that the upcoming vote will be part of the NFIB's next report card. Every legislator who votes with the NFIB's issues at least 70 percent of the time receives a small pewter trophy, inscribed with the words "Guardian of Small Business." More importantly for members of Congress, the 70 percent rating assures the NFIB's endorsement and campaign contributions (Hrebenar, Burbank, and Benedict 1999).

The NRA is almost ruthless in its use of elections to target members of Congress who do not vote its way. Following the 1993 NRA defeat on assault weapons, the organization targeted dozens of the 177 Democrats and 30 Republicans who voted for the assault weapon ban. The NRA took credit for the ouster of House Judiciary Committee chair Jack Brooks after he pushed anticrime legislation through his committee and voted for it on the floor (Nelson 2000).

It is important to keep in mind that members of Congress are not passive recipients of lobbyists' tricks and entreaties. In fact, legislators are actively engaged in seeking funds from lobbyists and more. Apart from PAC contributions, legislators often expect contributions from lobbyists' personal funds. Also, in recent years there has been pressure on groups to hire members of the majority party as their lobbyists and even their directors. There were a few instances when Republicans, as the majority political party, put pressure on groups to fire lobbyists who were Democrats. In one such instance, a House committee chair threatened to cut off access to a company with ties to his committee if it did not fire its Democratic lobbyist and replace her with a Republican (Ornstein 2004).

LOBBYING THE EXECUTIVE BRANCH

Lobbyists also target the executive branch—both the president and his bureaucratic agencies. Interest groups may lobby for specific changes in rules and regulations or to influence the appointment of an agency head. While access is as important in executive-branch lobbying as it is in lobbying Congress, contributions to assist that access are illegal. Therefore interest groups rely heavily on knowledge of public policies, solutions, and processes. The issues are often more technical and narrower than those dealt with by Congress. But they are no less important. A large majority of interests groups rate their lobbying efforts with agencies as just as important as or more important than lobbying Congress (Kerwin 2003). However, in sheer numbers, congressional lobbying still dominates. In one count of lobby efforts over a six-month period, interest groups, on average, lobbied on 11.1 issues per group in Congress and 1.4 issues in the executive branch (Furlong 2005). But economic organizations representing businesses and corporations are much more likely to lobby the executive branch than are public interest groups—which makes sense given the rather technical nature of executive-branch deliberation.

Furlong (2005) provides examples of the types of issues subject to lobbying in the executive branch: Medicare reimbursement for pathogen-inactivated blood, FDA-produced guidance documents for the reprocessing of medical devices, and Medicare/Medicaid reimbursement for treatment of obesity-related health conditions. In each case, it is easy to discern a particular group's interest and how the decision might affect the profitability of its enterprise.

To get their point across, interest groups can provide written comments on proposed rules, attend and participate in public hearings, contact agency officials, serve on advisory committees, or petition for rulemaking (Kerwin 2003). They can also use a variety of electronic mechanisms to communicate, including e-mail, bulletin boards, and chat rooms.

Interest groups often form coalitions to fight regulations, much as they do to fight legislation. When the Occupational Safety and Health Administration (OSHA) was drafting indoor air quality standards for a proposed ban on smoking in most work areas, the ADA, NFIB, and National Restaurant Association formed a coalition to fight ventilation system requirements (P. Stone 1994). In one study of approaches used by interest groups to influence rulemaking, more than 60 percent of the groups reported that they very frequently or always formed coalitions. Other mechanisms used very frequently or always were written comments (77 percent), informal contact with agency staff (55 percent), and mobilization of grassroots support (46 percent) (Kerwin 2003).

In one sense, the lobbying of midlevel personnel in the executive branch is easier than lobbying Congress: agency staff tends to be much more stable, and long-term relationships can be developed more easily with these staffers than with the more highly mobile congressional staff. It is also easier to get an appointment. When they are not able to sway an agency, lobbyists often go back to Congress. For example, Congress sided against HHS and with the United Network for Organ Sharing—a group of regional private, nonprofit organizations that harvest and allocate human organs—in passing legislation that blocked the much delayed HHS rules intended to alter the criteria for determining who receives organs.

Agency staffers know that lobbyists possess access-to-power weapons, and they are loath to simply ignore lobbyists' requests. Staffers may choose to resist and carry the fight forward, but they are likely to make a careful job of it when they know their administrative and political bosses are going to hear the other side of the story from lobbyists.

APPEALING TO THE COURTS

When all else fails, interest groups can turn to the courts. Litigation can be a powerful tool for influencing policy. Though often an expensive route for achieving change, it may be the last resort for a group unable to get satisfaction through the legislative and executive branches. As Berry (1984, 197) noted, "When an industry's profits are liable to be significantly reduced by a government policy, it becomes worth the cost of litigation for a trade association to challenge the policy in court." Berry also made the case that interest groups use the courts when they think the lack of popular support for an issue makes lobbying Congress or the executive branch fruitless. Interest groups can delay the implementation of a policy in the courts, sometimes hoping that, during the delay, Congress or the administration will change to a more sympathetic body.

In 2002, the AHA led a coalition in a suit against HHS to block implementation of a final regulation that would reduce the Medicaid "upper payment limit" for public, nonstate hospitals. The suit argued that HHS had violated federal administrative procedures by ignoring more than 200 comments that largely opposed the Medicaid revision. A year earlier, the AHA's threat to file a suit had led to a delay in the outpatient payment rule, saving hospitals hundreds of millions of dollars (Lovern 2002).

Interest groups can also go to court to prevent state actions that may harm their business and may spread to other states if not stopped. PhRMA has challenged state laws in Vermont, Maine, and Michigan that, according to the group, would violate the federal Medicaid statute and jeopardize the quality of health care that Medicaid patients need and deserve (PhRMA 2004b). These state laws called for manufacturers' "rebates" as a means to control rising drug costs for Medicaid—which might be viewed as threatening to drug companies' profits. PhRMA noted on its Web page that "as part of its advocacy on behalf of the millions of patients that the pharmaceutical industry serves, PhRMA occasionally, and reluctantly, determines that an issue can be resolved only through the courts" (PhRMA 2004b). Ironically, when this type of approach failed in several important cases against various states, PhRMA went back to Congress and got what it wanted. The MMA of 2003 took Medicaid drug purchasing away from the states and placed it in the hands of small area-specific pharmacy benefit managers—considerably more attractive negotiating partners for PhRMA than the states had proved to be.

Sometimes interest groups use litigation as a means to force administrative action, hoping that federal agencies will settle out of court rather than risk uncertain court decisions. Groups representing people with disabilities have been especially successful in these out-of-court settlements. For example, Vietnam War veterans and chemical manufacturers that produced Agent Orange, a suspected carcinogen, settled a massive class action suit out of court in 1984.

Interest groups choose (or avoid) the judicial route based on their political standing in the electoral process, the extent to which the group can frame its interests in terms of rights, and the demographic characteristics of the group's membership. Traditionally, groups turn to the courts if (1) they are politically disadvantaged or (2) they have organizational resources such as a full-time staff, attorneys, the money to pay the legal costs, and organizational networks closely coordinated with affiliated groups or other interest groups. The AMA fits the second definition. It has its own Litigation Center, which actively brings cases against hospitals, managed care companies, and federal and state governments (Lovern 2002). Groups that are often in conflict are more likely to use the judicial remedy than groups that engender no conflict. Interest groups are also more likely to use the courts when their areas of interest coincide with issues over which courts have clear jurisdiction (J. Walker 1991).

Finally, interest groups sometimes work with executive-branch agencies to bring "friendly" suits. One example is when the American Lung Association initiated a lawsuit against the Environmental Protection Agency (EPA), seeking to force the agency to review and tighten its air quality standards because of the effect of polluted air on people with asthma. The suit was friendly because the agency welcomed judicial confirmation of its ability to revisit existing standards (Wood 1999).

Health groups spend less time pursuing their goals in federal courts than do civil liberties groups, but do pursue this route on occasion. One reason for health groups to sue is to delay the implementation of regulations, a mechanism noted above. Starr (1982, 407) called this the "little known law of nature [that] seems to require that every move toward regulation be followed by an opposite move toward litigation." For example, the Association of American Physicians and Surgeons sued over the constitutionality of professional standards review organizations (PSROs). The AMA sued when the proposed utilization review regulations were issued, and again to block the health-planning law from being implemented. And the AAMC sued over regulations imposed on medical schools. Paint manufacturers said they might sue California over new, tougher rules that would require them to rewrite 7,000 formulas at a cost approaching a billion dollars (Associated Press 1999).

The use of courts as a venue for policy change intensified during the 1960s, when the federal courts expanded the rules of standing so that citizens' groups and trade associations could sue in court even if they had no direct economic interest in the case (Berry 1984). Lawsuits are generally not lobbyists' preferred strategy, however. Not only are they expensive and time-consuming, but they can also alienate legislators and may adversely affect an agency's annual budget allocation, which may or may not be the lobby's desired outcome.

GRASSROOTS LOBBYING

Interest groups recognize the importance of using their own members as constituent-lobbyists. Members of Congress value their constituents' views and weight them heavily in making their decisions. How better to influence a legislator's vote than by sending your message through her constituents? Though it seems only recently to have hit the big time, the grassroots strategy has been employed for decades. Skocpol (1992) told of the successful effort of the National Congress of Mothers in 1920 to write letters, visit members of Congress, and get publicity in local papers in support of a federal program to promote maternal health education (the Sheppard-Towner bill). To assist the women in their effort, the official National Congress of Mothers magazine included blank petitions on its last page.

Grassroots lobbying is important to legislators because it provides information about the preferences of their constituents; it is important to groups because it builds a coalition of support among their members (Hojnacki and Kimball 1999). With the technological and communications advances of the 1990s, reaching and organizing the grass roots has become an increasingly important part of lobbying efforts and one primarily orchestrated by lobbyists. Part of its importance is in persuading legislators that an issue "is really a constituent issue," said one lobbyist (Fritsch 1995). An example was the grassroots campaign conducted by the Health Benefits Coalition to oppose the patients' bill of rights. The coalition argued that the proposed legislation would cause firms to drop health insurance, producing more uninsured citizens. To bring the point home, the coalition aimed ads at key constituencies, attacking the bill's potential effects on the size of the uninsured population: "There are already 655,000 in the state of Washington without health insurance . . . If costs go up, 41,000 more people will be without health insurance" (Rubin 1999).

Interest groups take advantage of this constituent concern by organizing these local voters. Lobbyists and coalitions hire either their own "grassroots coordinator" or a firm that specializes in these activities. A grassroots strategy is particularly attractive to groups wanting to convince lawmakers that there is sufficient public support to change an existing law (Hojnacki and Kimball 1999). It also has the advantage of providing evidence of action that can help maintain and build group membership.

The first generation of large-scale grassroots activity involved flooding congressional offices with mail-in postcards. Later, interest groups motivated their members to correspond with their senators and representatives by writing letters or sending faxes and by meeting personally with legislators in their districts or in Washington. In a 1990 effort, the AMA initiated 100,000 letters to Medicare officials to protest budget cuts affecting physicians (Kosterlitz 1992). Four years later the AHA launched a million-dollar grassroots effort to get its 4,900 member hospitals and their workers to advocate community-based networks, employer mandates, and universal access (AHA Launches 1994). In 1994, during discussions of the Clinton reform proposals, groups representing drug manufacturers, insurers, and a myriad of health care providers blanketed Capitol Hill offices with postcards, letters, and telephone calls.

Coordinators prefer personalized letters from constituents to legislators but will settle for "patching" callers into the legislator's office. When a group representative finds someone answering his phone who is sympathetic to the message, the caller asks whether he would like to express his view to his representative in Congress. The call can then be patched in to the member's office at no cost to the constituent. Electronic mail is a newer variation.

Members of Congress say they can spot an orchestrated strategy and give it low weight in the political calculus, but they nonetheless give it some weight. And if the call, letter, or e-mail is from an "attentive" in the district, it will get recorded. As Rep. Jim Leach (R-IA) put it, "Whether or not it's generated by a lobbyist, if it's signed by a respected constituent, it's valued" (Fritsch 1995, A11).

In the 1993–94 health care reform debate, the NFIB, representing thousands of small-business owners, was very successful in mobilizing its members to write to and call their representatives and tell them about the potential harm employer mandates could inflict on their business. The NFIB bombarded members of Congress with faxes and mailings, targeted telephone campaigns just before key votes, and scheduled hundreds of meetings during members' visits to their local districts. "What the NFIB did in the local community was to give the issues a larger meaning," said one member of the House Energy and Commerce Committee who was heavily lobbied by NFIB members in his district. "Their information was literally corroborated by first-hand stories," he said (Lewis 1994, A9). In 2000, the Health Benefits Coalition specified what it expected from a grassroots campaign in a mailing to potential contractors, a document obtained by the *Wall Street Journal*. The coalition sought to encourage calls and letters from two groups in the districts of key legislators: grass tops (community leaders or other prominent constituents) and grass roots (employees and employers). They also wanted to generate carefully scripted "intercepts," or informal encounters, with members of Congress at public places such as county fairs and town-hall meetings.

In another case, in the late 1990s, the tobacco industry mounted an extensive grassroots campaign intended to result in a deluge of letters, phone calls, and signed petitions to members of Congress, expressing opposition to tobacco control legislation. Besides patching through to their members of Congress any callers who, on receiving a cold call, seemed sympathetic to the cause, the industry used a more devious mechanism. It prepared letters and petitions presenting the would-be signer with what seemed to be a form prepared by her member of Congress seeking local citizens' views. The voter then sent the signed petition to her U.S. senator in an enclosed business reply envelope, which was printed to suggest that the senator's office had paid for it, when in fact the tobacco industry had paid the postage. The U.S. Post Office was unamused: "It is imperative that you stop distributing Business Reply Mail addressed with the senators' names imprinted on the mail to avoid revocation of your permit," a Post Office official wrote to the actual permit buyer, Brown and Williamson Tobacco Company. A company spokesperson was unabashed, however. "If Senator Harkin, with all due respect, is getting petitions that are signed by voters from Iowa, the fact that we paid the postage, which is minimal, shouldn't make the difference," the spokesperson told the *Washington Post*. "This is what these voters think. I don't think it would have made a difference if we had put our logo at the top corner of the petition" (Marcus 1998).

Though grassroots efforts are popular, there is some sentiment that they have been overused. As noted above, if the effort is clearly programmed, with every postcard and phone call making identical pleas, the recipient may discount it. Former senator Lloyd Bentsen (D-TX) once derogatorily called an effort more "astroturf" than grass roots when, as chair of the Senate Finance Committee, he received reams of programmed responses (Toner 1994). But, one user of these strategies countered, "Some members of Congress probably would like people to write letters only with quill pens and parchment by candlelight, but that's not the world we live in . . . Having worked on the Hill for many members, you certainly know when you get calls and letters that are part of an effort; it's very obvious. But the bottom line is you count them and they certainly are an expression of opinion by a voter . . . No one is being forced to do this, to pick up the telephone and dial" (Marcus 1998).

Grassroots lobbying can also be applied effectively to the White House. In 1997, in response to a massive letter-writing campaign from the American Diabetes Association, President Clinton agreed to call for increased public funding for diabetes research. The letters pointed out that the proportion of government-sponsored research on diabetes was extremely low compared with that for other conditions, including arthritis, cancer, multiple sclerosis, and dementia (Wood 1999).

A common first step in developing a strategy to blunt the effect of a reform on a group's interests is to hire a pollster who can help the group "shape" its message to "resonate" with the public. In a poll commissioned by the Consumers Union that questioned the appropriateness of forcing citizens into HMOs, nearly half of the respondents said they would be willing to pay more money to choose their own doctor, and 91 percent said it was important to choose a specialist when needed (Rubin 1993). Surveys funded by a community-based primary care training consortium found that the public highly valued primary care and supported providing more federal dollars for the training of generalist physicians and nurses.

FUELING THE ELECTION ENGINE

Figure 3.1 shows the increase in financial contributions to members of Congress by health-related interest groups since 1990. In addition to the increase in dollars—a fourfold increase between 1990 and 2002—the figure illustrates the change in the party of choice. In 1990, when the Democrats had control of both houses, Democrats garnered 54 percent of total health contributions. In 2004, the Republicans, now the controlling party, did better—receiving 60 percent of total health contributions. Incumbents remained the preferred recipients of the funding, although incumbents were more likely to be funded

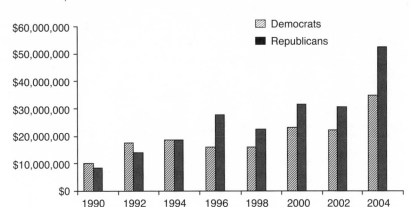

Figure 3.1.
Health Interests' Contributions to Members of Congress, by Party, 1999–2004.
Source: Data from Center for Responsive Politics 2005.

in 1990 than in 2004. In 1990, 83 percent of congressional funding by health interests went to incumbents; in 2004 the percentage fell to 68 percent (Center for Responsive Politics 2005).

As shown in figure 3.2, health-related interests' contributions have steadily risen in the House since 1990. Senate contributions vary from election to election, depending on which senators are up for reelection. In 2004, contributions in the Senate increased significantly.

Figure 3.3 illustrates both the continuity and change in the top health association contributors. Two of the largest associations representing providers, the AMA and the ADA, were among the top 20 contributors among health associations in each of the eight congressional sessions between 1990 and 2004. Also steady contributors were the ANA, the American Academy of Ophthalmology (AAO), and the American Optometric Association (AOA), which were in the top 20 health-related contributors for seven of the eight periods. The only time they were not in the top 20 was in 2002–3, when 11 of the top spots were taken by pharmaceutical companies. As figure 3.3 also illustrates, some groups participate heavily in contributions only infrequently, when they are urging a measure's passage or trying to stop passage of something they do not like. For example, the American Association of Orthopaedic Surgeons (AAOS) and the American Occupational Therapy Association (AOTA) appeared in the top 20 in only one session of Congress. The Association for the Advancement of Psychology (AAP) appeared in the top 20 in only two sessions.

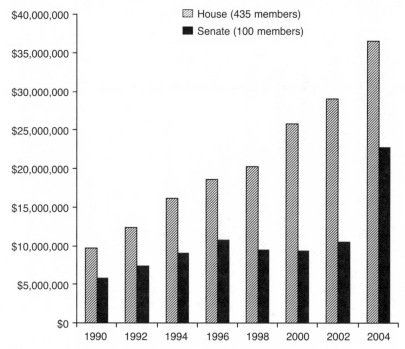

Figure 3.2.
Health Interests' Contributions to Congress, by house, 1990–2004.
Source: Data from Center for Responsive Politics 2005.

Political Action Groups

For interest groups, contributions to political action committees—the campaign-funding arms of an organization or group—are the price of admission. Initially, PACs existed only to give money to candidates. This, and much else, has changed. The first PAC was established in 1944 by the Congress of Industrial Organizations (CIO) to raise money for the reelection of President Franklin D. Roosevelt (Center for Responsive Politics 2005).

Political action committees come in several varieties. Connected PACs are affiliated or coexist with some parent organization; more than 80 percent of PACs fit this description (Wright 1985). Unconnected PACs have no sponsoring organization and tend to be ideological in nature, often promoting a single issue. Some PACs are associated with a single business. Leadership PACs are organized by members of Congress, particularly party leaders and committee

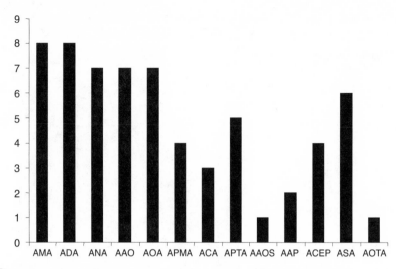

Figure 3.3.
Health Professional Groups in the Top 20 Contributors to Federal Candidates
and Parties, 1990–2004. AMA, American Medical Association; ADA, American
Dental Association; ANA, American Nursing Association; AAO, American
Academy of Ophthalmology; AOA, American Optometric Association; APMA,
American Podiatric Medical Association; ACA, American Chiropractic
Association; APTA, American Physical Therapy Association; AAOS, American
Association of Orthopaedic Surgeons; AAP, Association for the Advancement
of Psychology; ACEP, American College of Emergency Physicians; ASA,
American Society of Anesthesiologists; AOTA, American Occupational Therapy
Association.
Source: Data from Center for Responsive Politics 2005.

chairs. They receive money from various sources, including other PACs, and
dispense it to candidates (up to $5,000 per candidate per election) in ways
that help their party (and often enhance legislators' own prominence and
influence nationally or within their house or party). Legislators organizing
the leadership PACs cannot spend this money on their own campaigns, but
they can use it to pay general and overhead expenses that may also benefit
themselves. Mostly they spend the money on other candidates of their own
party, strengthening relationships with those who are elected and with whom
they will be serving in the next Congress.

Political action committees can be permanent or temporary, devised to
support or oppose a policy on the institutional agenda. They can also spend

money independent of candidates, without any explicit coordination or consultation with candidates. The purposes of PAC funding may be to obtain "access" to legislators or to secure a Congress more to their ideological liking. Under federal rules, PACs must report their activities to the Federal Election Commission (FEC), and contributions, as noted above, are limited to $5,000 to a federal candidate per election. But a member of Congress with a campaign fund and a leadership PAC can receive maximum contributions to both. State-level PACs do not report their activities and have no spending caps.

Until the mid-1970s, members of Congress got about two-thirds of their campaign money from individual donors. In the 1974 campaigns, PACs had only "bit" roles, providing less than 20 percent of House and Senate spending (Matlack, Barnes, and Cohen 1990); by 1998, PAC contributions made up 35 percent of House spending and 18 percent of Senate spending (Ornstein, Mann, and Malbin 2002). As campaigns became increasingly expensive and public concern grew over the large quantities of unreported contributions during the Nixon election, Congress passed a series of statutes in the 1970s that defined and institutionalized PACs. Following the 1974 revision of the Federal Election Campaign Act, PACs grew rapidly. Before then, 608 PACs were registered with the FEC. Two years later, the number had nearly doubled. By the early 1990s there were more than 4,000 PACs, a great many (1,795) of them associated with corporations (fig. 3.4). The number stabilized during the 1990s. In 2004 there were 4,184 registered PACs, most (39 percent) associated with corporations (Federal Election Commission 2005).

Some 249 PACs were associated with health issues in the 2003–4 federal election cycle. They gave more than $32 million to federal candidates in that election, almost two-thirds of it going to Republicans (table 3.3). Most of the health professions have PACs, including the Academy of Dispensing Audiologists, the National Association of Spine Specialists, and the Renal Leadership Council. The PAC associated with the American Medical Association—AMPAC—gave more than $2 million in 2003–4, 80 percent of it to Republicans. The Academy of Dispensing Audiologists gave $4,000—all of it to Democrats (Center for Responsive Politics 2005).

Political action committees can employ one of several strategies for distributing their dollars. They can seek to change the composition of Congress to make it more ideologically pleasing—as the director of the League of Conservation Voters candidly put it, "We want to see pro-environmental members of Congress elected" (Edsall 1996)—or they can maximize their access to legislators. The former strategy more often leads to the funding of challengers, the latter to favoring incumbents, particularly party leaders and

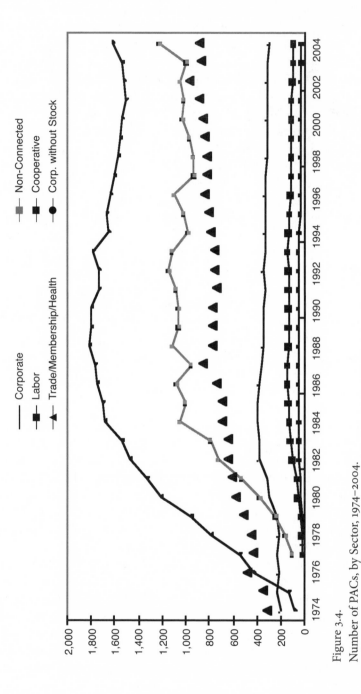

Figure 3.4.

Number of PACs, by Sector, 1974–2004.

Source: Federal Election Commission, Semi-Annual Federal PAC Count, various years.

Table 3.3
PAC Health Contributions to Federal Candidates, by Sector and Party, 2003–4

	Number of PACs	Total Spending ($)	Republicans (percent)	Democrats (percent)
Health professionals	105	16,713,589	65	35
Health services/HMOs	59	2,378,595	65	35
Hospitals/nursing homes	10	4,132,636	60	40
Pharmaceuticals/health products	75	8,459,510	70	30
Miscellaneous health	4	39,100	67	33

Source: Center for Responsive Politics 2005.

committee or subcommittee chairs. Given that challengers are usually cash-starved compared with well-placed incumbents, PACs have the potential to be better appreciated for their contributions to these upstarts.

Nevertheless, the lion's share of PAC money goes to incumbents. In the 2002 elections, health PACs gave 83 percent of their campaign dollars to incumbents (Center for Responsive Politics 2005). The appeal of incumbents is simple: access. By providing funding for those currently in office and likely to retain their seats, interest groups can maintain access to these policy players. Groups need access to affect details of policy that are important to them, and incumbents are in a better position to help groups with these details than are challengers. Sometimes conflicts appear between a group's Washington lobbyists who want access to incumbents and the group's members back home who think ideology is important and that the group's dollars should support like-minded challengers. Among incumbents, party leaders and members serving on committees important to the interest group are likely to receive the largest PAC contributions. Money tends to go to those who will actively support the PAC's goals. When given to a sympathetic legislator, the money may help transform her into an active advocate, or "horse." Indeed, Hall and Wayman (1990) found that PAC contributions are related to increased levels of committee participation. PAC contributions may also help shape campaigns, such as what issues are emphasized (Gais 1998).

Committee membership and seniority are especially important to PAC giving in House campaigns (Romer and Snyder 1994). In the Senate, PAC funding is more closely associated with party membership and voting record (Grier and Munger 1993). When no incumbent is running, interest groups often target dollars to attractive first-year legislators in the hope of getting more attention from them early in their careers. Some interest groups value ideology more than others. The ANA's PAC gave more than 85 percent of its contributions to Democrats in the 2003–4 election cycle, maintaining a consistent pattern of preference for the Democratic Party. Other groups are less loyal. The AMA, which divided its money between the two parties fairly evenly between 1990 and 2000, directed 80 percent to Republicans in 2003–4. The AHA is more variable, giving 70 percent to Democrats in 1990 but only 32 percent in 2003–4.

Sometimes PACs give to both sides. Some even give after the election, as a way of "buying off a mistake" (Sabato 1985, 92). The 1994 election, which ushered in a Republican majority in both houses of Congress, saw many PACs scrambling to retire the campaign debts of Republicans whose elections they had opposed. "When you back the wrong horses, you try to make a contribution as a token of good will," said one interest group's political director (quoted in Weisskopf 1995).

The timing of PAC giving can also be important. Not all money is given during the months just before or after an election. Money provided early in a campaign can give a candidate a legitimacy and visibility that scares off other possible candidates and increases the likelihood of even more campaign dollars from other sources. The ANA was the first major health association to endorse Bill Clinton in the 1992 election. Its support may have been rewarded with 12 seats on the 47-member professional advisory review committee to Hillary Clinton's health care reform task force. The AMA was not represented on the advisory review committee (Bendavid, Goldman, and Kaplan 1993).

The modern member of Congress collects money throughout her term, and PAC money can be provided at any time, such as before an important vote in a committee or on the house floor. Many PACs deny giving money for such "present needs" for a favorable vote or action. Rather, they say they give money for support they may need in the future or as good will that might come in handy later. Some people believe there is also a fair amount of "reward" or "thank you" money for votes previously cast in support of a group's interests. Some PACs admit to "punishment" money, refusing to contribute to a candidate or giving money to her opponent. One highly visible example of the punishment strategy was AMPAC's spending thousands of dollars in 1986 to unseat Rep. Pete Stark, chair of the Health Subcommittee of the House Ways and Means Committee. (The feeling was mutual. Stark once called the AMA "greedy troglodytes" [Noah 1993].) Nevertheless, such punishment is unusual and, in Stark's case, temporary. AMPAC donated to Stark's 1992 campaign. Eight years later, even as a minority party member, he still received a contribution of $1,500 from AMPAC (Center for Responsive Politics 2000).

The Sierra Club, a venerated environmental group (with 550,000 dues-paying members at last report, in the late 1990s), planned a hardball series of strategy moves for the 2000 election, identifying members of Congress it would support (several Democrats, but only two Republicans) and members it would specifically oppose: "We need to be even more focused in choosing places where we want to attempt to unseat anti-environmental opponents, and spend significant resources per race to do so," the club's political director wrote in a memorandum to his bosses on September 5, 1997, according to a *New York Times* reporter allowed to sit in on the Sierra Club's campaign strategy sessions (Berke 1998). The club spent $6 million on 15 House and 8 Senate races, according to the *Times*. It denies supporting or opposing specific candidates, however, fearful of running afoul of campaign laws, saying instead that it is simply educating citizens about how their representatives have voted.

Interestingly, there is very little evidence that PAC funding directly affects a legislator's vote on a given bill. Studies examining the linkage between PAC money and roll-call voting have found no relationship or a very modest correlation (see R. A. Smith 1995 for a summary of dozens of relevant studies). Two studies of AMPAC confirmed there was no evidence of vote buying. Rather, the PAC chose to fund members who were ideologically similar or in positions of power, particularly in the House (Gutermuth 1999; Wilkerson and Carrell 1999).

Soft Money and Issue Advocacy

Until the passage of the Bipartisan Campaign Reform Act in 2002, commonly known as the McCain-Feingold law, soft money was one of the most popular components of interest-group contributions. Soft money could be provided to political parties for voter mobilization and certain types of issue advocacy but not for efforts that expressly advocated the election or defeat of a federal candidate. The BCRA banned soft money and prevented special interest groups from running issue ads that mention a candidate during the 30 days before a primary election and 60 days before a general election. The law also doubled the amount of "hard" money individuals could provide to candidates.

Scarcely had the ink of the signature dried when several suits were filed claiming that portions of the law were unconstitutional. The AFL-CIO, the American Civil Liberties Union, and the NRA (strange bedfellows indeed) filed a suit claiming that the ban on issue ads before an election was an unconstitutional limit on free speech. Sen. Mitch McConnell (R-KY) and several groups filed a suit challenging the law's ban on soft money contributions. The U.S. Supreme Court ruled (5–4) that both the soft money ban and the issue ad restrictions were constitutional (Center for Responsive Politics 2005).

Political action committees and individuals may also spend money on "issue advocacy," a new phenomenon that sometimes comes in the form of advertising aimed at particular candidates but falling just barely short of calling for their defeat or reelection. Sometimes the ads are strong attacks on a candidate's views or record. When the contributions that pay for the issue ads are made through PACs, the contributions are tax deductible 'and the donor must be disclosed. But issue ads can also be sponsored by 527 groups (organized under Section 527 of the Internal Revenue Code), which operate separate from political parties to raise money for political activities, including voter mobilization and issue advocacy. These groups differ from PACs in three important ways: (1) there is no limit on how much their sponsors can donate, (2) the money given is not tax exempt, and (3) they report their receipts and outlays to the Internal Revenue Service (IRS), not the FEC. The third point is important in that the FEC outlays are easily tracked while the IRS has been slow to make information available (Roll Call 2003). The 527 groups advocate for issues rather than candidates. They must not specifically endorse or recommend voting against a particular candidate, but they can come very, very close—for example, by saying that a particular candidate, named in the ad, "has a lot to answer for on protecting the environment."

The 527 provision, although part of the 1974 campaign reform act, received little attention until 1996, when the Sierra Club and a few other mostly liberal groups discovered its powerful potential—unlimited donations and no requirement to disclose donor identity. IRS rulings in 1999 liberalized the provision's interpretation, while at the same time creating demand for an unregulated vehicle by cracking down on the Christian Coalition for running afoul of its tax-exempt status by advocating on behalf of candidates. The number of groups taking advantage of the 527 provision grew quickly in 1999 and 2000, especially among conservatives, including House majority whip Tom DeLay. Frequent users of the loophole spend millions of dollars this way. Smaller groups can raise and spend only small amounts to push their position on a particular issue. "We agree it's a loophole," a Sierra Club spokesperson admitted, adding that while his group would support legislation to eliminate it, the club would keep using the loophole until such legislation was passed. He told the *New York Times* that a handful of wealthy, anonymous donors had given about $4.5 million to the Sierra Club's 527 committee to use during the 2000 elections (Purdum 2000). The Center for Responsive Politics (2000) called issue advocacy ads "one of the most prominent loopholes in the nation's campaign finance laws today."

In 2000, legislation designed to increase disclosure about 527 groups was signed into law. It requires 527 groups to register with the IRS within 24 hours, to disclose the identities of its senior officers, and to report its receipts and disbursements every three months during an election year. Any 527 group that spends more than $25,000 a year must disclose contributors who give more than $200 and report any expenditure greater than $500. The information is to be made public and posted on the Internet (Dwyre 2002). By 2004, a loophole had been identified by which 527 groups could omit disclosure information as long as they paid a tax on the amount not disclosed. Some groups, such as the Sierra Club, operate both 527 groups and PACs. Other 527 groups are organized almost solely for election purposes and are not associated with interest groups.

In the 2003–4 federal election cycle, Section 527 organizations spent around $543 million. Most of the spending was by ideological groups and labor. Health interests spent less than a million dollars through 527 groups (Center for Responsive Politics 2005).

Another approach used by some groups is to organize as a 501(c)(4) committee or social welfare organization; these groups may engage in political activities as long as these activities do not become their primary purpose. Disclosure requirements for these committees are less restrictive than those for the 527 groups, and they are not required to report the identity of their donors (Dwyre 2002). One recent example of such a nonprofit group is United Seniors Association (also known as USA Next), billed as an alternative to the AARP. Some have argued that USA Next is the foil for groups that do not want to be directly identified with a position. Groups can provide large amounts of money to a 501(c)(4) nonprofit, which does not have to report its contributors and need only generally outline its expenditures. Drug companies and PhRMA are large donors to USA Next, which in 2005 sponsored a controversial series of television ads implying that the AARP supported gays and was against the military. At issue was the AARP's opposition to President George W. Bush's reform of Social Security (Tackett 2005). Just as for the 527 groups, the stepped up use of 501(c)(4) groups was an unintended consequence of the ban on soft money in 2003.

These uses of nonprofit groups or the spending of money embedded in corporate budgets have been dubbed "stealth campaigns" (Hojnacki and Kimball 1998), and they can be quite effective. In fact, differences between the politics of elections and the politics of policymakers are becoming much smaller. Interest groups wage campaign-like efforts to "win," and members of Congress are constantly running for election and collecting money to run. The days of behind-the-scenes lobbying among "gentlemen" are truly over and long forgotten in today's technology-savvy, no-holds-barred campaigns.

THE SUCCESS OF INTEREST GROUPS

Modern lobbying is more a campaign than a social event. Interest groups target members, hone the message, and decide on the best approach based on the target group and the message. Grassroots lobbying is usually done before committee action to help "soften up" the system by demonstrating public support. Direct lobbying is still focused on the committee and entails the lobbying of allies to encourage them to become advocates, or horses. Typically, interest groups combine grassroots and direct lobbying efforts aimed at supportive members of Congress and those who have not committed to a position. If the issue has no strong district ties, groups concentrate on direct contact (Hojnacki and Kimball 1999). In some sense, direct contacts can help close the deal on specific issues that cannot be dealt with by the grass roots. As one lobbyist put it, "The grassroots got this issue [vitamin labeling] on the radar screen, but it's the Washington lobbyists who are crucial to making a law" (quoted in Weisskopf 1995). The statement certainly is self-serving, but it also rings true.

There is some evidence that the money tends to be more persuasive in committee activities than on the house floor, because, in committees, visibility is lower, more decisions are made, and there are fewer members to persuade (Hall and Wayman 1990; Keiser and Jones 1986). Committee members can relatively easily and without much attention table a provision or make an amendment, without seeming to "sell out." They also have many choices to make about their level of formal and informal participation on an issue, ranging from merely attending a hearing or markup session to offering amendments and advocating on a group's behalf. If groups can tie their desired policies to strong public support, their chances of success are enhanced.

Some of the nation's strongest interest groups are weakened in their bargaining ability by their own members. For groups representing a large, diverse membership, developing and maintaining a policy focus that satisfies all members can be tough. Sometimes a group's leadership in Washington ("inside the beltway") does not reflect the rank and file. In March 1994, the board of the U.S. Chamber of Commerce reversed its one-year position supporting an employer mandate for health insurance when many of its members threatened to quit over the issue. Similarly, the AHA had supported a pay-or-play proposal (provide health insurance or pay government to do it) and then backed away from that position as the for-profit hospitals in its ranks opposed the government regulations they feared such a plan would engender.

The clearest example of an interest group's change of heart was on catastrophic health insurance, passed by Congress in 1988 with the support of the AARP. The AARP played an insider role in the passage of the law, working closely with Congress to fashion a law that would be palatable to its constituents (Torres-Gil 1989). The strategy backfired, however. A year later an embarrassed Congress repealed the law in response to a loud and insistent elderly population. Later, in the 1994 health care debates, the AARP approached controversial policy positions a bit more carefully. It refused to endorse President Clinton's proposal, preferring its members to transmit their views to their own representatives. In a statement clearly reflective of its earlier experience, the association's chair said, "When you have 33 million members, it's hard to say that every one of them feels any particular way" (Pear 1994). When later (August 1994) the AARP board endorsed two Democratic health care proposals and recommended its members support the bills, irate AARP members flooded the phone lines to the association's Washington headquarters, prompting the AARP to publish a full-page ad in the *Washington Post* explaining its reasons for the action (Ross 1994). In 2003, the AARP again surprised many observers by becoming an enthusiastic supporter of the administration's Medicare prescription drug bill, a much scaled-down version of the comprehensive package Democrats had called for. One motivation was the concern that with rising deficits, it was now or never for getting expanded drug coverage. A more direct inducement was the congressional leadership's agreement to reduce a House-passed head-to-head competition between Medicare and private plans to a limited demonstration project. And, by cooperating on the MMA, the AARP bought itself access to the GOP leadership when needed on future issues.

Dissatisfaction with an interest group's activity can also be exhibited in other ways, such as leaving the group. The insurance industry has seen much movement of this type, especially in the HIAA, the 300-member association of insurance companies. Five large companies left the association between

1990 and 1993, a reflection of the different interests of large and small insurers on such issues as managed competition. Larger insurers supported the idea, but small insurers feared they were more likely to be forced out of business if they could not select enrollees or price policies based on risk.

Hundreds of different health-related interest groups participate in health policy making today, collectively affecting a range of programs and policy issues. There are many new consumer groups and an increasing number of groups representing corporate medicine, such as prepaid health plans, hospital chains, walk-in clinics, and home care companies. Relman (1980) referred to this body as the "new medical-industrial complex." There have also been huge increases in the number of businesses and other non-health-related corporate entities involved in health policy making and in groups representing providers and corporate interests, which tend to have substantially more resources.

It would be completely misleading to overstate the difficulties of interest groups in today's competitive policy world. They have kept many issues from reaching the agenda and have seriously delayed and modified policy action on many others. Political scientists have long recognized the power to keep issues from being discussed and recognized as problems. For example, the excess of hospital beds was widely acknowledged and the cost implications well understood. But federal funds continued to be available to build more hospitals, largely because of the ability of provider lobbies to keep the issue off the agenda. Big business has successfully kept reforms of ERISA at bay, and teaching hospitals have protected graduate medical education dollars for years, despite the need for cuts in federal health spending and the desire to give states more flexibility in making policy decisions formerly concentrated in Washington. Groups have also been successful in delaying or stalling national health insurance, hospital cost controls, employer mandates, patients' managed care rights, and tough quality controls on physicians and hospitals, and they have reduced the size of other initiatives, including federal subsidies for HMOs. Ergonomics rules were delayed for years and later abandoned because of interest-group pressures.

CONCLUSION

Interest groups are powerful actors in health policy making, arguably second only to Congress. Yet not all interest groups are equally powerful, and even the powerful are not dominant on all issues and at all times. These groups are most likely to affect bills when the issues are nonsalient, narrow and specialized, and without public support, and when the groups employ a multipart strategy that includes contributions, direct and grassroots lobbying, and coalition building. Similarly, strategies that target a few specific changes can focus attention in a way that broader consumer groups cannot.

Changes in Congress, the presidency, the bureaucracy, the media, the public, and technology have affected interest groups' efforts and success rates, in some cases to reduce their influence. Some analysts now believe that interest groups have more access than influence (Heinz et al. 1993), and others note that their influence, at least on the big issues, has declined (Nexon 1987; Petracca 1992). But this view of declining power is not universally held. One widely respected journalist bemoaned the increasing power of interest groups (and the press) and the concomitant weakening of Congress, the presidency, and the political parties (Broder 1994c). Some academics agree that the overall influence of lobbyists and interest groups has increased over the past 30 years (Jacobson 1987). And President Clinton, in his September 22, 1993, address introducing his health care proposal, acknowledged his concerns about special interests that would "bombard" Congress with information and stoutly disagree with policies of change. Events proved him correct.

What both sides of the debate might agree on is the instability of the modern policy world, including interest groups. The presidency, Congress, even the courts undergo changes in focus, institutional organization, rules, and energy over time. These changes affect interest groups. The public is notoriously fickle, strongly supporting one policy or evidencing concern for one problem, only to move on to other policies and problems a short time later (Downs 1972). Interest groups themselves are far from stable; the 1993–94 health care debate highlighted changing positions and support over the months of high-level public attention to the issue.

Interest groups tend to take advantage of technological advances and changes in campaign finance statutes to update their approaches and present their positions. Most, if not all, interest groups use the Internet and e-mail to maintain their constituencies and get their message out to policymakers and the public. When changes are made in one aspect of campaign finance—be it soft money or Section 527 committees—the groups adjust their funding streams to other entities. They also adjust their funding strategies, if not their positions, when political changes occur in Congress or the White House.

The success of interest groups, in health and other areas, is in the details—the often complex, many times largely ignored, aspects of the law or regulation that can affect millions of dollars in reimbursement or the ability of health professionals to ply their trade independently. The expertise and intensity of interest groups' involvement in the complex details are often persuasive. It is at these margins of public policy that groups can most effectively use their lobbying strategies and PAC dollars, often without the benefit of public or media scrutiny.

Some worry that interest-group spoils go predominantly to the wealthiest of groups—those not only able to contribute generously to campaigns but also able to afford the most targeted, most professional media campaigns, electronic services, and informational assistance, including polling and focus groups. While all groups can use the Internet—and small groups may have an advantage here—the Internet is a passive form of lobbying and is probably most effective when part of a larger lobbying campaign.

In this atmosphere, then, health-related interest groups seek to inform and influence national policymakers to act (or refrain from acting) in ways that benefit their membership. The field is crowded and the stakes are high. One public relations staffer described health lobbying this way: "In all the issues we've worked on, we've never, ever found an issue that so many different constituencies were so instantly interested in. On health care, the interest level is immediately there and it is very deep. You don't have to explain to people why they should care" (Rubin 1993, 1084).

As more and more health care groups come to realize that they too must be players to protect their interests, the number and variety of these groups will continue to grow. Balance may yet be achieved as the cacophony fades into background noise. Poor people will likely have to count on health care interests with a stake in serving them to press the concerns of lower-income groups about access, quality, and financing. Whatever measures are taken to reduce the influence of PACs and campaign spending on health care policy making, interest groups will still find a welcome on Capitol Hill, at the White House, in the health care agencies of the executive branch, and often in the courts. Those who become health lobbyists are likely to enjoy a successful and well-supported career. Plying their trade, they will work in an institution that is as integral a part of the system of health care policy making as Congress itself and those who actually provide health care.

4

Bureaucracy

IN THE 1965 negotiations over Medicare, one of the most important players, Wilbur Cohen, was a bureaucrat. As a long-time staff member in the Federal Security Agency, the Social Security Administration, and the Department of Health, Education, and Welfare, Cohen had had a hand in virtually every national health insurance proposal since the 1930s. He was well known on Capitol Hill for his knowledge of both Social Security and health insurance. Sen. Paul Douglas (D-IL) once said that "a Social Security expert is a man with Wilbur Cohen's telephone number" (R. Harris 1966). Cohen helped draft the administration's bill on Medicare, consulted with members of Congress on proposed bills, and was asked to summarize various proposals to the key committees. When Ways and Means Committee chair Wilbur Mills decided to combine several proposals into a "three-layer cake" (the layers were later known as Medicare Parts A and B and Medicaid), he asked Cohen to draw up legislative language to pull the pieces together, along with an analysis of the costs, within 12 hours.

Cohen was more than a substantive expert. He was involved in meetings in the White House and on Capitol Hill to assess the standing of proposals and develop strategies to achieve legislative success. He was one of a small group of strategists who developed a plan in 1956 that prompted congressional action by persuading a well-placed legislator to sponsor a bill and elicited wide public concern about the health of elderly people through a media campaign sponsored by the labor unions (Marmor 1970, 30). Standing outside the Senate chamber during debates on the measure in 1965, Cohen heard rumors that labor unions were supporting an amendment the administration opposed. He called the labor representative, found out the rumor was wrong, and was able to hold the votes of liberal senators that might otherwise have been lost (R. Harris 1966).

Cohen served as a broker between the president and congressional committees and among interest groups (Marmor 1970). He reported regularly to the president and transmitted the president's views back to legislators. The president assigned Cohen the responsibility for working with interest groups, most notably the American Medical Association and the American Hospital Association, in implementing the newly adopted Medicare program.

Although Cohen had more access and visibility than a "typical" bureaucrat, he epitomized the importance of bureaucratic expertise and guidance to both the president and Congress. In 1965, the presidential staff was small and typically dominated by political, rather than policy, experts. Lyndon Johnson, like presidents before him, relied on the staffs in the executive agencies to put presidential preferences into legislative language and to produce statistics and rationale to support it. Congress, too, relied on the federal departments in the mid-1960s. Clapp (1963, 129) called the executive branch "a leading source of information for the legislator." Executive-branch officials worked closely with congressional committees, providing them with briefings, speeches, useful documents, and strategy suggestions. Though more responsive to members of the president's party, agency personnel were generally available to assist any lawmaker in drafting legislation and often provided research to help back up their position, even if it did not reflect the thinking of the department.

In the 1960s, Congress typically gave considerable discretion to the agencies in implementing the law. Wilbur Cohen negotiated actively with interest groups on many aspects of the implementation of Medicare. In the Public Welfare Amendments of 1962, Congress specified that the federal government would match 75 percent of the cost of services "prescribed" or "specified" by the secretary of HEW, words that gave HEW enormous discretion in deciding the nature of the program—and its cost (Derthick 1975).

In 1965, federal health spending exceeded $3 billion, with most going to the "other" category (not falling in the other four program areas—Medicare, Medicaid, Veterans, and Defense health), including research and training. HEW was the major health agency, accounting for 4 percent of all federal outlays (excluding Social Security). It was divided into eight agencies: Administration on Aging, Food and Drug Administration, Office of Education, Social Security Administration, Public Health Service (PHS), Vocational Rehabilitation Services, St. Elizabeth's Hospital, and Welfare Administration.

1981

President Ronald Reagan was highly skeptical of the loyalty and ability of the 366,000 federal public employees working in Washington. Even though Jimmy Carter had served in office only four years, following an eight-year Republican occupation of the White House, there was a general view that the federal departments were filled with Democrats hostile to Reagan's desire to reduce the size and power of government. President Reagan's skepticism led him to adopt a very careful hiring policy, putting in place cabinet and sub-cabinet appointees and other top officials who were often highly ideological and very loyal to him. Extreme cases involved an Environmental Protection Agency director and an Interior Department secretary who were forced to resign early in their assignments over questionable decisions and clear preferences toward business. The Reagan administration reached down further into the operations of the agencies, filling a higher proportion of noncareer senior executive positions, than any other modern presidential administration.

In addition to "stacking the deck" with like-thinking employees, the White House also encouraged these appointees to use their administrative powers to advance White House objectives (Salamon and Abramson 1984). They were encouraged to reinterpret the conduct of agency business to the greatest extent possible, reduce regulatory actions, and reduce the adverse effects of regulations on business. There were layoffs in many agencies, called reductions in force, or RIFs. Some 12,000 federal employees lost their jobs through RIFs in fiscal years 1981 and 1982.

In 1981, the relationship between the executive agency staff and Congress was very different from that in the days of the Johnson presidency. With the dramatic increase in congressional staff, there was less call on agency staff to assist in drafting laws and less need for agency help in plotting political strategies. Some agency expertise was still needed, however, particularly in statistics, evaluations, simulations, and informed estimations of the effect of current and proposed programs. A congressional staff person, usually new to the job and often to the issue, could rely on a seasoned agency expert to help in preparing speeches, testimony, committee reports, and sections of the bill. To gain expertise, a congressional committee would often "borrow" federal agency employees for temporary assignments. Such an arrangement benefited all parties. For Congress, it was an opportunity to get top-flight expertise; for the staffer on loan, it was an opportunity to affect policy directly; for the agency, it was a way to build good will and strong bonds with congressional members and staff.

In 1980, a new Department of Education was formed, and HEW became the Department of Health and Human Services. HHS had four operating agencies: the Public Health Service, Social Security Administration, Office of Human Development Services, and Health Care Financing Administration. By 1981, HHS accounted for some 13 percent of total federal outlays, with overall spending of nearly $90 billion. Federal health spending was more than $66 billion, with health care services and Medicare making up more than 90 percent of the total.

1993

The federal bureaucracy facing Bill Clinton was similar in size to that in the time of Lyndon Johnson and Ronald Reagan. The number of public employees had grown between 1965 and 1993, but largely in the state and local sectors, which had increased by more than 40 percent. The health bureaucracy played a key role in Hillary Clinton's health care reform task force. But the key decisions about the makeup of the Clinton health package were made in the White House. Donna Shalala, HHS secretary, took a back seat to both the first lady and White House advisor Ira Magaziner. Magaziner directed and coordinated the efforts of the 500-member task force assembled in the early months of the Clinton presidency. Federal agency personnel were actively involved in the task force deliberations but were outnumbered by congressional staffers and outside advisers. Some 137 HHS staff members participated in the health care reform work groups—about one-third of all the government employees (including congressional staff and representatives of other federal agencies) in the groups and more than one-fourth of the total work-group membership. While White House officials were busy crafting a comprehensive health plan, HHS officials, working with Congress, drafted a $1.4 billion entitlement program to provide vaccines to state Medicaid programs for uninsured children, enacted in the summer of 1993.

Vice President Al Gore headed an effort to make government more efficient, called the National Performance Review. The effort produced hundreds of recommendations designed to save $108 billion over five years. In the first year, the review claimed to have reduced the federal workforce by 71,000 positions and saved $47 billion. Early in his presidency, Bill Clinton announced that he intended to provide more flexibility to states in launching innovations in Medicaid and Aid to Families with Dependent Children. The HCFA soon set about implementing the policy, which broadened the scope of the research and demonstration waivers and allowed states to ignore some Medicaid and AFDC rules to try out new approaches and policies in 1993 and 1994.

In 1993, HHS accounted for some 18 percent of all federal spending—more than $280 billion. Health care services and Medicare made up 95 percent of the total federal spending on health. The four operating agencies in HHS were now the Public Health Service, Social Security Administration, Health Care Financing Administration, and Administration for Children and Families (replacing the Office of Human Development Services).

2005

In the early years of the new millennium, the expertise and the nonpartisan nature of federal bureaucrats and their agencies were questioned in a highly public manner that would have been alien and unrecognizable to Wilbur Cohen and other federal bureaucrats of previous decades. Some of the nation's most venerable health institutions—the Food and Drug Administration and the Centers for Disease Control and Prevention (CDC)—and the staff overseeing Medicare (Wilbur Cohen's legacy) were subjected to media criticism and divisive congressional hearings.

In 2005, the CDC concluded in a widely reported study that obesity was not nearly as dangerous as was once thought and that being a little plump might actually be healthy. A few months after release of the study, the CDC director acknowledged its flaws. The result was widely fluctuating estimates of the number of deaths per year from obesity. In 2004, that number was estimated to be 365,000; then the CDC report of 2005 claimed there were only 25,814 obesity-related deaths per year. But two months later, on its Web site, the CDC gave the number as 112,000 (Marchione 2005).

The FDA was embarrassed in 2004 when several popular drugs it had approved turned out to have major adverse side effects that had been ignored by the agency. In one case involving certain antidepressants, an FDA staffer was prevented from presenting findings to an FDA advisory committee that the drug caused some children and teenagers to become suicidal (G. Harris 2005). Another FDA official was prevented from providing evidence to an FDA committee that Vioxx, a popular pain medication, increased the risk of heart attacks or strokes. The manufacturer later voluntarily took the drug off the market, based on findings from its own internal studies (Spake 2004). Finally, in 2005, FDA staff findings about possible links between blindness and Viagra, the popular drug for treatment of erectile dysfunction, were ignored by the agency, until an article linking the two was published in a medical journal (M. Kaufman 2005). These instances of the FDA's inaction were widely covered in the media and were the target of congressional investigations and calls for reform in the agency. Central to the suggested reforms was a new office for drug safety.

The Centers for Medicare and Medicaid Services was in the hot seat when, during the activity surrounding passage of the Medicare Modernization Act in 2003, the CMS actuary was pressured to reduce the cost estimate for the measure in order to secure its passage. Both Democrats and conservative Republicans were very concerned about the impact of MMA spending on the rising deficit. A few months after passage of the law, the actuary recalled that the administrator of CMS had threatened to fire him if he reported to Congress that his cost estimates for MMA were one-third higher than the $400 billion estimated by the Congressional Budget Office (Schuler and Carey 2004). It turned out that the CMS actuary was right: a few months into 2004, the costs for the new law were estimated at more than $700 billion—only to rise closer to $1 trillion in the following years.

In a related public health area—the possible occurrence of mad cow disease (bovine spongiform encephalopathy, BSE) in the United States—another federal agency was criticized as being too close to its regulated industry, perhaps endangering the lives of American citizens. The Department of Agriculture waited seven months to report positive test results for a cow suspected of having BSE. When the test results came to light, the agency blamed poor communication—the laboratory results were never reported up the agency hierarchy. Some in Congress have called for removing the food safety agency from the confines of the Department of Agriculture (McNeil and Barrionuevo 2005).

Finally, in 2005, FEMA was roundly criticized for its slow and uncoordinated response following the massive hurricane that hit the Gulf Coast.

What is one to make of these events—just a sample of recent administrative difficulties in Washington? One conclusion concerns the importance of whistleblowers, or staff who come forward to politicians and the media with evidence that might be important to the public interest. A second important point is the role of the 24-hour media, always looking for scandals or missteps (or apparent scandals or missteps), in widely publicizing these events. A third point is the apparent need for more transparency in federal administrative activity. While the work of most bureaucrats and agency advisory groups is not generally conducive to public viewing, the results of this work are important, and many think these results should be made public by the agencies—rather than by a muckraking press or disgruntled whistleblowers. The final point is that the importance of federal agency staff in the operation of government is now recognized by political interests and is perhaps used in ways that Wilbur Cohen might have vehemently objected to. The importance of bureaucrats in conducting the business of government remains essential. But the public's opinion of the collective bureaucracy and the agencies in which bureaucrats serve may be worsening—a situation that could pose future problems for the legitimacy of and trust in the nation's public workforce.

UNDERSTANDING THE PUBLIC BUREAUCRACY

The president, members of Congress, and the courts, the traditional triumvirate of power in the United States, tend to overshadow another group of policymakers, one that is clearly more important in the day-to-day operation and working of government: the public employees who work for federal, state, and local governments. There are more than 21 million public employees, 13 million of them working at the local level. Roughly 4 in 10 Americans work for or have a family member who works for government (28 percent) or a nonprofit agency that contracts with government (14 percent) (Light 1999). Although the term *bureaucracy* encompasses both public and private sector organizations that are large, hierarchically organized, and highly specialized, in common parlance *bureaucracy* has come to mean publicly funded agencies and offices. Public sector employees are called, usually derisively, bureaucrats.

Bureaucracy conjures up images of inefficiency, waste, and red tape. Yet the evidence is not so clear cut. For example, *red tape,* clearly understood in the abstract, is difficult to pin down. Appleby (1945, 64) described red tape as "that part of my business that you don't know anything about." A study by Herbert Kaufman (1977) concluded that though citizens object to the weight of red tape, everyone likes some portion of that weight. What is red tape to one person is, to another, an important consideration that could not be omitted. Many local officials consider regulations associated with the rights of people with disabilities to be excessive, expensive, and unnecessary, but to individuals who are disabled these requirements are essential. In their study of red tape, Bozeman and DeHart-Davis (1999) narrowed its definition to include rules, regulations, and procedures that remain in force and entail a compliance burden but do not advance the legitimate purposes the rules were intended to serve. Burdensome—yet effective—rules such as those protecting people who are disabled would not qualify as red tape under this definition.

Public administrators have much lower standing in the United States than in European and many Asian countries. In part this is a function of history. There is no mention of administration or bureaucracy or federal agencies in the U.S. Constitution, and the modern administrative state developed only recently, somewhere between the two Roosevelt administrations (Morone 1990). In many European countries, the bureaucracy developed before the system of government and plays a strong institutional role in developing and implementing policy. The rather weak position of U.S. public bureaucracy is also explained by Americans' reverence for individualism and democracy—notions that run counter to bureaucracy and its quest for efficiency and effectiveness, not accountability.

Political Appointees versus Careerists

The top-level policy-making jobs in federal and state governments are generally filled with appointees of the chief executive: president or governor. At the federal level, the president fills more than 2,000 positions in federal departments—from department secretary and deputy chief of staff to assistant administrator. He also names members of the Federal Communications Commission and other independent commissions. Some 470 of these top jobs require Senate confirmation (Light 1999). In some states, governors make many appointments; in others, appointments are limited. Public appointees tend to be short-timers in both federal and state government; the mean tenure for a Washington political appointee is about two years. When the president leaves, so do these people, to be replaced by appointees of the new administration. Heclo (1977) dubbed public appointees "birds of passage," who understand they will not be around long and must act quickly if they expect to accomplish anything. Most public employees are civil servants, personnel who are hired and rewarded on a merit system and whose tenure does not rely on any one political party or officeholder.

Robinson (1991) gave examples of conflicts that can arise between political appointees who are pursuing a presidential goal (in the 1980s it was holding down costs) and careerists who want to continue or expand programs they consider worthy. The Reagan administration wanted to drastically reduce support for professional standards review organizations. One career agency official dedicated to keeping the PRSO program launched a campaign lobbying Congress on its value. Though his supervisors knew what he was doing and objected to it, they could not stop him.

Sometimes members of Congress try to separate careerists from the political aspects of a department by contacting them directly. According to Robinson (1991), some congressional committees sent packages of materials to the HCFA with instructions that political appointees were not to see the material. The committee wanted technical assistance but did not want to release the information to political appointees of the opposite party.

Bureaucratic Power

When we think of power, defined simply as the ability to act or produce an effect, we generally do not think of the bureaucracy. But we would be wrong to overlook it. As Norton Long (1949, 257) noted more than a half-century ago, "The lifeblood of administration is power." Public employees are armed with the ability to influence legislation, interpret it, implement it, and evaluate it. They work closely with most of the central actors in the policy-making process and make linkages among them. They have their own motivations and act accordingly.

Bureaucratic power has long rested on expertise. No matter how many staff members Congress and the president may add, that staff will likely not be expert in every programmatic aspect of an issue. Agencies staffed with personnel whose job it is to deal with the details of a program, and who likely have been doing so for many years, will still have the advantage. Bureaucratic expertise is "indispensable for the effective operation of any modern political system" (Rourke 1984, 15). Sparer and Brown (1993) provided evidence of how state Medicaid staffs use their expertise to guide policy development. Minnesota's Medicaid staff helped draft legislative language, lobby, and otherwise "quarterback" for the state's prenatal initiatives, children's health plan, and innovative and comprehensive MinnesotaCare Plan, first adopted in 1992.

Similarly, New York State's Medicaid staff helped launch an innovative home care program by acting as intermediaries among elected officials, industry representatives, and client advocates, drafting legislation, testifying before legislative committees, and "generally pushing for action in a contentious area" (Sparer and Brown 1993, 294). The staff's knowledge of the programs and their strengths and potential were the basis for staffers' standing in the policy debate.

State and federal bureaucrats also have the advantage of staying power. Executive-branch political appointees come and go, and congressional and state legislative staffers are highly transient, but careerists, by definition, stay. They stay and learn and remember. They comprise the institutional memory of what was proposed and adopted in earlier years—a valuable commodity in an area such as health, where many "new" proposals have actually been introduced several times over.

Bureaucratic power also rests on what Francis Rourke (1984) called political mobilization and Norton Long (1949) called political astuteness—the ability of an agency to garner support from the recipients or beneficiaries of the agency's programs. As Rourke (1984, 48) put it, "In the United States, it is fair to say, strength in a constituency is no less an asset for an administrator than it is for a politician, and some agencies have succeeded in building outside support as formidable as that of any political organization." One example of a politically astute health agency is the National Institute of Mental Health, which has enjoyed support from mental health practitioners across the country and successfully separated itself from the other national institutes, becoming independent in 1966 and later forming the basis for the Substance Abuse and Mental Health Services Administration (SAMHSA), an agency within HHS.

We need to keep in mind that power does not reside solely in the top leaders of an organization; rather, as Long (1949, 258) said, "It flows in from the sides of an organization . . . it also flows up the organization to the center from the constituent parts." Power is not just a friendly lunch between the department secretary and the chair of the House Energy and Commerce Committee. It is also the friendship between congressional committee staff and a staffer at the CMS's Office of Legislation and Policy, and the support from interest groups and program recipients who want to make certain that Medicare and Medicaid are well staffed and well funded—a goal shared with the agency personnel.

Agencies often try hard to obtain positive and strong public support. They do it with good service, good media relations, advertisements, education campaigns in public schools, and public involvement in commissions, boards, or contests. They especially seek the strong support of "attentives," those people and groups who directly benefit from or otherwise support an agency's mission. The National Institutes of Health (NIH), for example, is supported by the research community of health-professions schools and laboratories, high-tech industries, and broad-based organizations supporting specific diseases (such as the American Cancer Society). In the case of the NIH and other agencies, many of these groups benefit from research dollars available from the agency, directly or indirectly. Some agencies have a specific, highly targeted clientele, such as veterans. Organizations of veterans have been extremely vocal and effective in maintaining programs and increasing funding for the Department of Veterans Affairs.

Some observers believe bureaucrats are becoming more powerful. Morone (1993) noted that bureaucrats are playing a greater role in formulating health care and are implementing laws with less deference to Congress. Others disagree. Rourke (1991) argued that the role of expertise has diminished in recent years as public confidence in experts has declined. Think tanks and nonprofit groups, often advocating certain points of view, have proliferated in Washington and the states and provide white papers, policy analyses, and applied research that compete with bureaucratic advice. There are simply too many experts—and they disagree too often. Whether it is conflicting "expert" testimony on the psychological profile of the defendant in a murder trial, the disagreement of scientists over the extent of the problem caused by destruction of the ozone layer, or the disagreements of statisticians over the prevalence and incidence of HIV/AIDS or the impact of obesity on morbidity and mortality—the point is the same: whom is the public to believe? Possibly both sides of the argument on the importance of bureaucrats are right. On detailed, complex issues, much is delegated to the bureaucracy. On less salient, less complex issues, Congress may be less willing to delegate authority to the bureaucracy.

The Political Environment

The political environment of government agencies can vary enormously. James Wilson (1989) categorized agencies into four types based on whether the benefits they provide are narrow or wide and the costs they impose are narrow or wide. For agencies providing narrow benefits and imposing narrow costs (benefits to a few, costs shared by a few), their political environment can be categorized as interest-group politics, best described as having interest groups on both sides of an issue. A good example of this interest-group agency is the Occupational Safety and Health Administration: labor and business often clash over the agency's actions, and the agency finds it hard to please both sides in its activities and its choices. At the other extreme, some agencies that distribute broad benefits and impose broad costs have little interest-group involvement, and these may be called majoritarian agencies. The CDC is one such agency. Reduced interest-group participation might seem enviable at first glance, but it could prove problematic in times of budget cutbacks, when the agency can find it hard to muster outside support.

An agency granting broad benefits while imposing narrow costs is not in an enviable position, since the interest groups paying those costs might coalesce to oppose agency goals. Members of the broad group of beneficiaries seem, individually, to have little at stake in the benefits, but those suffering the costs are big losers. The FDA is a perfect example of this type of agency, called an entrepreneurial agency. Its mission is to protect the broad public interest. But doing so means battling with food and drug manufacturers who are financially harmed by agency actions. With millions of dollars at stake, the effort and costs of marshalling powerful coalitions to fight the agency are a good investment for the pharmaceutical industry. Indeed, the FDA has long suffered from the criticism that it pays too much attention to the industry and not enough to consumers.

In the final category of agency politics are those agencies whose benefits accrue to a few and whose costs are widespread. Health personnel agencies such as the Bureau of Health Professions are examples of these client agencies. Their programs directly benefit medical and nursing schools, with costs widely spread across most of the population. Such an agency is a good candidate for "capture" by interest groups, because the goals of the agency and the goals of the groups are likely to be closely aligned. Opponents are hard to find and are unlikely to invest the effort to form an interest group to oppose the agency's actions, since the costs are so small to each payer.

Bureaucratic Behavior

Rationality is an important goal of public administration. Rationality has many meanings, but Waldo's concept (1955) of rational action is appropriate to public administration: action correctly calculated to realize given desired goals with minimal loss to the realization of other desired goals. Not all decisions are rational, of course, because few decision makers have the full information, time, and resources necessary to know with certainty the consequences of each alternative. Public decision makers are under time and resource constraints. Full knowledge about the alternatives and their consequences is nearly impossible. Instead, public decision makers "satisfice," or make the best decision given the constraints. Simon (1945) described a "satisficing" decision maker as one who does not examine all possible alternatives, ignores most of the complex interrelationships of the real world, and makes decisions by applying relatively simple general rules. Simon also described this decision maker as applying "bounded rationality" to decisions. Knott and Miller (1987) argued that rationality is impossible because of the dysfunctions in bureaucratic structure. Characteristics of bureaucracy—specialization, trained expertise, hierarchy, and rules—combine to produce a variety of bureaucratic dysfunctions, including trained incapacity, goal displacement, and rigidity cycles.

Simon (1960) talked about two types of decisions: programmed and nonprogrammed. Programmed decisions are those that recur frequently and can be handled by standard operating procedure (SOP), the rules of operation followed by all employees in the same situation. SOP can be viewed as a way to limit bureaucratic power and to force staff to conform to organizational goals (Rourke 1984). It is also the only practical way to run a large organization. The regional offices of federal agencies make many decisions every day about what is acceptable and unacceptable behavior from grantees and recipients. SOP helps ensure uniformity among these offices and their counterparts in Washington. The emphasis on SOP is not arbitrary or necessarily convenient. As Guy Peters (1981, 76) put it, federal agencies "are responsible for public money and act in the name of the people and must therefore be accountable to the public. Accountability, in turn, may force the bureaucrat to protect himself against possible complaints, and the protection comes through adherence to rules and procedures."

Nonprogrammed decisions are those that Simon (1976, 6) described as "novel, unstructured, and consequential." They cannot be handled with SOP but must be dealt with using the staff's discretion. Decisions related to the drafting of regulations, allocation of resources, and implementation of new programs are examples of nonprogrammed decisions.

In nonprogrammed decisions, bureaucrats must balance many concerns— those of their own professions, their political bosses, their funders (Congress), and the public. Bureaucrats are also cognizant of their own agency's reputation and mission. In many cases there are conflicts among several of these "masters" and the agency's own mission that are important to that agency's survival. In health, the NIH is an example of an agency with a strong sense of mission—biomedical research—that has remained constant over decades. In contrast, the PHS has seen its mission change from caring for merchant sailors, to environmental and preventive medical activities, to responsibility for care delivery to targeted populations, preventive care, and health personnel. Although agencies must be somewhat flexible to survive, such major organizational personality changes can strip an agency of its identity and leave it floundering. The NIH, by contrast, holds so strongly to its mission that it has repeatedly resisted efforts by powerful health committee and subcommittee chairs to add new agencies with a statistical and social science focus. When one was slipped in—the National Institute on Aging—its director (despite his own training as a psychiatrist) quickly realized that his agency must focus on the biological aspects of aging rather than social science concerns, if it was to thrive in the NIH environment.

The Food and Drug Administration is an agency that is frequently conflicted. Presidential and congressional goals are often not the same as the goals of industry or the public. In the 1980s the FDA responded to the calls of AIDS activists to speed up approval of HIV/AIDS drugs. In 1989, legislation was enacted making the FDA commissioner a presidential appointee, subject to Senate approval. In 1992, Congress passed a law setting performance goals for approval of new drugs in exchange for new industry fees to supplement the FDA's budget. The law has dramatically shortened review time: from an average of 24.2 months in 1991 to 14.2 in 2002 (Adams 2005a). But critics argue that the drug company funding has made the agency more accountable to the industry and less concerned about the public's interest—a clear conflict in mission.

PUBLIC BUREAUCRACY AND THE POLICY PROCESS

In the early years of public administration, the roles of politicians and public employees were seen as distinct and clearly defined. Elected officials were responsible for making political decisions or policy; appointed officials handled administrative matters and the implementation of political actions. In contrast, today's public bureaucrat is involved in all aspects of policy making: setting the agenda, formulating solutions, and implementing the policy, including translating sometimes vague congressional directions into concrete, workable programs.

Setting the Agenda

Bureaucrats, according to Kingdon (1995), are communities of specialists who provide information and statistics that define problems in a way that can move the issues to the forefront of public attention. They can make the dimensions and severity of a problem known to Congress, the White House, and the press. Kelman (1980) attributed the addition of occupational safety and health to the presidential and congressional agenda to a bureaucrat in an HEW research unit who worked on occupational safety and health issues and whose brother wrote speeches for President Johnson. The brother occasionally slipped occupational safety and health issues into the president's speeches. The staff for the secretary of labor, looking for new legislative proposals, noticed the references in the president's speeches and proposed legislation on the issue in 1968.

Robinson (1991) recounted how a midlevel civil servant in the HCFA was assigned to answer a letter to the president from a retired single teacher in California who discovered that her state medical insurance was not available to retirees and that she was not eligible for Medicare. The letter alerted the staffer to a problem that could be solved with a change in the Medicare statutes to include state and local employees. He persuaded others in the HCFA, the White House, and eventually Congress. His proposal, prompted by the teacher's letter to the president, became law.

Formulating Health Care Policy

The Medicare Prospective Payment System flowed from more than a decade of HCFA-sponsored research and demonstration projects to develop a more effective administrative mechanism for controlling health care costs. The HCFA funded eight state demonstration projects in 1975 to try out mandatory and voluntary programs to control health costs. Seven years later, Congress required the HCFA to develop a legislative proposal for prospective Medicare payments to hospitals, skilled nursing facilities, and other providers. Following the advice of a task force composed of HCFA staff and experts from outside the government, the HCFA administrator proposed a hospital prospective payment plan based on the latest prospective payment system (PPS) demonstration project, operating in New Jersey. The plan was enacted virtually intact by Congress three months after it was submitted (Morone and Dunham 1985).

A more recent example of a federal agency taking the lead in launching a new policy approach is the HCFA's agreement in 1997 to an innovative plan to pay hospitals around the country not to train doctors. The idea came from the Greater New York Hospital Association and was approved by the HCFA administrator Bruce Vladeck. When members of Congress complained that New York was getting special treatment, Vladeck, a former New York hospital executive, challenged Congress to make the program national. "If other people think it's a good deal, they have the power to make it more available," he said (E. Rosenthal 1997).

When Congress considers measures to provide insurance for the uninsured, it needs to know how many Americans are uninsured, where they reside, and why they are uninsured. HHS can provide that information. The agency is even more successful in helping develop a policy agenda for the administration than for Congress. Robinson (1991) noted that 89 percent of executive-generated Medicare legislation in 1987 could be traced to the HCFA. Borins (1999) found that 71 percent of state and local "cutting-edge" innovations were initiated by bureaucrats. Only 18 percent were initiated by politicians.

Implementing Health Policy

Implementation may be defined as the activities directed toward putting a program into effect (C. Jones 1984), or what happens after laws are passed that authorize a program policy, benefit, or some other tangible output (Ripley and Franklin 1986). Guy Peters (1981, 77) argued that, to a great extent, "the 'real' policy of government is that policy which is implemented, rather than that policy which is adopted by the legislature." Yet implementation is an area not widely understood—even by policymakers. Nathan (1993, 122) called it the "shadow land," the neglected dimension of U.S. governance. A report of the National Commission on the State and Local Public Service (1993) described implementation as the short suit of U.S. government. So much time is devoted to what should be done that little energy remains for the questions of how to do it. The commission thought that the public's frustrations about government stem from unsuccessful implementation—the failure of government to turn promises into performance.

Implementation begins when Congress, through a series of instructions—sometimes specific, sometimes less specific—delegates to federal agencies the policy it wants carried out. The federal agency then follows those instructions. Though seemingly straightforward, many things can happen to impede successful implementation:

— Agencies responsible for implementation may lack the enthusiasm, the staff, the expertise, or the resources to carry out their responsibilities.

— The congressional instructions may be so vague that the federal agency must make many important assumptions, such as designating which state programs are "acceptable" or what is "reasonable cost."

— Multiple congressional goals or conflicting instructions may make it difficult for agencies to carry out their assignments.

— Interagency rivalries may cause problems, with agency staffs fighting one another over interpretation of the law and resource issues.

— The recipients of a program (for example, state or local governments) may be uncooperative or demanding of different interpretations.

— The number of people involved may slow the process: if several federal agencies and several state and local agencies must serve as "clearance points," the eventual outcome will be adversely affected.

— Time can be a problem; for complicated measures, such as clean air and clean water, the process of collecting information, writing draft regulations, and encouraging public comment can add years to the process of rulemaking.

— State and local agencies, communities, or recipients of the program can slow implementation if they disagree with any aspect of it.

An example of a program that was poorly implemented owing to lack of resources was the National Center for Health Care Technology (NCHCT), authorized in law in 1978 but without any appropriations. The agency limped along for several months with borrowed staff and offices. Finally, a small amount of money was shifted from another HHS agency. A short time later, the center's mission was transferred to the National Center for Health Services Research (NCHSR), which later became the Agency for Health Care Policy and Research (AHCPR). Downs (1967) would say that the NCHCT never overcame the initial survival threshold necessary for a thriving agency.

Congress gives broad discretion to federal agencies to implement its laws, for a variety of reasons: it is impossible (and unwise) for Congress to write a law in such detail that it can be put in place immediately; sometimes lawmakers do not want to deal with a touchy or difficult issue, and passing it on to federal agencies lets them off the hook; the complexity of many issues prevents Congress from understanding them sufficiently to write details; and the experimental nature of policy making is promoted by allowing bureaucratic discretion. It is easier for administrators to change or revise a troublesome provision than for Congress to reconsider the matter.

Sometimes the delegation of authority is quite broad. In implementing Medicare, for example, HEW officials had to determine what Congress meant by "reasonable costs" of providing hospital care. Because hospitals were crucial to the success of the new program, Social Security officials agreed to depreciation and capital development provisions that were quite generous and contributed to rapidly increasing hospital costs in the 1970s (J. Feder 1977). The law setting up OSHA stated that the agency should foster healthful working conditions "so far as possible" and deal with toxic substances "to the extent feasible" (Thompson 1983, 219, 221).

The Health Insurance Portability and Accountability Act of 1996 called on Congress to enact comprehensive national standards for the privacy of medical records by August 1999. If Congress did not act by that time, the secretary of HHS was required to issue regulations. Congress did not reach an agreement. The first-ever national standards to protect patients' personal medical records were issued by HHS in December 2000. As another example, federal officials decided to include Viagra in the Medicare prescription drug benefit package in 2003—and were roundly criticized as a result. "Bureaucrats, isolated from fiscal reality, have made a thoughtless decision that will accelerate Medicare's demise," complained a spokesman for Citizens Against Government Waste (CAGW 2005b).

Health and Human Services' Bureau of Maternal and Child Health exercised a great deal of discretion in the development of guidelines for sexual abstinence education. Title V of the Personal Responsibility and Work Opportunity Reconciliation Act of 1996 set out eight precise guidelines that states must follow to get funding. However, the rules, devised by the Bureau of Maternal and Child Health, did not place equal emphasis on each of the eight factors—and in fact funded state projects as long as the projects were not inconsistent with any aspect of these factors. As a result, the state programs vary enormously and many states ignore parts of the law they do not support (Vergari 2001).

States, too, give health experts plenty of leeway in conducting their business. Medicaid officials in New York State placed a limit on the number of physician and dentist visits and laboratory procedures that the program would reimburse. A state court invalidated the regulations as "unauthorized by law," but the legislature later adopted the limitations and they were carried out (Sparer and Brown 1993, 288). In day-to-day implementation of state and federal Medicaid policy, state officials' discretion can lead to big interstate differences in the provision of service delivery (C. Weissert 1994).

Congress does not treat all agencies equally. The amount of discretion afforded an agency depends on several factors, including the agency's resources (such as political support, expertise, and leadership) and its tolerance of other actors, especially interest groups. Meier (1985) described agency decisions as falling within or outside a zone of acceptance. If the agency decision falls within the zone of acceptance to Congress, the president, and the courts, the agency will be given more autonomy. Agencies dealing with salient, noncomplex issues are more likely to have smaller zones of acceptance, and Congress is more likely to intervene. Sometimes Congress has little choice but to provide discretion to agencies, especially on complicated, politically volatile issues, but it can still provide specific guidance. For example, while delegating to the HCFA the authority to set new physician fees in the Resource-Based Relative Value Scale (intended to increase payments to primary care physicians), Congress placed two constraints on the agency's decisions: the payment levels had to reflect production costs and had to be "budget neutral" (Balla 1998). In some cases, the enabling legislation describes in detail what information should be collected. OSHA not only is obliged to rely on what is already known about health and safety aspects of substances and activities but must also create and use new knowledge when what is available is insufficient. Different statutes require different criteria for risk assessment and require different information to be collected—even for the same agency. Sometimes the criterion is "no known or anticipated adverse effects"; sometimes it is to ensure that "unreasonable risk" is eliminated, but using the "least burdensome requirements" (Kerwin 2003, 59).

Congress can set deadlines for agencies' actions (although they often do not meet them). It can also impose "hammers," which call for provisions in the statutes that will take place only if the agency fails to issue its own regulation. These provisions are not the desired policy of Congress but rather ways to pressure the agency to act quickly (Kerwin 2003).

The congressional tendency to limit agency discretion flourished in the 1980s, thanks to the distrust between a Democratic Congress and a Republican White House. The Democratic Congress wanted to make certain its version of a piece of legislation was implemented by including detailed instructions, definitions, and guidance in the law. Congress decided it liked this detailed brand of legislation so well that even when a Democratic president took office in 1993, the micromanagement continued. Such direction of the agencies had become not only possible but commonplace, because Congress now had the staff to oversee agency activity. One example of this micromanagement was a congressional order to add another layer of bureaucracy in the AIDS office.

"There isn't a scientist in the country who thought that [this personnel change] would give us better science," complained HHS secretary Shalala, "but it certainly responds to a political need" (Broder and Barr 1993).

Issuing Regulations

The single most important bureaucratic task in implementation is issuing rules and regulations for carrying out the law. Broadly speaking, regulation is government restriction of individual choice so as to keep conduct from crossing acceptable boundaries. Examples include prohibitions against selling unsafe drugs, operating an unsafe workplace, and polluting the nation's air and water. Regulations are made explicit in rules designed to implement, interpret, or prescribe law or policy. A more colorful definition, from former U.S. Supreme Court justice Oliver Wendell Homes, is that "a rule is the skin of a living policy . . . Its issuance marks the transformation of a policy from the private wish to public expectation" (Kerwin 2003, 2). In one year (1998–99), 4,752 final rules were issued by federal agencies (Skrzycki 2000a).

Given the importance of rulemaking, it is not surprising that agencies must follow procedures set forth in federal law—in this case, the federal Administrative Procedures Act. This act requires notice when a department plans to issue a rule. The notice must be published in the *Federal Register,* the official notification document of the federal government. Interested parties are then allowed an opportunity to participate in the proceedings by presenting written or oral information. Hearings are often held on salient rules of great interest to many people. Final regulations are then published. Some agencies are required by law to hold hearings and base final rules on the evidence in the record. Others must convene advisory groups to aid in the drafting of regulations. A 1996 federal law requires that if a regulation under development has substantial implications for a significant number of small businesses, the agency—especially if the EPA or OSHA—must convene a panel to develop information and secure recommendations from affected interests. The panel reports to the agency, which in turn is expected to incorporate the information into the regulation or supporting analyses (Kerwin 2003).

When an issue enters the regulation-writing stage, it does not cast aside politics. Rather, interest groups understand the bureaucracy to be one more venue for achieving policy goals. A simple way to affect the process is to comment on the proposed rule. Agencies must read and respond to these comments in their final regulations. For the 2000 rule establishing privacy standards for medical records, HHS received more than 52,000 comments (HHS 2000). Legislation delegating to the HCFA the assignment to set new Medicare physician payment levels under RBRVS required the agency to publish preliminary payment levels in the *Federal Register*, giving physicians ample opportunity to comment. Nearly 100,000 physicians did so (Balla 1998). Again, agencies respond to these formal and informal comments. Rules issued by HHS in March 1996 on disclosure of provider incentives by HMOs enrolling Medicare and Medicaid patients were suspended four months later following a "torrent of criticism" from regulated organizations (Pear 1996).

Though many regulatory decisions are complex, detailed, and of interest to only a few affected groups, some do have broad public interest. In 1994, when OSHA published draft rules that would ban smoking in the workplace, more than 700 organizations and individuals wanted to testify. The hearings continued for three months (Swoboda and Hamilton 1994).

The assumption is that agencies will do whatever Congress asks and do it well. This is not always the case. For example, in 2000 the EPA issued new water pollution rules only hours before President Clinton was expected to sign a bill that included a provision killing the rules. "EPA's arrogance under this administration has risen to new heights," protested Bud Shuster (R-PA), chair of the House Transportation and Infrastructure Committee (Wald and Greenhouse 2000).

There is often considerable delay between legislative enactment and the issuance of final regulations. One such delay occurred in hospital outpatient services under the Medicare PPS. In a 1986 law, Congress directed the HCFA to develop a PPS for hospital outpatient services. The regulations were finally issued in July 2000. The delays were due to the complexity of the issue, opposition from providers, and the demands of other, more politically expedient issues that had a higher priority in the HCFA's allocation of staff responsibility (Matherlee 2000). A delay measured in decades is a bit unusual, but multiyear delays are common. For example, in 1994 the EPA said it would propose an exposure rule for hexavalent chromium by March 1995. Five years later, the rule had not yet been drafted (Wald and Greenhouse 2000). It took HHS six years to issue the rules noted above on the 1990 federal law requiring disclosure of provider incentives by HMOs enrolling Medicare and Medicaid patients.

In contrast, the pace of regulatory initiation sometimes picks up as a president gets ready to leave office. President Carter issued more than 200 regulations in the final weeks of his term. Similarly, President Clinton's administration issued scores of regulations in its final week, including well over 50 from the EPA (McCoy 2000). Two important sets of health rules were among those issued in the final weeks of 2000: rules ordering ergonomics programs at worksites and rules setting time limits for health insurers to make treatment decisions.

A new president is sometimes reluctant to strike down regulations that have worked their way through laborious and legally defined processes. Indeed, the Supreme Court overturned an effort by President Reagan to eliminate a rule ordering air bags or passive-restraint seat belts in cars. The EPA under President George W. Bush sought to soften regulations promulgated during the Clinton years that required companies to install additional pollution controls when expanding or modernizing older power plants. The new regulations allowed utilities to make improvements without adding pollution controls. Several states sued the EPA, challenging the changes (Heilprin 2004). Rule changes between administrations became easier with passage of a 1996 law, the Congressional Review Act, giving Congress the power to kill final rules put in place within the preceding six months (Skrzycki 2000b). Democrats in Congress, joined by a few Republicans, tried to use the Congressional Review Act to challenge a regulation on mercury in 2005, but were unsuccessful. To send a regulation back to the EPA, majorities of both houses and the president have to agree on the change.

Sometimes presidents use the regulatory route to set policy without going to Congress. The EPA under President George W. Bush issued regulations setting up a cap-and-trade approach for sulfur dioxide and nitrogen oxide emissions and looser standards for emissions of mercury. The changes were not minor. For example, coal-fired power plants emitting mercury were given 11 additional years to make significant cuts under the regulation (C. Drew and Oppel 2004). One problem with heavy reliance on regulatory policy is that the regulations are often challenged in court.

In past years it was common in political science to talk about agencies being "captured" by special interests, an event most likely to occur for agencies that provide benefits to a narrow group of interests—a client agency—such as the Department of Veterans Affairs. The idea was that, since the agency's survival depended in large part on the support of its constituents, it could not be impartial but would accommodate the needs of its constituents, regulating to protect their interests. In recent years, empirical studies testing the capture theory have debunked the idea for most regulatory agencies. In fact, the studies have shown how, over time, agencies continue to regulate an industry vigorously rather than becoming increasingly sympathetic to it (Meier 1985; Quirk 1981). Other research has highlighted a more pluralistic interest-group model in which many groups form advocacy coalitions but find their influence curbed by external pressures from other actors and groups and by an agency's internal structure, professionalism, and leadership (Gormley 1982; Meier 1985).

The courts do not get involved in writing regulations, but they do respond when a group or person challenges the legality of a regulation. The Administrative Procedures Act provides for judicial review of any agency action by a person or corporation wronged by the agency or with a grievance. Under this act, citizens can use the courts to prod agencies into action. When federal agencies fail to issue regulations expeditiously or within congressional deadlines, they may get sued and the plaintiffs may prevail. Some federal agencies see their regulations taken to court with some regularity. For example, the EPA's and OSHA's regulatory products are routinely challenged in court. In fact, with only one exception, every health standard issued by OSHA in the past 30 or so years has been challenged in court (Kerwin 2003). A health-related regulation issued by the Equal Employment Opportunity Commission was blocked in 2005. The rule would have allowed employers to reduce or eliminate health benefits for retirees when they reached age 65 and became eligible for Medicare. Some 10 million retirees could have been affected by the regulation. The district court ruled that the provision was contrary to congressional intent and the Age Discrimination in Employment Act (Pear 2005c).

Where the Rubber Hits the Road

Simply issuing regulations does not get an agency home free. Bureaucrats must encourage, cajole, and otherwise urge the entities to which the money will flow for the provision of service to act in an expeditious way faithful to the law and regulations. Sometimes, getting a high level of compliance is not easy. Because much of the money goes to state and local governments, they are the primary focus of much of this activity. Control by federal bureaucracy over state and local officials is quite limited. Washington agencies can urge, educate, provide their state and local counterparts with financial incentives, or threaten them with the loss of federal grant money, but they cannot force perfect compliance or timeliness. The relationship can best be described as bargaining, under which, by offering a grant, the federal government achieves only the opportunity to bargain with the states: "Instead of a federal master dangling a carrot in front of a state donkey, the more apt image reveals a rich merchant haggling on equal terms with a sly, bargain-hunting consumer" (Ingram 1977, 499). What the "consumer" can shop around for is a better political deal from another part of the federal government—often Congress or the president. (In fact, the opportunity for such relief greatly impedes states' implementation of desired federal activities [Hill and C. Weissert 1995].)

In the late 1980s, the HCFA may have viewed California as something of a stubborn donkey when the nation's largest state balked at implementing 1987 nursing home standards adopted by Congress. California argued that its state standards were better than those proposed by the HCFA and that imposition of the federal standards would cost the state nearly half a billion dollars. After the HCFA threatened the state with the loss of federal Medicaid dollars, California's Republican governor appealed to the Republican president. A short time later, the state and the HCFA reached a compromise. The agency eased its demands that states use a lengthy and complicated survey process in return for California's agreement to begin inspecting nursing homes using HCFA guidelines. California did not win in the long run, however. While Sacramento and Washington argued, a group of providers went to court over implementation of the law and forced California's Medicaid program to pay an extra $2 per day per bed to meet the nursing homes' costs of complying with the law.

A more recent example of HCFA attempts to move states along was the State Children's Health Insurance Program (S-CHIP). The S-CHIP legislation was passed in mid-1997, and soon thereafter President Clinton expressed dismay to HCFA director Nancy-Ann Min DeParle that the states were not making more progress in signing up children for S-CHIP and Medicaid. In early 1998, the president ordered eight federal agencies to report back to him in three months on their plans to enroll more children. The group drafted a report offering more than 150 action steps. Meanwhile, the HCFA issued communications to state Medicaid agencies and S-CHIP officials urging them to step up their efforts to sign up children. The agency encouraged states to avoid inappropriate denials of Medicaid applications and made specific recommendations for increasing Medicaid and S-CHIP enrollments. The HCFA actively worked with individual states to monitor local offices' practices and make appropriate changes. Finally, in August 1999, the president instructed the HCFA to conduct comprehensive onsite reviews of Medicaid enrollment and eligibility processes in all states. Federal officials were assigned to interview state officials and check case files (Thompson 2001).

More popular with states are efforts in which federal health officials work with them to reach a compromise solution. The EPA has led the way in innovative cooperative ventures, including those that give states more discretion in complying with federal law. For example, one program, the National

Environmental Performance Partnership System (NEPPS), is designed to give states with strong environmental programs more flexibility, both in program operations and in spending authority. The agency has also tried to involve stakeholders, including states, in writing the regulations. However, implementation of this initiative was hampered by lack of buy-in by EPA staff and continuation of old oversight practices (Scheberle 2005).

Regulatory Agencies

In addition to "line" agencies within HHS—such as the Social Security Administration, CDC, and CMS, whose primary responsibility is program management—there are agencies whose entire role is to regulate economic or social activities. The three main regulatory agencies with authority over health issues are the Food and Drug Administration, the Federal Trade Commission (FTC), and the Occupational Safety and Health Administration. A fourth regulatory agency, the Environmental Protection Agency, deals with environmental issues.

The Food and Drug Administration

The FDA is probably the best-known of the federal health agencies, certainly of the federal regulatory agencies. It regulates food, pharmaceutical drugs, medical devices, and dietary supplements. In the 1980s and 1990s, the FDA was frequently in the news for targeting smoking among young people, the ill effects of passive smoking, and efforts by cigarette makers to hide the adverse effects of their products. In recent years its attention has been on drug safety and, most recently, on bioterrorism. It has around 10,000 employees and a $1.8 billion budget (Adams 2005a). By one estimate, its jurisdiction covers more than 20 percent of every consumer dollar spent in the United States (Stolberg 2002b).

The FDA's interest in drug safety flows from its establishment in 1906, when one of its top concerns was patent medicines. The 1937 Food, Drug and Cosmetic Act required manufacturers to prove the safety of a drug before the FDA would allow it on the market. In 1958, an amendment to that law, known as the Delaney Amendment for its sponsor Rep. James Delaney (D-NY), required the FDA to bar the use of any food additive that caused cancers in either humans or laboratory animals. In 1992, federal law allowed the FDA to assess user fees on drug companies to reduce the time to review and approve new drugs. In 1997, Congress mandated faster reviews of clinical trials, review of drugs within 60 days of submission of an application, and reporting of the recommendations of advisory panels within 90 days of receiving applications.

The FDA is no stranger to controversy. Given its nature as an agency whose decisions are broad and interests are narrow, this makes sense. Its mission is to ensure the safety of the nation's food and drugs, but in doing so it must regulate some of the most powerful companies and interests. The battles are many over genetically modified foods, regulation of cigarettes, dietary supplement labeling, and prescription drug safety.

Since the 1990s, battles have been waged between companies wanting to produce genetically modified foods and consumer groups that oppose those foods. The latter group has generally lost, but often in a noisy fashion. In 1992 (at the strong urging of President George H. W. Bush), the FDA ruled that genetically modified food products would be treated no differently than foods produced through traditional methods. The decision was especially controversial because it was against the advice of nearly two-thirds of the FDA's own scientific panel, and later congressional reports criticized FDA oversight of genetically modified food products as too lax.

Under a Democratic administration little changed. In 1993, FDA rules required the industry to keep the agency informed of new products but did not require firms to label products as genetically modified. In 1994 the FDA banned farmers from labeling milk as free from a genetically modified growth hormone that is used to increase milk production. In 2000 the agency required companies to notify it within 120 days of a genetically modified food going to market. Although a survey of consumers in 2000 found that an overwhelming majority were in favor of mandatory labeling of genetically modified foods, there is still no such policy (Hord 2001). The FDA sent a letter to the Oregon legislature in 2002 stating that it was against an upcoming ballot measure in the state on the mandatory labeling of all foods that contained genetically modified components, because the measure would interfere with national food producers (Weise 2002).

The FDA launched a high-visibility effort in the 1990s to regulate cigarettes and dietary supplements. It lost both causes. In 2000, the U.S. Supreme Court, in *FDA v. Brown and Williamson*, ruled by a 5-4 vote that the FDA did not have the authority from Congress to regulate tobacco products. In 1994, the agency fought unsuccessfully against passage of the Dietary Supplement Health and Education Act, which gives manufacturers the right to advertise potential benefits of herbs as long as the FDA cannot prove the product is unsafe and the ads do not claim the products can prevent, treat, or cure disease (Stolberg 1998).

The FDA has regulated the advertising of prescription drugs since 1962. In 1982 it declared a moratorium on direct-to-consumer advertising. Three years later, it lifted the moratorium but stipulated that ads directed at consumers must meet the standards required for information targeted to professionals. In 1997 the FDA allowed prescription drugs to be advertised on television and radio along with a list of major health risks associated with each drug. In 2004 the agency recommended that the ads describe the side effects in formats that are easy to read and understand (Michigan Consumer Health Care Coalition 2005).

Drug safety came to the fore in the early years of the new century as the FDA seemed to be slow to alert the public to approved drugs that had unexpected and unwanted side effects. There was some concern among agency staff that certain antidepressant drugs could cause some children and teenagers to become suicidal, but the official raising the issue was not allowed to present his findings and concerns before an FDA advisory committee. Agency officials said they did not want to confuse the committee with differing agency interpretations (G. Harris 2005). In one case in 2004, the FDA rejected a citizens' petition to remove a powerful cholesterol-lowering drug from the market, only two months before a study published in the American Heart Association's journal reported on its serious side effects, including kidney disease and kidney failure (M. Kaufman 2004). In another case, FDA staff raised concerns about the safety of Vioxx, a popular painkiller, that were ignored until the drug company voluntarily withdrew the drug from the market (Adams 2005c).

Off and on during its existence, the FDA has been accused of being captured by the pharmaceutical industry. In recent years the criticisms have arisen again. Indeed, the number of FDA warning letters to drug companies about inappropriate advertising fell from a peak of 157 in 1998 to 23 in 2004. And in the past five years, the FDA has intervened in several product liability cases, arguing that the drug companies should not be held accountable for patients' being unaware of adverse side effects not mentioned on drug labels (Adams 2005b). As box 4.1 describes, the FDA has actively fought reimportation of drugs from Canada and Europe—to protect the nation from possibly unsafe drugs or to protect the drug industry from lower-priced competition.

The FDA has often had an adversarial relationship with Congress, which has watched over its decisions, and its budget, very carefully. One reason

Box 4.1

Reimportation and the FDA

The Federal Food, Drug, and Cosmetics Act (FFDCA), as amended by the Prescription Drug Marketing Act of 1988 (PL 100-293), prohibits the re-importation of prescription drugs manufactured in the U.S. by anyone other than the original manufacturers (though the FDA rarely enforces this prohibition for small amounts—up to 90 days supply—intended for personal use). As such, the FDA has long sought to discourage states and localities from promoting re-importation. Citing the Supremacy Clause in a letter to the Deputy Attorney General of the State of California, for example, William K. Hubbard, then Associate Commissioner for Policy and Planning at the FDA, argued that "the drug importation scheme set forth by Congress preempts the State of California (or any city or county within the State) from passing conflicting legislation that would legalize the importation of certain drugs from Canada in contravention to the FFDCA." Several states (Illinois, Iowa, Maine, New Hampshire, Oregon, Vermont, and Wisconsin) have sought permission from the federal government to implement legal re-importation programs. All have been rejected, because, according to Acting FDA Commissioner Lester M. Crawford, "such state pilot projects are not authorized under current law and present added safety concerns," A HHS appointed Task Force on Prescription Drug Re-importation recommended maintaining current federal policy in this area. Although the FDA has issued several warning letters to state and local government officials, the agency has yet to prosecute cities and states implementing re-importation programs. Given limited resources and significant popular and political support during the 2004 election cycle, the agency instead chose to highlight the dangers of imported drugs through "import blitz exams" of mail shipments to U.S. consumers and inspections of medications purchased over the Internet along with enforcement actions against the "middlemen" in re-importation transactions—Internet and storefront operations that assist U.S. consumers in ordering prescription drugs from Canadian and other foreign pharmacies.

Several states, including Minnesota and Wisconsin, have gone ahead with their re-importation programs anyway. Both states have inspected participating pharmacies, signed performance agreements, and listed prices for hundreds of medications on their websites. Under the Minnesota and Wisconsin programs, residents mail or FAX prescriptions, medical history forms, and order forms to one of the three state-approved pharmacies where a licensed Canadian physician reviews the information submitted and writes new prescriptions that are shipped at prices averaging 35 percent less than U.S. price.

New Hampshire and the multistate I-SaveRx Program also link residents to state-approved pharmacies. Washington simply links residents to pharmacies approved by other states. Several local governments have also established re-importation programs, including: Springfield, MA; Boston; San Francisco; Columbia, SC; Washington, D.C.; and Montgomery County, MD. Like Washington State, most simply link residents to Canadian pharmacies that have been inspected and approved by Minnesota and Wisconsin. In August 2004, Vermont filed a lawsuit in U.S. District Court against the FDA for failing to approve its proposal to establish a pilot program covering 20,000 state employees, retirees, and their families who would be able to buy prescription drugs from Canada.

Reprinted from William Weissert and Edward Alan Miller, "Punishing the Pioneers: The Medicare Modernization Act and State Pharmacy Assistance Programs," *Publius: The Journal of Federalism*, 35, no. 1: 115–41, 2005. With permission of Oxford University Press.

for the skeptical treatment might be that unlike the budgets for other health agencies, the FDA budget is approved by the agriculture appropriations committees—thus competing for funding with crop insurance, commodity price supports, and other agricultural issues (Adams 2005b).

The FTC, OSHA, and EPA

The Federal Trade Commission was established in 1914 to prohibit unfair competition and prevent unfair and deceptive trade practices. In health, the agency battles anticompetitive restraints in the health care market and challenges false and misleading health care claims. In 1982, the FTC won a U.S. Supreme Court case upholding its regulation of physicians. For example, in 1993 the commission barred the California Dental Association from preventing certain classes of price advertising (such as discounts for senior citizens) and prohibiting the advertising of special patient services. In the 1997 BBA, after fierce provider lobbying, Congress granted antitrust protection to groups of providers who wanted to form preferred provider networks, which would function much like managed care organizations. In 2000, the FTC took on the pharmaceutical industry: it filed complaints against two drug companies for allegedly delaying the generic versions of drugs and subpoenaed records from 90 other drug companies to see whether they were using similar delaying tactics (Gerth 2000). In recent years, the FTC has been vigilant in monitoring Internet advertising of prescription drugs, bringing enforcement action when an online pharmacy makes false or misleading claims about the product or the service it provides.

The Occupational Safety and Health Administration was established in 1970 with passage of the Occupational Safety and Health Act. Its director also holds the title of assistant secretary of labor. OSHA's rulemaking power is broader than that of most other regulatory agencies. For example, OSHA can adopt temporary emergency rules outside the Administrative Procedures Act procedures, and in its first two years it was allowed to promulgate consensus industry standards as rules (Meier 1985). OSHA may undertake rulemaking processes on its own initiative or in response to an individual petition.

The Occupational Safety and Health Administration is a federal agency that Democrats love and Republicans hate. Democrats think OSHA protects working men and women, and Republicans think it targets businesses and treats them unfairly. In its early years, OSHA concentrated mainly on safety issues, until a House committee directed the agency to shift its emphasis from safety to health standards enforcement (Thompson 1983). The relationship of OSHA with Congress and businesses has been rocky. In OSHA's first six years, 100 or so bills were introduced each year that would have restricted the agency, many involving exemptions of farms and other small businesses from OSHA rules. The courts have also been engaged in agency activities. OSHA fared very poorly in the Reagan and George H. W. Bush administrations, which targeted the agency for cuts and reduction in its monitoring activity. However, under the Clinton administration, the agency stepped up its enforcement of workplace safety laws and strongly supported a major revision of the Occupational Safety and Health Act, the first since its initial passage in 1970. With the return of a Republican administration in 2001, OSHA once again became the focus of efforts to reduce its scope and reach through congressional legislation, but the effort has been unsuccessful in the Senate. OSHA has moved in recent years toward more voluntary compliance and partnership programs with small businesses, corporations, and industries, including the construction industry.

The primary regulation in the environmental area comes from the Environmental Protection Agency, which regulates air pollution, water pollution, hazardous wastes, and pesticides. During the George H. W. Bush administration, the role of developing environmental regulations was shared by the EPA and the President's Council on Competitiveness, whose purpose was to make certain that new regulations issued by the government were not unduly burdensome to business and industry or injurious to the national economy. In the case of regulations for Title V of the 1990 Clean Air Act Amendments, the council proposed more than 100 changes to the draft regulations. In 1992, President Bush ordered the EPA to make the changes in the proposed rule that were sought by the council. The resulting final rule took up 63 pages in the *Federal Register,* and industry, state, and environmental groups sued the EPA over nearly 60 parts of the rule (Bozeman and DeHart-Davis 1999).The EPA, like the FDA, is a highly visible, important agency that affects businesses, environmental proponents, energy interests, states and localities, and the general public. Under Democratic administrations, the agency often runs afoul of business and energy interests. Under Republican administrations, the critics are largely states and localities and environmentalists. According to Scheberle (2005), the rate and nature of state environmental litigation against the EPA since 2002 are remarkable. There has been an unusual number of suits and they relate to making the agency more aggressive in enforcing its own regulations on coal-fired plants or imposing new regulations on carbon dioxide emissions.

THE MANY MASTERS OF THE BUREAUCRACY

In recent years, political scientists have argued among themselves about bureaucratic accountability and control. Some (Calvert, Moran, and Weingast 1987; Fiorina 1981; Weingast and Moran 1983) argued that Congress is the real master of the bureaucracy. Its long-standing ability to authorize programs, appropriate agency funding, approve executive appointments, and monitor activities has been amplified in recent years by its tendency to micromanage the implementation of programs through detailed legislation. Thus, say these scholars, Congress is clearly chief puppeteer, holding most of the strings. A counterargument is that the president is the primary overseer of the bureaucracy, through the appointment process and budgetary and regulatory direction (Moe 1985; Rockman 1984; W. West and Cooper 1989–90). Others have argued that the existence of so many masters undercuts the power of any one and that the bureaucracy is relatively autonomous because Congress and the president are simply too busy or too bored to adequately oversee its activities (J. Wilson 1989).

Hammond and Knott (1996) concluded that there are conditions for which each argument seems to fit. One institutional actor cannot determine the policy outcome, they argued; rather, the results are the product of interactions among the president, the House, the Senate, and the congressional committees.

The Bureaucracy and Congress

Congress is important to federal agencies because it authorizes the legislation that sets up the programs, outlines the duties of the federal bureaus, and appropriates funds to carry out the programs and staff the agencies. With these laws, Congress must decide how much discretion to give agencies—whether to "hardwire" or "softwire" the process (D. Epstein and O'Halloran 1994). When Congress hardwires the program, it provides detailed directions to the agency; when it softwires, it gives the agency considerable discretion in carrying out its will. Either way, the idea is to curb bureaucratic "drift," the gradual shift of the bureaucracy's activities away from the original congressional intent.

Congress can provide oversight in two ways. In setting up the agency, key and enabling coalitions can make certain structural choices and arrangements to ensure that current and predicted future needs are met. These choices, in turn, affect the ability and willingness of future legislators to influence the administration to further their own ends (Horn 1995). This is called an *ex ante* approach. Congress can also conduct *ex post* activities that change the authorization or appropriations in ways that best suit the congressional interests of the moment. The problem with this second approach is that the transaction costs are very high. Congress might find it more efficient to set up an agency agenda "to perform like on automatic pilot," making precisely those decisions it desires (Calvert, Moran, and Weingast 1987, 500). Congress does not have to closely monitor or scrutinize agency proceedings.

We must keep in mind, however, that Congress is made up of 535 elected officials who often act in their own self-interest—apart from the institutional function of oversight. These individual choices of legislators to engage in agency oversight are less studied and understood. Hall and Miler (1999) argued that these individual actions are taken, often in the form of signals to the agency, to aid supportive interest groups. Sometimes these signals are subtle, such as letters to agency heads, and sometimes they are played out in hearings and in the press. Personalities can come into play as well. For example, Sen. Phil Gramm (R-TX), chair of the Senate Finance Committee's health subcommittee, was annoyed with the White House for not providing him with the Medicare budget projections he had requested. Gramm said he would hold up confirmations of HHS appointees until he got the numbers he had asked for. Then he lashed out at HCFA administrator Bruce Vladeck, saying he was going to make his life "miserable" (Crain Communications 1997). Congressional committees are the primary interface with federal agencies, and the interaction can be intense, confrontational, and protracted. For example, the FDA has a long history of being the target of congressional wrath, sometimes for being too lenient and sometimes for being too strident (C. M. Johnson 1992).

In 2004, Rep. Maurice Hinchey (D-NY) introduced legislation stripping $500,000 from the FDA chief counsel's office budget as punishment for the agency's assertion in a number of court proceedings that its labeling determinations preempt state law. He accused the FDA of using the courts in a "pattern of collusion between the FDA and the drug companies and medical device companies in a way that had never happened before" (quoted in Lasker 2005). The bill did not go beyond the introduction stage, but the message was sent. A final example was in 2005, when Sen. Tom Coburn (R-OK) put a hold on the nomination of Lester Crawford as commissioner of the FDA in an effort to make him obey a 2000 law that Coburn had sponsored. The law required the FDA to change condom labels to give more information on the "effectiveness or lack of the effectiveness in preventing" sexually transmitted diseases (L. Johnson 2005).

Few headlines are likely on hearings held to determine which agency is to administer a program or feasible scopes of work and timetables. But the spectacle of hapless bureaucrats cringing before an arm-waving member of Congress is inherently photogenic, and the legislator gets to take an active role in casting blame on someone else. Much of the congressional oversight fits the "fire alarm" analogy discussed in chapter 1: all it takes is one senator to become concerned about a program and press conferences will be called, hearings held, and the agency generally brought to task. In 1994, several senators were unhappy about the progress of a new program to supply vaccine to the nation's poor children. Sen. Dale Bumpers (D-AR), at a Senate Appropriations health subcommittee hearing, lambasted the CDC for assigning to the General Services Administration (GSA) the responsibility for storing the nation's supply of vaccine. The agencies' spokespersons tried to convince the senators of the safety of the plan and the competence of the GSA to manage it, but the Appropriations Committee voted to cut off funding for the program unless federal officials could prove they could safely implement it. A few weeks later, the administration scrapped the GSA warehouse and launched a private sector program to supply vaccines.

Congress often relies on agencies such as the EPA and CMS for information on proposed legislation. Lawmakers are particularly interested in the impact on costs, jobs, and other programs and how the current proposal differs from the status quo. Provision of such information is not usually major news, but it became so a few months after passage of the MMA in 2003 when, in testimony before Congress, Medicare's chief actuary recounted how the former CMS head had ordered him not to release cost estimates that were higher than the administration's public estimates (Schuler 2004a). While cost estimates are very sensitive to crucial assumptions and might understandably vary, the actuary flap provided an opportunity for Democrats to rail against the White House for misleading Congress and for Republicans to claim that such misestimation was no big deal. This does illustrate the importance of bureaucracy-generated numbers for both policy and political purposes.

Though the bureaucracy is responsive to the concerns of Congress and others, Congress is often unresponsive to the bureaucracy and unwilling to acknowledge agencies' needs and capabilities. Despite its willingness to oversee and even ridicule administrative implementation efforts, Congress does little "up front" to make certain that implementation goes smoothly. As one FDA official noted, "Comforting the bureaucracy isn't very important on the Hill" (quoted in C. M. Johnson 1992, 105). Derthick (1990), in a case study of two programs in the Social Security Administration, highlighted the congressional lack of concern over administrative problems. Congress has little interest in the capabilities of the implementing agency or department or in problems that might arise between agencies or between federal agencies and their state and local counterparts. "It does not occur to presidential and congressional participants that the law should be tailored to the limits of organizational capacity. Nor do they seriously inquire what the limits of that capacity might be" (Derthick 1990, 184). Congress changed its mind several times in the months preceding implementation of the Supplemental Security Income (SSI) program. On December 31, 1973, the day before the law was to take effect, the president signed a bill that increased benefits and changed the program for a last time before the checks were mailed. In 1997, Congress enacted the Food and Drug Administration Modernization Act, which required the FDA to initiate dozens of new administrative policies and procedural regulations. The act was seen as a sweeping reform of one of the nation's oldest public health laws and received bipartisan and industry support. Nevertheless, Congress provided no new resources to carry out the tasks set forth in the measure (Merrill 1999).

Another example of congressional lack of concern about agency capability is the 1997 BBA, which made major changes in Medicare and other health programs but without providing the implementing agency, the HCFA, with the additional resources to deal with the issues. The BBA created several new health insurance options for elderly people under Medicare; changed formulas for reimbursements to home health agencies, hospital outpatient departments, ambulances, physical therapists, nursing homes, and HMOs; and set up a major new health insurance program for children (S-CHIP). At the time of the law's enactment, the HCFA was already woefully understaffed. It was responsible for some 900 million Medicare claims, double the number of only a decade earlier. Yet over that decade, the agency had not received additional funding for administration and actually saw the number of employees decline (Pear 1998). But that did not keep Congress at bay. In oversight hearings in 1998, Rep. Bill Thomas (R-CA) told Medicare officials, "You have added a new parameter. We come up with what we believe is proper policy, often based on your recommendations. Then after it's enacted into law, you tell us you can't do it." The private sector was similarly critical. The government is "an unpredictable and uncertain partner," said Thomas D. Miller, chief executive of the Lutheran Hospital of Indiana (both quoted in Pear 1998, 24). By 1999, Congress had added more staff to the HCFA, but the dissatisfaction continued.

Sometimes Congress seems to act as though it wants its agencies to fail. Kerwin (2003) gave one example. The Department of Transportation, which was assigned the task of establishing mandatory alcohol testing for public transportation workers, was denied additional funds or personnel for that purpose. When the department sought to get another agency to loan some of its staff for the effort, the House Appropriations Committee intervened, pressuring the second agency to rescind its offer of help. Why? Congress wanted to show Transportation that it was serious when it said it would provide no more money to the agency. More recently, senators from 13 states introduced legislation in 2004 to exclude their states from a demonstration project that could affect Medicare premiums. The MMA authorized six demonstration projects combining the traditional Medicare program with private insurance plans for the purpose of determining premiums. The senators were concerned that beneficiaries who remained in traditional programs in the demonstration areas could have higher premiums than beneficiaries not in demonstration areas (Lipman 2004). Apparently, what was right for the country was not necessarily right for these senators' states—making implementation more difficult.

The Bureaucracy and the Presidency

One of the assignments given to the president in the Constitution is to make certain the laws are faithfully executed, notably by the bureaucracy. The president can do this in several ways. The first, and perhaps most important, is through the appointment of agency leadership. Second, the president has some leverage over agencies through the development of his budget—though Congress must finally dispose of the budget. The president has leverage in an agency's priorities, and its goals are expected to reflect those of the president. An agency will generally want to receive a maintenance, if not increasing, budgetary allocation, and so, with some exceptions at the individual level, the agency leadership brings its considerable weight to bear in testimony and meetings with Congress to pursue a program favored by the president. Finally, the president has leverage over agencies through the role of White House staff, particularly the Office of Management and Budget. The OMB oversees the issuance of regulations and agency policies that affect the budget.

Selection of agency heads can be difficult when strong supporters back candidates that are closely aligned with the industry regulated by the agency. Cases in point were the 2001 selection of Ann Veneman as head of the U.S. Department of Agriculture and of Linda Fisher as deputy director of the EPA. Veneman had served on the board of directors of Calgene (a company bought by Monsanto) and Fisher was the head lobbyist for Monsanto. The controversy surrounded the issue of genetically modified foods—a primary concern of Monsanto, the giant of the biotechnology industry. Genetically modified foods are in the regulatory domain of both the EPA and the FDA. The special difficulty in naming the head of the FDA was evident when it took 20 months for President George W. Bush to name an FDA director who was acceptable to all sides (Stolberg 2002a). Some presidents use agency positions to reward cronies or former campaign workers. In 2005, George W. Bush was criticized for naming political operatives with little or no experience to top posts in FEMA.

The relationship between the president and the federal bureaucracy is often adversarial, at least on the part of the president. Harry Truman was reported to have complained, "I thought I was President but when it comes to these bureaucrats, I can't do a damn thing" (Nathan 1983, 3). Richard Nixon in his second term tried to control the bureaucracy by putting Nixon loyalists in key policy-making roles in federal agencies. Ronald Reagan adopted a jigsaw puzzle management approach, whereby information was given to career bureaucrats only in pieces so they would not be able to see the larger picture (Pfiffner 1987). There has also been a trend toward installing political appointees further and further down the policy chain as a way of ensuring compliance (Rourke 1991). But there is little evidence of deliberate bureaucratic sabotage. Rather, career bureaucrats tend to want to please newly elected presidents, even those with whom they may not agree. As James Wilson (1989, 275) put it, "What is surprising is not that bureaucrats sometimes can defy the President but that they support his programs as much as they do."

Of course, presidents can take a proactive role in setting up offices and using bureaucrats to advance campaign promises or dearly held policy goals. For example, George W. Bush set up new faith-based offices in 5 federal agencies nine days after his inauguration. Subsequent executive orders added offices in 10 more agencies, each with a director and staff and with a mission to increase the capacity of faith-based organizations to compete for grants at all levels of government. Administrative rules were issued to overturn restrictions on religious institutions receiving federal dollars, on the use of government money to build and renovate places of worship, and on using religious beliefs as a criterion for recruiting and retaining staff (Gais and Fossett 2005).

Once a measure becomes law, the president's interest often wanes. Only on rare occasions will the president get involved in writing regulations or other implementation processes—for example, when a regulation is controversial, highly valued by an important interest-group ally, or potentially counter to other goals, such as cost cutting. There are some exceptions, however. Jimmy Carter, in 1978, concerned about inflation, ordered a weakening of the regulations protecting workers from cotton dust (Thompson 1983, 22). Similarly, the Reagan and Bush administrations of the 1980s were concerned about the impact of environmental and health regulations on businesses. President Clinton took on implementation of S-CHIP as a major focus—meeting with governors, setting up high-level interagency task forces, using the media to highlight the importance of the issue, and offering technical assistance to states in signing up children for S-CHIP and Medicaid.

Although the bureaucracy is clearly in the domain of the president, savvy bureaucrats cultivate congressional leaders of both parties. "Every program I had was bipartisan," said former HHS secretary Donna Shalala. "I was passionate about supporting the President's policies but I was bipartisan in administering the department" (CMS 2005).

The Bureaucracy and the Courts

The judiciary plays an important role in bureaucratic policy making, a relationship that Judge David Bazelon called "an involuntary partnership" (Rosenbloom 1981, 31). The courts oversee bureaucratic actions to make certain they are not violating due process, legislative intent, individual liberties, or equal protection of the law. Many regulatory agencies spend years developing legal theories, collecting data, and preparing analyses that will stand up in court (W. West 1984).

In the past decade, courts have stepped up their oversight of administrative regulatory decisions, often questioning both the process and the substance of administrative activities, abandoning their traditional deference to bureaucratic expertise. One example is a 1999 U.S. Court of Appeals ruling that prevented the EPA from implementing the clean air standards it had established two years earlier. The three-judge panel found that the EPA was violating the delegation of power by making policy and usurping the authority of Congress (Judis 1999).

The courts are also concerned with what Rand Rosenblatt (1993, 439) called "rights-enforcing roles," a tendency to consider recipients' entitlement to benefits as a right rather than a privilege that may be withdrawn or diminished at any time. This emphasis on beneficiaries' rights has led to greater concern about the use of agency discretion over Medicaid, cash assistance, housing assistance, and other federal programs and to more specific court guidelines for action. In 1999, the U.S. Court of Appeals for the Ninth Circuit upheld a lower court finding that Medicare beneficiaries have a constitutional right to receive written notices and hearings on any denial of medical services. Apart from the intrusiveness of the courts in daily management issues, these decisions usually cost governments money, often millions of dollars. In this case, the Clinton administration argued that the appeals process required by the district court could impose significant administrative and financial burdens on health plans, raising costs by $4.70 per person per month, for a total of $343 per year (Pear 1999).

One of the most far-reaching court cases affecting the administration of a health program, and one costing states a great deal of money, was *Wilder v. Virginia Hospital Association*. In this 1990 U.S. Supreme Court case, the Court found that hospitals and nursing homes were the intended beneficiaries of the Medicaid law and had standing to sue in court. The case reaffirmed the rights-affirming role adopted by earlier courts but surprised many observers by extending standing to providers. The statute also "creates a 'binding obligation' on a government agency to do something" (R. E. Rosenblatt 1993, 459). Following the Supreme Court's lead, courts in a number of states, including Washington, New York, and Michigan, found state reimbursements were less than "reasonable and adequate" and ordered higher state spending, totaling $70 million per year in Michigan alone. Other state agencies settled out of court with nursing homes and hospitals, at a cost to Oregon, for example, of $65 million over two years. (The federal provision initiating these cases, known as the Boren Amendment, was repealed in 1997 as part of the BBA.)

One criticism of this increased judicial activity, also dubbed "imperial judiciary" (Glazer 1975), is that court mandates have come to dominate federal and state agency activities, particularly for those agencies most likely to be sued in court. The EPA, for example, must choose among competing priorities, and, with few exceptions, court mandates take top priority, even ahead of congressional directives. O'Leary (1989) concluded that courts have reduced the discretion, autonomy, power, and authority of EPA administrators. She also concluded that the emphasis on responding to courts increases the power and authority of attorneys within the EPA while decreasing the power and authority of scientists.

For the states, one of the most troublesome court rulings concerns the interpretation of the federal Employee Retirement Income Security Act. The courts have ruled that the 1974 law preempts state laws that relate to employee benefit plans, including their health coverage. However, recent court cases have narrowed the sweep of the ERISA preemption, making it clear that ERISA does not preempt all types of state health care legislation. A Supreme Court case in 2004 was a setback in some ways. The Court overturned a Texas law that allowed enrollees of HMOs and other insurers to sue in state court, claiming that ERISA preempts the state law (Butler 2004).

Agencies are not simply victims of the courts; they also use the courts to uphold their pronouncements or punish those who violate federal regulations. The EPA, for example, has brought civil suits against companies that fail to comply with the Clean Air Act. Some state agencies use the courts to get increased funding from their legislatures (Rosenberg 1991). If agency directors' pleas for more money for a program fall on deaf ears in the legislative appropriations process, they may encourage a court order mandating spending to ameliorate the situation with the needed funds.

Is There a Winner?

Some scholars have pointed out that in recent years, the federal agency role in intergovernmental relations has increased and Congress's role has decreased. Probably nowhere is that illustrated more than in health, where federal agencies are actively engaged with the states to implement positions that are not always in line with congressional wishes. The EPA staff is engaged with states in negotiating performance indicators; the HHS staff determines whether states have met performance standards, and which deserve bonuses and which sanctions. The CMS has been criticized for not stopping states from "gaming" Medicaid through what is known as Medicaid maximization strategies and for allowing states to use waivers to spend Medicaid and S-CHIP dollars on adults who should not be eligible under the law. The CMS has encouraged states to enact waivers and is highly engaged in their negotiation. The Clinton and George W. Bush administrations have strongly encouraged the use of waivers—to the point that little legislative change is needed; states can make the adjustments they desire by working with federal bureaucrats. Thus, according to Gais and Fossett (2005, 510), "Waivers also allow presidents to pursue controversial policy goals without seeking approval from a slow and divisive legislative process." These authors also note that waivers allow a president to help political friends (and punish enemies) and neutralize congressional scrutiny by encouraging state delegations to support their states' waiver requests.

THE HEALTH BUREAUCRACY

The primary health agency in the federal government is the Department of Health and Human Services, and at least 15 other federal agencies have health care–related outlays. In 2005, HHS's budget was more than $543 billion (excluding Social Security), of which more than 90 percent was spent on health (OMB 2005). Federal health spending accounts for nearly one-fourth of total federal spending, up from 3 percent in 1965 and 12 percent in 1981 (table 4.1). HHS administers the two largest categories shown in table 4.1—Medicare and Medicaid—and most of the "all other" category, which includes everything from the federal employees' health program (which HHS does not administer) to maternal and child health, information technology, programs directed to rural areas and public hospitals, and immunizations and epidemiology.

The oldest federal health agency is the Public Health Service, whose lineage dates back to the 1798 Marine Hospital Service. It became the PHS in 1912.

Table 4.1
Federal Health Spending in 1965, 1981, 1993, and 2004

	Spending (billions of dollars)			
	1965	1981	1993	2004
Federal health spending, total	3.1	77.8	259.9	566.6
Medicare*	—	39.2	130.6	269.4
Medicaid	0.3	16.8	75.8	176.2
Veterans	1.3	7.0	14.8	26.8
Defense health	—	4.8	15.2	30.4
All other	1.5	10	23.5	63.8
	Spending (percent)			
Health spending as percentage of total federal spending	2.6	11.5	18.4	24.7
Federal health spending as percentage of gross domestic product	0.4	2.5	4.0	4.9

Source: Data from the Budget of the United States Government, Fiscal Year 2006 (OMB 2005).
*The Medicare numbers reflect the net after paid premiums.

The agency was originally concerned with the provision of medical care to merchant seaman and later took over the responsibility for quarantining those with infectious and communicable diseases. The PHS is no longer a department within HHS but a unit under the Assistant Secretary for Health (see the organizational chart of HHS, fig. 4.1). Other early federal health agencies were the National Hygienic Laboratory, established in 1887 (which became the National Institutes of Health in 1930); the Food and Drug Administration, established by law in 1907; and the Children's Bureau, established in 1912. These early agencies were primarily concerned with public health. The interest in children's issues—evidenced by establishment of the Children's Bureau and passage of the Sheppard-Towner Act of 1922, providing funding to states for personal health services to pregnant women and to children—was a turning point in the federal government's duties and responsibilities, a turn away from public health and toward personal health services.

Until the 1950s the United States had no overall, comprehensive health agency but rather departments operating independently, reporting to Congress and the White House. The Department of Health, Education, and Welfare was created in 1953. President Truman had attempted to create this consolidated agency for several years but had been thwarted by interest groups, including the American Medical Association. The AMA agreed not to oppose HEW when President Eisenhower promised that the government would "stay out of medical affairs" and that the AMA could choose the department's special assistant for medical affairs (R. Harris 1966, 65).

The Health Care Financing Administration was created in 1977 to combine Medicare and Medicaid under one administrative agency. In 1980, HEW became the Department of Health and Human Services, when the Department of Education was created. Today's HHS has a workforce of more than 65,000 people and is made up of 11 major line agencies, each with a set of programs authorized in legislation. They range from the large and highly visible—including the Centers for Medicare and Medicaid Services, the Food and Drug Administration, and the National Institutes of Health—to those less well-known to the public and to Congress, such as the Agency for Healthcare Research and Quality, the Substance Abuse and Mental Health Services Administration, and the Health Resources and Services Administration (HRSA). The largest of these agencies is the CMS (until 2001 the HCFA); it oversees the Medicare and Medicaid programs, which provide benefits for more than 85 million people and, with the HRSA, runs the Children's Health Insurance Program.

Although the CMS is the largest of the agencies within HHS, it is also the one most disliked by Congress and the president. In part this is because of

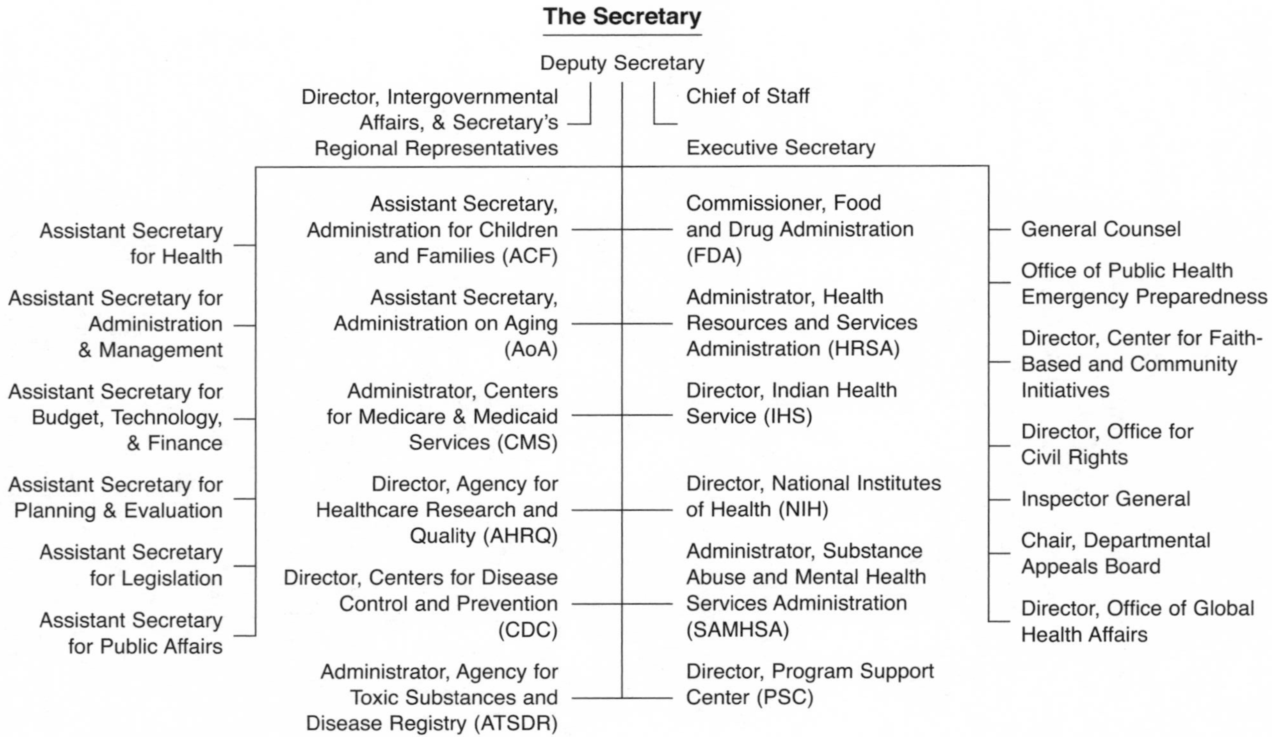

The Secretary

Deputy Secretary

Chief of Staff

Executive Secretary

Director, Intergovernmental Affairs, & Secretary's Regional Representatives

- Assistant Secretary for Health
- Assistant Secretary for Administration & Management
- Assistant Secretary for Budget, Technology, & Finance
- Assistant Secretary for Planning & Evaluation
- Assistant Secretary for Legislation
- Assistant Secretary for Public Affairs

- Assistant Secretary, Administration for Children and Families (ACF)
- Assistant Secretary, Administration on Aging (AoA)
- Administrator, Centers for Medicare & Medicaid Services (CMS)
- Director, Agency for Healthcare Research and Quality (AHRQ)
- Director, Centers for Disease Control and Prevention (CDC)
- Administrator, Agency for Toxic Substances and Disease Registry (ATSDR)

- Commissioner, Food and Drug Administration (FDA)
- Administrator, Health Resources and Services Administration (HRSA)
- Director, Indian Health Service (IHS)
- Director, National Institutes of Health (NIH)
- Administrator, Substance Abuse and Mental Health Services Administration (SAMHSA)
- Director, Program Support Center (PSC)

- General Counsel
- Office of Public Health Emergency Preparedness
- Director, Center for Faith-Based and Community Initiatives
- Director, Office for Civil Rights
- Inspector General
- Chair, Departmental Appeals Board
- Director, Office of Global Health Affairs

Figure 4.1.
The Organization of the U.S. Department of Health and Human Services.
Source: Health and Human Services, Department of, 2005b.

the arcane rules that surround Medicare and Medicaid. "The legislation . . . for HCFA, is essentially flawed," said Donna Shalala, former head of HHS. "It's contradictory, it's rigid, and they [Congress and the president] blamed HCFA for what was a bad piece of legislation" (CMS 2005).

Though some view the bureaucracy as an unchanging leviathan, nothing could be farther from the truth. In the past four years, HHS has added an office of public health emergency preparedness, office of global health, and Center for Faith-Based and Community Initiatives. As table 4.2 illustrates, the health bureaucracy changed with some regularity over a 40-year period, with consolidations, reorganizations, and agency elimination regularly reframing the bureaucracy over time.

Table 4.2
Chronicle of Bureaucratic Change: A Sample of Activity, 1965–2005

Year	Action
1966	National Institute of Mental Health (NIMH) becomes independent of other NIH institutes
1968	HEW reorganized from eight operating agencies to six
	Health Services and Mental Health Administration (HSMHA) and Social and Rehabilitative Services (SRS) created
	PHS broken into three units
	PHS removed from the surgeon general to the assistant secretary for health and scientific affairs
	NIMH becomes part of the HSMHA
	Consumer Protection and Environmental Health Service (CPEHS) established within HEW
	FDA placed under CPEHS
1970	CPEHS eliminated
	Environmental Health Service (EHS) created
	FDA restored to operating agency status
1972–73	EHS disbanded
1973–74	Major reorganization of HEW
	NIH, FDA, CDC (Communicable Disease Center, established 1946), Health Resources Administration (HRA), and Health Services Administration (HSA) subsumed under PHS, which is under Assistant Secretary of Health and Scientific Affairs (ASHSA)
	SRS and Social Security Administration (SSA) remain autonomous and report directly to HEW secretary
	HSMHA divided into three parts: CDC, combining CDC and National Institute for Occupational Safety and Health (NIOSH); HRA; and HSA
	NIMH renamed Alcohol, Drug Abuse, and Mental Health Administration (ADAMHA)

Table 4.2 *(cont.)*

1977	HCFA created by taking Medicare and Medicaid financing away from SSA and SRS
	PHS financing responsibilities given to HCFA
1980	HEW split into HHS and Department of Education
1982	HRA and HSA combined into Health Resources and Services Administration (HRSA)
1983	Agency for Toxic Substances and Disease Registry (ATSDR) created
	Prospective Payment Assessment Commission (ProPAC) created
1986	Physician Payment Review Commission (PPRC) created
1989	Agency for Health Care Policy and Research (AHCPR) created, subsuming the National Center for Health Services Research
1995	ATSDR. FDA, HRSA, Indian Health Service (IHS), NIH, and SAMHSA reorganized, each as separate operating divisions within the Public Health Service
1997	ProPAC and PPRC combined to create the Medicare Payment Advisory Commission (MedPAC)
1998	AHCPR renamed Agency for Healthcare Research and Quality (AHRQ) and mission defined as research to improve the quality of health care, reduce its cost, and broaden access to essential services
	CDC renamed Centers for Disease Control and Prevention
2000	National Institute of Biomedical Imaging and Bioengineering created as part of NIH
2001	HCFA renamed Centers for Medicare and Medicaid Services

Source: National Archives and Records Administration, various years.

Note: All abbreviations not spelled out in the table are included in the book's abbreviations list.

Among the federal health agencies, the CMS is by far the biggest spender, by itself accounting for outlays of more than $448 billion in fiscal year 2004 for Medicare, Medicaid, S-CHIP grants to states, fraud and abuse control, and administrative expenses. The distant second in health agency spending is the NIH, the principal biomedical research agency of the government, with appropriations of nearly $28 billion in fiscal year 2004 (OMB 2005). The NIH is made up of 27 institutes and centers, listed along with their dates of establishment in table 4.3.

The National Cancer Institute receives the most funding, some $4.7 billion in 2005; the National Institute of Nursing Research, one of the newest, received only $134 million in that year, though it surpassed the even newer National Center for Complementary and Alternative Medicine, funded at just $117 million. The National Institute of Mental Health was funded at $1.4 billion; the National Eye Institute, $653 million; and the National Institute on Deafness and Other Communication Disorders, $382 million (NIH 2005).

The National Cancer Institute is the oldest institute, created in 1937, predating the formation of the NIH by seven years. Its organization is more

Table 4.3
Institutes and Centers within the National Institutes of Health,
by Date of Establishment

1937–50

National Cancer Institute (1937)

Center for Scientific Research (1946)

National Heart, Lung, and Blood Institute (1948)

National Institute of Allergy and Infectious Diseases (1948)

National Institute of Diabetes and Digestive and Kidney Diseases (1948)

National Institute of Dental and Craniofacial Research (1948)

National Institute of Mental Health (1949)

National Institute of Neurological Disorders and Stroke (1950)

1951–70

NIH Clinical Center (1953)

National Library of Medicine (1956)

National Institute of Child Health and Human Development (1962)

National Institute of General Medical Sciences (1962)

National Center for Research Resources (1962)

Center for Information Technology (1964)

John E. Fogarty International Center (1968)

National Eye Institute (1968)

National Institute of Environmental Health Sciences (1969)

National Institute on Alcohol Abuse and Alcoholism (1970)

1971–90

National Institute on Drug Abuse (1973)

National Institute on Aging (1974)

National Institute of Arthritis and Musculoskeletal and Skin Diseases (1986)

National Institute of Nursing Research (1986)

National Institute on Deafness and Other Communication Disorders (1988)

National Human Genome Research Institute (1989)

1991–2005

National Center on Minority Health and Health Disparities (1993)

National Center for Complementary and Alternative Medicine (1999)

National Institute of Biomedical Imaging and Bioengineering (2000)

Source: National Institutes of Health 2005.

autonomous than that of the other institutes, with the director reporting directly to the president, through the OMB, bypassing the NIH director and HHS secretary (S. Epstein 1979). The unusual organizational system was put in place by 1971 federal legislation launching a national effort to cure cancer. As Samuel Epstein noted in *The Politics of Cancer,* the effort was sold to Congress in a campaign that claimed the cure for cancer was imminent and only a massively funded national effort was needed to conquer the disease by America's 200th birthday. The National Cancer Institute's autonomy was so important that it should be "removed from the 'bureaucracy' of NIH" and be free to find the cure for cancer (Epstein 1979, 326). This organization suited President Nixon, who was suspicious of federal agencies and preferred a direct relationship with the rejuvenated and well-funded agency. The National Cancer Institute remains the only institute directly accountable to the president. The cure for cancer still evades us.

One of the most recent changes in the federal health agencies was the recasting and restructuring of the National Center for Health Services Research, first, in 1989, into the Agency for Health Care Policy and Research, with a new mission, then in 1999 into the Agency for Healthcare Research and Quality (AHRQ), again with a new mission. The AHCPR was formed to showcase and more generously fund health services research on the outcomes of diagnostic and therapeutic interventions. One of its most controversial concerns was the development of clinical practice guidelines, a task that soon ran into political problems when the agency issued a set of guidelines for the public in December 1994 that said, in effect, that most of the back surgery performed in the United States was unnecessary. In 1996, the agency ended its clinical guidelines program.

The new agency title, AHRQ, includes the word *quality* to highlight its new responsibility to coordinate all federal quality-improvement efforts and health services research, and it drops *policy,* which the agency thought created the misconception that it determined federal health care policies and regulations. The agency's restated mission is "to improve the quality, safety, efficiency, and effectiveness of health care for all Americans" (AHRQ 2006).

In 2001, the Health Care Financing Administration changed its name to the Centers for Medicare and Medicaid Services, reflecting more clearly the major programs under the agency's domain.

CONCLUSION

In the United States, unlike in many other countries, a life of public service in the executive branch has never been highly regarded. Rather, bureaucrats are often the butt of jokes, cartoons, and snide remarks from friends, family, and customers. Nevertheless, bureaucrats are key actors in forming, implementing, and evaluating policy in health as in almost every other area of public concern. Bureaucrats provide the expertise and institutional history that are essential to Congress and the presidency, which may have ideas but little sense of how they might actually work in the real world.

The linkage that bureaucrats provide between truth and power is essential. Nevertheless, the health bureaucracy, like its legislative and presidential counterparts in other areas, is suffering under a public skepticism about government and government programs. Its role as scapegoat, especially useful to members of Congress, state legislators, and presidential candidates, has hurt the health bureaucracy in the public's perception. Many people worry that the unattractiveness of the public sector will repel the best and brightest young people and lead to a weakening of government expertise. With so many baby boomers nearing retirement, these concerns may be realized very soon.

In health, bureaucrats have helped draft major legislation such as Medicare and Medicaid, have offered solutions such as diagnosis-related groups (DRGs), and have been responsible for implementing every national health program since 1887. They regulate the operation of the health care industry, safeguard the health of the nation's workplaces, and protect consumers from unsafe foods and drugs. At the state level, they oversee the insurance industry, license health care professionals, and monitor provider services and facilities. Bureaucrats work closely with Congress, the president, and interest groups but are also policy actors in their own right, with their own preferences and goals, their own expertise and political support. Federal bureaucrats are also key intergovernmental actors, working closely with state and local officials and nonprofit groups to achieve policy goals and allocate funding. Some scholars contend that this component of bureaucratic power has strengthened in recent years with increased use of waivers, rules, demonstration projects, and selected interpretations of congressional direction. Gais and Fossett (2005) worry that what they call "executive federalism" can use these tools to pursue presidential goals and build coalitions with political friends at the state level in a way that exploits state differences and political ties to the detriment of broader intergovernmental effectiveness.

Yet the wide availability of expertise, the technological advances that allow members of Congress to obtain data quickly and in an accessible form, the proliferation of specialized health lobbies armed with detailed information and technical analyses, the difficulties in attracting smart new employees, and budgetary constraints—all may adversely affect a stronger bureaucratic role in policy making.

Political partisans have long recognized the importance of bureaucracy but have often attempted to work around or ignore what they cannot control. Scandals that give rise to questions about the independence of federal agencies from political interests and interest groups are troubling markers of what may be an undermining of the public's and Congress's faith in public servants working in Washington and around the country.

5

States and Health Care Reform

A LOOK BACK

1965

IN THE early 1960s, state governance was largely embarrassing. Governors were generally elected every two years or were allowed only one four-year term, and they had little power when they did assume office. Thanks to citizens' concerns about vesting too much power in a few persons, states had successfully spread decision making over a spate of agencies, commissions, and boards that were not directly accountable to anyone. When Daniel Evans, on taking office as governor of Washington in 1965, called a cabinet meeting, 60 people came (Sanford 1967). Legislatures were even more poorly prepared to deal with state problems. Legislative pay was a pittance, there were no or very few staff members, and the legislature was in session for only a few days every other year. Many states were run by special interests. In some states, railroad interests dominated; in others it was power companies or racetracks, oil or insurance companies.

Cities were often ignored by legislatures composed largely of members representing rural parts of the state. In 1960, more than six million people lived in Los Angeles County and fewer than 15,000 lived in a rural county in northern California's mountains, yet each was represented by one state senator. In Vermont, a town with a population of 38 had the same representation as the city of Burlington, with 35,531. Translated into legislative control, 11 percent of the people in California could control the state senate; 12 percent of the people in Vermont could control the state house of representatives (Grant and Omdahl 1993). The reason for this maldistribution was twofold. First, many states had not changed their legislative district lines, or redistricted, for decades. In 1963, 27 states had not redistricted their legislatures in 25 years, and 8 states had not redistricted in more than 50 years (Sanford 1967). The Vermont house had not redistricted since 1793. Second, many states copied the federal legislative model, with an upper house based on geographic units; the obvious geographic units were counties, and states often assigned one senator for each county.

State officials often ignored the problems inherent in states' legislative structures. As Sanford (1967, 35, 36–37) put it, "The states . . . have failed to advance with their citizens into the modern world . . . When twentieth-century growth began to overtake us, the machinery of state government was outmoded, revenue resources were outstripped, and the state executive was denied the tools of leadership long supplied the President of the United States."

Despite their lackluster leadership, states were key players in health in the early 1960s, serving as the primary providers of mental health and (with local government) public health services. By 1965, change was in the air. States were scrambling to reapportion their legislative bodies to respond to the U.S. Supreme Court decisions in *Baker v. Carr* (1962) and *Reynolds v. Simms* (1964), which applied the principle of one person, one vote, to both houses of every state legislature. In 1967, more than half the states had constitutional revisions on their ballots to reorganize the legislature, make changes in the executive branch, improve the judicial branch, and change the relationship between the state and local governments.

Between 1965 and 1975, states underwent a remarkable transformation. Their legislative, judicial, and executive offices became vibrant and responsive. Their state employees were energized, and state capitols became places where exciting programs were launched and carried out, thus attracting many of the brightest and best young people to Albany, Lansing, and Tallahassee. Changes were made in state constitutions to unshackle local government and to balance the state's tax system so it would weather economic difficulties and maintain equity among its citizenry. States began to tackle the tough issues they had often avoided in previous years—from the environment to economic development, from education reform to controlling health care costs.

1981

By the start of the 1980s, state legislatures had greatly improved their staffing and more adequately represented all citizens of the state. The legislatures had more women and minorities and, compared with the 1960s, greater partisan competition, with Republicans picking up seats in the South and Democrats in the North. There was a tremendous jump in the number of women serving in state legislatures between 1969 and 1980, from a total of about 300 to nearly 800 (S. Patterson 1983). Membership in legislatures for ethnic and racial minority groups also increased during this time, although their proportion of all legislators was small—about 4 percent. State after state strengthened the powers granted to governors, giving them stronger budgetary authority, longer terms of office, and the ability to serve multiple terms, to appoint more cabinet members, and to have a strong line-item veto (Beyle 1989). Overall, states had made a remarkable, though not widely heralded, recovery in their ability to deal with tough problems. Indeed, in the mid-1980s, the Advisory Commission on Intergovernmental Relations (ACIR 1985, 364) described states as moving from fallen arches to arch supports of the system. The ACIR noted that states were "more representative, more responsive, more activist and more professional in their operations than they ever have been."

Furthermore, states were becoming the sources of innovative policies, particularly in health. In the 1970s and 1980s, states became concerned about the rapidly increasing costs of health care to their budgets and instituted reforms such as rate-setting systems, negotiated contracting, and diagnosis-related groups. They also adopted risk pools for health insurance, right-to-die acts, and mandatory seat belt laws.

1993

The makeup of state legislatures in 1993 was much more representative of the population in gender and occupation than in earlier decades. More than 20 percent of the 7,424 state legislators were women—five times as many as in the 1960s (Thaemert 1994). In five states—Arizona, Colorado, New Hampshire, Vermont, and Washington—women held more than one-third of the legislative seats. In others, women were still somewhat rare. In Alabama, Kentucky, Louisiana, Oklahoma, and Pennsylvania, women made up less than 10 percent of the total (the percentage of U.S. Congress members that were women in 1993). But overall, compared with the U.S. House of Representatives and with previous years in the states, female representation in state legislatures in 1994 was greatly enhanced (table 5.1). State legislatures had fewer attorneys, business owners, and farmers than in the 1960s and more legislators whose legislative service was a full-time job. Some 15 percent of all state legislators were full-time—up from 3 percent in 1976.

In 1992, a sitting governor was elected to the presidency—the first time since Governor Franklin Roosevelt was elected in 1932. Bill Clinton, governor of Arkansas, not only understood state governance but also was actively involved as a spokesperson for states through the National Governors Association (NGA), which he had headed and for which he served as leader in the development of several policy positions—including those on welfare reform and health care.

States had become increasingly active players in the health care field. Ideas discussed in Washington, D.C., in 1993–94 were already in place in several innovative states; other states were considering ideas such as a single-payer system, generally viewed as too radical for national consideration. The role of states in health care reform was more than a parochial concern; it was a central issue in congressional hearings, news conferences, and Sunday morning television talk shows. Washington clearly could not monitor and implement the program on its own. It needed states.

Table 5.1

Women Serving in U.S. Congress and Senate,
as Percentage of Legislators, 1975–2005

	1975	1981	1994	2000	2005
U.S. House	4.4	4.4	11.0	12.9	15.0
U.S. Senate	0	2.0	6.0	9.0	14.0
State houses	9.3	14.0	21.8	23.5	23.3
State senates	4.5	7.0	17.3	20.0	20.3

Sources: Ornstein, Mann, and Malbin 2002; Center for American Women and Politics, Eagleton Institute of Politics, Rutgers University; *CQ Weekly,* Jan. 31, 2005.

2005

In 2005, most states were emerging from several fiscally difficult years during which demands from citizens had outstripped the revenues coming into state coffers. In 2002–4, states found themselves cutting back on programs—including one of the largest, Medicaid—and sometimes adding new taxes on their citizens. But the economy improved in 2005, and states looked once again at ways to help provide health insurance to their citizens, protect their public health operations from possible bioterrorist attack, and improve their health infrastructure and citizens' access to it.

Although the president was a former governor—the fourth of the past five presidents—states saw little immediate benefit. Domestic spending was a target of cuts as the president sought to reduce taxes and to wage an expensive war on terrorism at home and abroad. In areas ranging from medical malpractice to environmental protection, Washington, D.C., proposed preemptive legislation and even came up with new ways to "make states pay" for their own innovations.

Perhaps because of the national threat to federalism, governors, state legislators, and state attorneys general were active political players, leading the way in areas where Washington could not come to an agreement—regulation of managed care, medical malpractice, controlling drug costs, curtailing greenhouse gases, to name a few. States moved ahead with policies while Congress continued to argue. Finally, in the early years of the new millennium, the U.S. Supreme Court followed the pattern of earlier years and issued a series of decisions that favored state sovereignty and constrained federal power. Medicaid reform was again a top concern for the NGA and for other groups as federal cuts in the massive program loomed. States pursued new waivers in Medicaid to find ways to both cover the uninsured and hold down costs—a difficult, if not impossible, task.

While academics and pundits continued to argue about why a universal health policy was more desirable than individual state actions to cover the health needs of their own citizens, states continued to act. Even under fiscal duress, Utah and Maine, for example, came up with innovative programs to expand health care coverage, often working with the private sector. Other states, such as Florida, came up with ambitious plans to revamp Medicaid by providing recipients with a voucher-type program that would be managed without state bureaucratic direction. Still other states targeted clean air and clean water and quietly implemented programs that in some cases were more stringent than tough international protocols. As Washington, D.C., continued to amass federal deficits and cut domestic programs, the states responded to their citizens and learned from each other.

OVERVIEW

States have a broad role in health. One analyst called the scope of state activities in the health area "truly awesome and capable of reaching into almost every facet of health care delivery" (Clarke 1981, 61). States are responsible for the funding and coordination of public health functions, the financing and delivery of personal health services (including Medicaid, mental health, public hospitals, and health departments), environmental protection, regulation of providers of medical care and the technology they employ, regulation of the sale of health insurance, and the state's rate setting, licensing, and cost control. States provide health insurance for their own employees and retirees and play a pivotal role in educating and credentialing health care professionals.

State institutions are similar to national entities in their structure and purpose. However, several differences are important in understanding why state and federal policies can be so divergent, including, at the state level, direct democracy, the requirement for a balanced budget, and the very muted role of the press in state capitols. States differ from one another in very significant ways, including in their willingness to enact innovative legislation and in their implementation of Medicaid programs. In recent years, states have provided innovative solutions to a wide range of health problems yet are constrained by federal law from making some changes (especially by the Employee Retirement Income Security Act, which limits states' ability to make comprehensive state reforms).

FEDERALISM AND INTERGOVERNMENTAL RELATIONS

To understand states and health policy, one must understand federalism and the intergovernmental relations that define states' roles and responsibilities in health and other areas.

In its earliest years, the United States was governed by the Articles of Confederation, which set up a weak national government and strong states. The national body (unicameral, with equal representation from the states) had no power to tax, enter into commercial treaties, retaliate against discriminatory foreign trade policies, or enforce the provisions of existing treaties. Congress relied on states to act, and it needed state cooperation to discharge any functions. There was no national government, but rather the United States "consisted solely in the congregation of envoys from the separate states for the accommodation of certain specified matters under terms prescribed by the federal treaty" (Diamond 1985, 30). The states issued their own money and had their own trade policies with other states. When there were interstate disagreements, Congress was virtually powerless to deal with them.

While acknowledging that the confederation did not work, the delegates to the Constitutional Convention of 1789 were not yet ready to establish a fully national government. They compromised in the wording of the Constitution, which divides responsibilities between the two levels of government. Certain functions, such as interstate commerce and national defense, were assigned to the national government; others, such as the selection of presidential electors who would choose the president, were left to states. The strongest language in favor of states came in the Tenth Amendment: "powers not delegated to the United States by the Constitution, nor prohibited by it to the states, are reserved to the states respectively, or to the people." Yet the Constitution authorizes the national Congress to "provide for the general welfare" and to "make all Laws which shall be necessary and proper" for executing this and other powers given to the legislature. The commerce clause is also crucial: anything defined as interstate commerce, or crossing state lines, is in the federal domain. Finally, the supremacy clause clearly states that if federal and state laws are incompatible, the federal law prevails.

Federalism was the key means by which the Founding Fathers sought to ensure that power was not concentrated in one set of government officials. Instead they wanted to establish a balance of powers so that one level of government would have a "check" against the undue power of another. They set up a system of government in which both governments were sovereign and powerful. As James Madison described it, "The federal and State governments are in fact but different agents and trustees of the people, constituted with different powers and designed for different purposes" (Publius [1787–88] 1961, 294).

The broad parameters allocating powers between the national and state governments soon led to the important role of the courts in defining those powers. The first major decision on this, *McCullough v. Maryland* (1819), was made when Maryland leaders questioned the power of the federal government to establish a national bank in Baltimore, a power not specifically listed in the Constitution. This celebrated decision established the notion of "implied powers": the national government was not limited to those powers clearly outlined in the Constitution; Congress could also become involved in areas that were "implied" in such vague phrases as "providing for the general welfare" or "necessary and proper." By so broadly construing the intent of the Constitution, the Supreme Court allowed the responsibilities of the federal government to encompass a broad array of activities and programs. Until the 1990s, the Court generally came down strongly on the side of the federal government.

An important point to keep in mind about federalism is that it is a system of rules for the division of public policy responsibilities among a number of autonomous government entities (Anton 1989). In the United States, these entities are the national and state governments. The autonomous nature of the relationship is crucial: states are not administrative units of Washington, D.C.; rather, they have their own responsibilities and duties, many of them overlapping those of Washington. The relationship was once described as cooperative federalism, with federal and state governments interacting to achieve common goals. The metaphor commonly used is of a marble cake, with the government units representing the halves of the cake and programmatic activities, such as education, welfare, and health, "marbling" through them.

The states were the dominant actors in federalism in the country's first century. With the Civil War came a nationalizing effect, expanded later during Franklin Roosevelt's New Deal and still further by Lyndon Johnson's Great Society. States had become key actors in implementing an activist federal domestic agenda, largely thanks to federal grants that provided incentives for state action in social programs, transportation, urban development, special education, community development, and job training.

Ronald Reagan, in his vision of "New Federalism," preferred a different view of the relationship between federal and state governments. His call for a sorting out of responsibilities, whereby the national government would handle only those functions purely national and the states would handle most other areas, was similar to dual federalism, a system with another cake metaphor: a layer cake, one layer representing the responsibilities of one government, the other layer those of the other government, with little cross-layer mingling. The models differ in the extensiveness of the federal role; they share the view, established in the Constitution, of state sovereignty.

Federalism has another important policy strength: improving the possibility of policy innovation. States can try out new ideas and techniques or philosophies that, if successful, can later be adopted by other states or on a national scale. Indeed, states are regularly referred to as the "laboratories of democracy." Compared with the federal government, states' smaller size and proximity to the people make them proving grounds for innovations in policy and governance. Moreover, the likelihood of finding a significant innovation is greater with 50 different states devising different policy programs than if we relied on the action of one federal government.

The important role of states is established in the U.S. Constitution and ratified by history. As in most dynamic relationships, changes occur over time. In the 1960s and 1970s, Washington was very strong and states rather weak in capacity and resources. In the 1980s and 1990s, the federal government was fiscally constrained with a $3 trillion budget debt, while the states were reasonably fiscally secure and administratively capable of taking on problems, including health care. In the early years of the twenty-first century, states were constrained by falling revenues and increasing demands, while Congress, free from pay-as-you-go budget restraints, reduced taxes and increased defense and homeland security spending, and ignored calls for Medicaid reform and fiscal relief.

Congress and the president cannot "make" states do anything. However, they can provide incentives through federal grants, or punish states that do not act in a desired way by withdrawing federal dollars, or simply preempt state actions. Preemption must be based on some constitutional purpose such as interstate commerce or protecting the public welfare. And preemption is increasingly being used, even by a conservative Congress and president.

Federal Grants

During the nation's first century, government at any level did very little. The people did not particularly want government services, and governments had few taxes through which to raise the resources to provide services. The federal government's role was largely restricted to "war and danger" and some limited pork-barrel funding. States were more active, particularly in economic development activities: they built roads and bridges, dredged canals, set forth civil and property rights and family and criminal laws, and provided education (D. B. Walker 2000). For the federal government, a turning point was the imposition of the income tax in 1913; finally, it had resources. And with the coming of the New Deal, Franklin Roosevelt's effort at overcoming the Depression, it also had a cause. The federal government wanted to help citizens find jobs and bring home a salary, setting them on the road to financial recovery. Yet it could not do this solely from Washington. Rather, it was easier for Washington to give grants to states and localities so they could provide the services. Thus, in the 1930s, began the age of the federal grant. Between 1933 and 1938, 16 federal grant programs were enacted.

Not until the 1960s and 1970s did federal grants reach their heyday. Again, the federal government wanted action: to alleviate poverty, to equalize educational opportunities, to clean the nation's air and water, and to ensure adequate health care for underserved populations. But, again, this could not be done from Washington. In the 1960s, Congress enacted hundreds of new federal grants: 150 in 1965 alone. Between 1965 and 1970, the dollars provided in federal grants doubled; the total doubled again between 1970 and 1975, and nearly doubled again over the next five years (table 5.2). The growth after 1990 was substantial: an increase of $131 billion between 2000 and 2005 alone. However, much of the growth was concentrated in one program—Medicaid.

Other federal grants go to programs ranging from highway beautification to Head Start, from water purification to prevention of terrorism. Federal health programs include block grants for substance abuse, mental health, and maternal and child health; funding for AIDS programs through the Ryan White Comprehensive AIDS Resources Emergency (CARE) Act; and funding for anti-bioterrorism activities. These grants totaled $8.6 billion in fiscal year 2004—less than 5 percent of the federal Medicaid allocation that year. Health grants accounted for nearly half of all federal grants in 2005—up from about 6 percent in 1965 (fig. 5.1).

Federal grants were a boon to states and localities, since they provided the

Table 5.2
Federal Grants, 1965–2005

Year	Amount of Grant (billions of dollars)	Percentage of State and Local Expenditures	Percentage of Federal Outlays	Constant Dollars (billions, 2000)	Grants to Individuals (percent of total)
1965	10.9	15.5	9.2	$56.7	34.1
1970	24.1	20.1	12.3	105.3	36.2
1975	49.8	24.0	15.0	157.7	33.6
1980	91.4	27.4	15.5	192.6	35.7
1985	105.9	22.0	11.2	163.1	47.3
1990	135.3	18.9	10.8	172.1	57.1
1995	225.0	22.8	14.8	247.9	64.2
2000	284.7	22.1	15.9	284.7	64.1
2005	425.8	—	17.2	377.9	65.4

Source: Data from the Budget of the United States Government, Fiscal Year 2006 (OMB 2005).

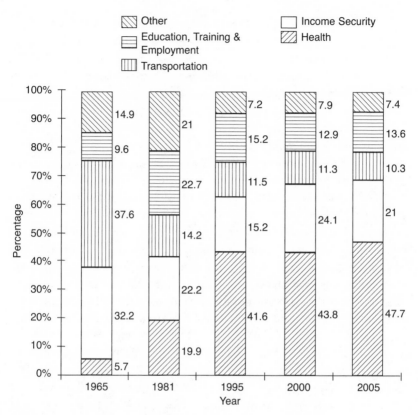

Figure 5.1.
Federal Grants by Function, as Percentage of Total Federal Grants, 1965–2005.
Source: Data from Budget of the United States Government, Fiscal Year 2006.

resources to pay for services that could not, or would not, be offered without the additional money. They also helped professionalize state and local work-forces in many areas, including health. States increased the salaries of their employees and challenged them with innovative and much needed programs, funded in part by federal dollars. Finally, federal grants equalized services in a way that states could not accomplish on their own. Medicaid, AFDC, and other federal grants are designed especially to assist poor states, or states with poor citizens and few natural resources to tax.

Most federal grants are categorical: money is provided to states and locali-ties and must be used for rather specific functions, from funding clinics for patients with black lung disease to providing curriculum assistance to the health professions. Sometimes the grants are competitive; states and localities submit proposals, and only a small number receive funds. More often, the grants are distributed to all states or localities based on a formula that includes such "need" measures as counts of poor persons, rural highways, waterfront land, or dilapidated housing.

In 1966, a new type of grant came into existence, a block grant, which allowed states and localities more discretion over how the dollars could be used. Generally, Congress would specify the policy area in which the funds could be spent, but states or localities could decide, within those broad categories, which programs best fit their own needs. The first block grant was in health, legislated in the Partnership for Health Act in 1966. Other health-related block grants were for maternal and child health; alcohol, drug abuse, and mental health; and preventive health care. The most recent block grant was the State Children's Health Insurance Program (S-CHIP), enacted in 1997. States and localities typically like block grants, but Congress is generally less enthusiastic; it is much harder for members of Congress to take credit for programs funded under this grant device, and oversight is difficult. Block grants usually suffer from these political flaws in their struggle for funding. The substance abuse, mental health, and maternal and child health block grants have not increased substantially since their inception. A recent block grant—Temporary Assistance for Needy Families (TANF)—is a case in point. Congress was unable to come up with a multiyear reauthorization and relied on temporary extensions for more than three years—in the process leaving states and the program recipients with considerable uncertainty.

Regulatory Federalism

In the 1980s, when federal budgetary restraints began to take hold, new federal grant spending became a liability, and federal regulation—whereby states and localities could be coerced into acting in certain ways—became more appealing. Regulations and requirements have long been a part of federal grants, going back to the Hatch Act of 1939, which prohibited partisan political activity by federal employees and by state and local employees funded with federal grant dollars. Nevertheless, the past few decades have seen a new type of regulation in which Washington enlists state and local governments in national efforts on behalf of particular disadvantaged groups or to advance certain policies such as environmental protection. Four types of intergovernmental regulation are popular: crosscutting requirements, crossover sanctions, partial preemption, and direct orders or mandates.

Crosscutting requirements are general policy provisions that apply across all federal grants in such policy areas as discrimination, wage rates, and environmental protection. David B. Walker (2000) identified 62 crosscutting requirements. One example is the Drug-Free Workplace Act, which requires all federal contractors, grant recipients, and state agencies receiving contracts or grants of $25,000 or more to certify that they will provide a drug-free work environment. Most of the existing crosscutting requirements were enacted more than a decade ago.

Crossover sanctions are newer regulatory mechanisms that impose a financial penalty in one area based on defects in another. Particularly popular is imposing penalties in the highway trust fund if states do not make desired federal changes. Early crossover sanctions dealt with transportation matters (such as lowering the speed limit and changing the minimum drinking age), but more recent laws have tied the loss of a state's highway trust-fund monies to nontransportation issues such as the control of junkyards and clean municipal air. One of the most recent crossover sanctions calls for states to strengthen their standard for drunk driving or lose 2 percent of their federal highway trust-fund money. States now face well over a dozen different financial penalties under which they can lose from 5 to 100 percent of their highway trust funds for failure to comply with federal requirements. Occasionally the sanction is connected with a nonhighway funding source. For example, the 1992 Synar Amendment punishes states that do not meet negotiated targets for reducing tobacco sales to minors through a 40 percent reduction in their substance-abuse block grants. A new twist on the crossover sanctions was introduced in 2005, when the Senate version of the highway bill called on states to adopt stiff penalties for repeat offenders, those with very high blood-alcohol levels, and those whose licenses had been suspended for drunken driving but who drove anyway. States that failed to enact legislation setting forth specific penalties for these three groups would see up to $600 million diverted from highway construction to programs aimed at highway safety (Wald 2005).

With partial preemption, the national government establishes rules and regulations calling for minimum national standards for a program. States can administer the program if they follow the standards; in states that fail, or do not wish, to do so, federal agencies will administer the program. This type of intergovernmental mandate is often used in the environmental area in such laws as safe drinking water, surface mining, and clean air amendments. It also applies to state occupational health and safety: half the states have chosen to administer that program; half have chosen not to do so. The Health Insurance Portability and Accountability Act of 1996 contained partial preemption provisions. The law included new access, portability, and renewability standards for group and individual market insurers. If states do not pass laws that enforce these provisions, the federal Department of Health and Human Services must do so (Ladenheim 1997).

In direct orders or mandates, the federal government orders lower governments to take certain types of action. More than 50 percent of all federal statutes preempting state and local authority enacted over the nation's 200-year history were adopted during the past two decades. Particularly troublesome for states is the tendency for Washington to mandate without federal financial assistance to pay for the newly required service. Many of these mandates are in the area of environmental protection. Though states pay some of these environmental costs, they mainly shift the burden to local governments. The effect on smaller jurisdictions can be devastating. An Environmental Protection Agency mandate requiring localities to monitor a particular substance in sewage discharge cost a small North Carolina town of 3,000 residents more than $30,000 a year—an amount equal to a 6 cent increase in their property tax. The 1990 Americans with Disabilities Act is another unfunded mandate that costs states and localities billions of dollars. The Drug-Free Workplace Act of 1988 also imposed substantial costs by requiring all federal grantees and contractors (including, of course, states and localities) to ensure that their workplaces were drug-free and that they offered antidrug programs for employees (Gais and Fossett 2005). But the largest federal mandate is Medicaid: Congress has substantially broadened the scope and reach of the program over the past decade. Though the federal government shares the cost of Medicaid with the states, changes made in Washington force states to fund their share of the program expansion.

One of the first measures to pass the Republican-controlled Congress in 1995 was a bill to limit unfunded mandates. The 1995 law provided that any proposed bill is out of order if it will cost state and local governments more than $50 million. The provision can be overruled with a majority vote. Mandates in place in 1995 were not affected by the law. Though clearly a step forward, in the opinion of many state and local officials, the law does not guarantee that unfunded federal mandates will end; in fact, as many as two-thirds of the major mandates that Congress imposes on states are exempt from the law. Also, one assessment of the early implementation of the measure found that passage of significant new mandates and preemptions continued. In fact, state and local governments' biggest success may have been in changing how the mandates were to be implemented rather than whether they should be enacted (Posner 1997).

Perhaps one of the most contentious intergovernmental regulatory areas in which state cooperation is essential is environmental protection. In the 1970s and 1980s, the federal approach to environmental protection could be characterized as "command and control." Congress and the EPA set standards and expected states to meet certain goals and undertake certain activities. More recently, the EPA has worked cooperatively with states, often by providing incentives. One example of this "easing" of federal oversight is the federal policy on underground storage tanks. The potential problem of leakage from tanks containing petroleum products or other hazardous substances emerged in the mid-1980s. In 1984, Congress amended the Resource Conservation and Recovery Act (RCRA) to require the EPA to establish a regulatory scheme that helps reduce the threat of these tanks to public health and safety. The EPA developed rules in 1988 requiring that the owners of all new and existing tanks must respond to any leaks, including remediation if necessary. The agency set a 10-year deadline for removal or upgrading of the underground storage tanks. When it became clear that these efforts were expensive (particularly remediation), Congress established a trust fund to be used to reduce the economic hardship of compliance. As part of the regulations associated with this trust fund, the EPA offered states the option to set up their own underground storage programs, including the ability to disburse funds. To be recognized by the EPA, state programs must set up state remediation funds and meet the agency's financial responsibility requirements. Half the states have set up EPA-recognized programs, and almost every state has established some type of fund for underground storage tanks (Berrens et al. 1999).

The story does not end there, however. In 2000, the EPA began to issue fines against businesses and organizations for failing to meet the 1998 deadline for removal or upgrading of tanks. However, as had become clear, state enforcement of the federal regulations was not uniform. More than 85 percent of the storage tanks were in compliance, but in some states the rates were much lower. For example, Ohio reported that only 16 percent of its tanks had been fully upgraded. Texas failed to report any data to the federal agency. The fault may not lie fully with the states, however. The federal Leaking Underground Storage Tank Trust Fund, funded by taxes on petroleum companies, contained $1.3 billion in 2000, but federal law allowed the EPA to draw only $70 million a year from the fund—roughly the amount earned annually in interest. The money is used to clean up spills rather than enforce current regulations.

Congress has refused access to the remaining trust funds, which have been used as part of the effort to reduce the federal deficit (Zielbauer 2000).

In the 1990s there were other examples of new, more cooperative forms of federal-state relationships. The EPA launched the National Environmental Performance Partnership System (NEPPS) in the mid-1990s specifically to improve relationships with the states. It gives states with strong environmental programs more flexibility and allows the EPA to give more attention to weaker state programs. One aspect of the NEPPS is performance partnership agreements, which allow states to combine funds from one or more categorical grants to address a specific state environmental priority. Another innovation, called Project XL (excellence and leadership), kicks in when a plant wants to expand or relocate. The EPA works with states and localities to give that plant the needed flexibility while ensuring environmental protection goals (Kraft and Scheberle 1998). These efforts may be small steps—and may not be entirely successful—but they do represent a recognition of the need for federal-state cooperation in an area where regulation may not be the only answer.

In recent years, a new wrinkle in federal grants has emerged—the tying of federal grant dollars to specific performance standards or outcomes. The TANF block grant, enacted in 1996, required states to increase the proportion of adult TANF recipients who were engaged in "work-related activities." If states failed to meet this performance standard, their block grants were cut. Other performance measures relating to out-of-wedlock births and job retention rates provided bonuses for states that were the most successful at lowering birth rates and boosting job retention (Gais and Fossett 2005). The No Child Left Behind law set similar performance standards in the education area.

Political scientists have long recognized that states respond to incentives such as federal matching grants or funds to establish a program or office. While states complain about mandates, there is some evidence that they do respond to them—in fact, more so than to incentives. Sometimes lesser approaches also work. The federal government can "signal" to states to act through messages and instructions. HCFA/CMS officials were often very engaged with their state counterparts to instruct them on legal ways of maximizing Medicaid access and even promising lenient treatment in the federal quality-control process for states' mistakes in determining Food Stamp eligibility. Gais and Fossett (2005) reported that not all states responded to these efforts, but many did and enrollments rose quickly.

Federal officials can also signal to states by considering legislation in Washington but failing to enact it. For example, following Congress's failure to enact a ban on late-term or "partial birth" abortions in 1996, half of the state legislatures gave the issue serious consideration and many acted in 1997 (M. Allen, Pettus, and Haider-Markel 2004). Similarly, states enacted a series of regulations on managed care while Congress failed to enact such legislation in session after session. Another example where states have acted and Washington has not is another key area that highlights the importance of federalism: medical malpractice.

Although Republican ideology is typically more supportive of stronger states and a reduced federal government presence, ideology and politics often interfere with federalist beliefs. For example, although President George W. Bush came to the White House directly from the governor's mansion in Texas and, in his campaign, had argued for smaller government, he was strongly supportive of federal legislation to limit jury awards for pain and suffering in medical malpractice court cases. "It's a national problem that requires a national solution," he told a group of health care professionals (Stolberg 2002b, A16). Support for this position is especially noteworthy given that more than half of the 25 states with no damage caps have constitutional provisions that bar legislation limiting recoveries by plaintiffs in civil cases (Jost 2003). Supporters of federal malpractice laws say there are no problems with such preemption in an area where states have traditionally prevailed. They cite the federal government's primacy in interstate commerce as constitutional justification (Adams 2003a)—an assertion that might be challenged should federal law be enacted.

A second example of preemption, in a related area, during the George W. Bush administration concerned specific types of medical liability involving prescription drugs and medical devices. The Justice Department contended that consumers cannot recover damages for injuries from vaccines and medical devices approved by the FDA. While the administration initially said that FDA approval set the minimum standard and that states could provide "additional protection to consumers," in 2004 the Justice Department argued that FDA approval "set a ceiling as well as a floor"—preempting a state law or state court finding that a drug or devise is unsafe (Pear 2004b).

Disregard for federalism issues cuts across party lines. In 2005, Democrats sponsored legislation in the Senate to "force" states to report the names of companies with 50 or more employees who received government-funded health care (namely Medicaid). The measure—designed to pressure Wal-Mart to improve employee health coverage—may be politically pleasing to federal legislators but flies in the face of federalism. In fact, Maryland enacted a bill that would have required Wal-Mart to spend more on employee health benefits. Similar bills were introduced in several other states (Joyce 2005).

Most observers of federalism would describe the U.S. model as nationally dominant—that is, with the national government having assumed preemptive power. However, increasing state activism and institutional capacity has given support to the role of states as laboratories of democracy—in health and other policy areas. But the final arbiter of decisions related to which governmental level does what is the U.S. Supreme Court. Since the country's beginning, the Court's decisions have served to shape the contours of federalism and allocation of power.

The U.S. Supreme Court

By 5-4 majorities, the U.S. Supreme Court, beginning in 1992, began to reconsider the distribution of power between federal and state governments. In *New York v. United States* (1992), the Court resurrected the Tenth Amendment's residual powers clause to invalidate a provision of a federal law requiring states to "take title" to their low-level radioactive wastes. In a 1995 case, *United States v. Lopez,* the Court failed to buy the notion that a federal law banning the sale of firearms close to school grounds was justified under the interstate commerce clause. It was the first time in six decades that the Court found Congress exceeding its power under the interstate commerce provision. In *Seminole Tribe v. Florida* (1996), the Court defended the sovereign immunity of states by striking down a federal law that authorized private suits against states in federal court (the Eleventh Amendment states that the judicial power of the United States shall not be construed to extend to any suit in law or equity, commenced or prosecuted against one of the United States by citizens of another state). A 1999 ruling in *Alden v. Maine* extended state immunity from private suits to state courts.

Some observers view these developments with alarm, as indicating that the Court is committed to expanding state sovereignty at the expense of the federal government's policy-making and enforcement authority. However, others believe the decisions, while important, are more of an adjustment than a "sea change" (Brisbin 1998). Indeed, the Court did not always rule "in favor" of states. Several examples:

— In *Bush v. Gore* (2000), the Court found in a 5-4 vote that states may not, by later arbitrary and disparate treatment, value one person's vote over that of another, a decision that overruled the Florida Supreme Court and stopped a recount underway that might have resulted in a different president sitting in the Oval Office in 2001 (Savage 2001).

— In *Tennessee v. Lane* (2004), the Supreme Court upheld Congress's power to subject states to monetary liability under certain provisions of the Americans with Disabilities Act.

— In *Gonzales v. Raich* (2005), the Court ruled that marijuana consumption and cultivation was a matter of interstate commerce, and thus the "necessary and proper" clause authorizes regulation of that commerce even if there is also a purely intrastate noneconomic activity—overturning language in a California statute legalizing medical marijuana use.

What does this mean? It highlights the fact that the Supreme Court, much as the Founding Fathers desired, is the final arbiter of federalism. Sometimes the Court rules mostly in favor of Congress and the federal government, producing a strong national-level voice. Sometimes it rules in favor of states, providing a stronger balance of interest. There is some evidence that the Rehnquist Court rulings were designed in part to help balance federal and state interests. Justice Antonin Scalia, among others, has noted the duty of the Supreme Court to maintain "a healthy balance of power between the states and federal government" (Conlan and De Chantal 2001). It must be noted as well that most of the federalism rulings of the Rehnquist Court were 5-4—making the post-Rehnquist changes to the Court especially important to federalism scholars and students.

State Suits against the Federal Government

Over the country's history, the states have often utilized their ability to sue the federal government, but recently suits have been proliferating, particularly in environmental matters. (Education is also a popular area, with a few states suing over the No Child Left Behind legislation, which they see as an unfunded mandate.)

Three states (Connecticut, Maine, and Massachusetts) filed suit in federal court in 2003 claiming that the EPA had a mandatory duty to regulate carbon dioxide emissions, the first time states had sued the federal government over global warming. Later that year, 12 states, 14 environmental groups, New York City, and the City of Baltimore filed suit in an effort to force the EPA to regulate greenhouse gas emissions from new motor vehicles (Scheberle 2005). Also in 2003, attorneys general for 12 states, several citizens, and some environmental groups sued the EPA over a program that sets up a market for coal-fired plants so that polluters can purchase pollution allowances from plants that hold emissions below their cap. These plaintiffs argued that the program—called cap and trade—can lead to more pollution in certain areas of a state and that mercury should be regulated through the application of state-of-the-art pollution control rather than trading (Morandi 2005).

UNDERSTANDING THE DIFFERENCES BETWEEN FEDERAL AND STATE GOVERNMENTS

The ways in which states differ from and resemble the federal government—and one another—affect their policy making in health and other areas. States are similar to the federal government in their organization, structure, and policy-making processes. They are different in three key areas: budget constraints, direct democracy, and media coverage.

State government is structured and run much like the federal government. Every state has a state constitution that contains a bill of rights and provisions setting forth the structure and function of the state and local governments. Every state has three branches of government, and 49 have two houses. Like Congress, state legislatures are organized by the dominant political party, and 49 states have bipartisan membership (only Nebraska is unicameral and nonpartisan). Every state has a governor with duties roughly analogous to those of the president, including administering state government and initiating a policy agenda. Like the president, governors appoint members of a cabinet, although in some states several important cabinet positions are elected or appointed by commission. Every state has a judiciary that includes both trial and appellate levels.

The duties of the three branches of government are nearly identical at the federal and state levels. In both, the legislature passes laws, provides appropriations, and oversees the executive branch. Federal and state legislatures are organized by parties, use committees as key decision makers, and have nearly identical flow charts illustrating "how a bill becomes a law." In both, the chief elected official of the executive branch sets the agenda, oversees the running of the government, and handles relationships outside the capitol. The judiciary at both levels of government determines the constitutionality of laws, adjudicates violations of law, and protects the well-being of individual citizens. Both levels of government are lobbied by interest groups and receive money from PACs. And, importantly, both types of government are sovereign and operate by virtue of the power of the people. Each citizen is subject to at least two governments, under which some rights are identical and some are very different.

States and the federal government differ in their revenue sources and their spending priorities. The big spending area for states has traditionally been education (both kindergarten through twelfth grade [K–12] and higher education). However, in recent years, Medicaid has nearly overtaken K–12 spending nationally and has exceeded it in many states. Across the nation in fiscal year 2003, elementary and secondary education accounted for 21.7 percent of state spending; Medicaid, 21.4 percent. Higher education makes up nearly 11 percent of state budgets; transportation, 8.2 percent; corrections, 3.5 percent; and public assistance, 2.2 percent (National Association of State Budget Officers [NASBO] 2004).

Both states and the national government use the income tax as a major source of revenue. For the states, however, it is one of several lucrative taxes and is second to the sales tax in its revenue generation. Sales taxes (both general taxes and taxes on specific items such as gasoline, cigarettes, and liquor) make up around one-third of a state's tax revenue; individual income taxes account for 37 percent. The states also obtain substantial revenues from corporate income taxes, lotteries, motor vehicle and operators' licenses, and gift and estate taxes (NASBO 2004). The federal government relies overwhelmingly on the income tax, which accounts for nearly two-thirds of the total revenue (OMB 2000).

Balancing the State Budget

One of the important things to understand about states is that, unlike Washington, D.C., states cannot operate in a deficit. In 49 states, by constitution or statute, the state budget must be balanced at the end of each fiscal year (only Vermont allows a deficit by law, and it discourages it by custom). Unlike the federal government, states have capital budgets for financing infrastructure projects such as roads and buildings. States also have many special accounts, often funded with earmarked taxes, which are not subject to the limitations and have semiautonomous agencies that can use their own borrowing authority. Most states are prohibited from borrowing money for operating expenses such as payrolls or benefit checks. This provision has caused difficulty for many states, particularly in times of economic downturn, but it has also forced them to make tough choices much earlier than do their Washington counterparts and to stay within limited resources in meeting their citizens' needs. If, midway through a fiscal year, state officials realize that the budget will not be balanced (that is, spending is exceeding expected revenues), they must either cut an existing program or enact a tax. (There are, of course, some stopgap measures such as delaying a payment to state employees and welfare recipients, but these delays usually raise little money and are often unpopular.) Having to choose between program cuts or tax increases is not popular, and legislators prefer to make careful choices in the initial budget to avoid getting into this unwelcome situation.

States can and do enter a new fiscal year with a budget surplus, but for political reasons, officials are generally careful not to carry over too much money—the media and citizens will demand tax cuts, even though surpluses can be useful in tiding over the state in future years. To avoid some of the "feast or famine" choices facing them, most states have established "rainy day" funds: a certain small proportion of state revenues set aside in good economic times to help fund possible shortfalls in tighter economic times.

Finally, 28 states operate under some form of state tax or expenditure limit (TEL). Following the passage of Proposition 13 in California in 1976, which limited the growth in state property taxes, a number of states adopted similar tax or spending limits. For example, Michigan's TEL, adopted in 1978, limits state revenues to 9.49 percent of the prior year's personal income. Recently, there has been a second wave of state TELs, prompted in large measure by national antitax groups such as the Americans for Tax Reform. These TELs not only limit tax collection and spending (or both) but often also include supermajority requirements (no tax or spending legislation may be enacted unless there is a greater than 50 percent majority in the legislature) and voter approval requirements (voters must approve all new or increased taxes). Table 5.3 shows the mixture of TELs in the states. While most are constitutional, many are in statute. Spending limitations are much more common than tax limitations. Eleven states with TELs require approval by a supermajority (usually two-thirds or three-fourths) of the legislature to raise taxes. South Dakota has no TEL but does require a two-thirds vote of the legislature to raise taxes. A few states require public approval as well. In Colorado, all tax increases must be approved by a vote of the people (NASBO 2002). TELs constrain legislators' choices (as they are intended to do) and are not applied to the U.S. Congress.

Direct Democracy

Democracy is much more direct in many states than at the national level. In some states, citizens can initiate, endorse, or recall a law or elected official.

Table 5.3
States with Tax or Expenditures Limitations

State	Constitution	Statute	Tax	Spending	Supermajority
Alaska	X			X	
Arizona	X			X	X
Arkansas	X		X		X*
California	X			X	X
Colorado	X	X	X	X	
Connecticut	X			X	
Delaware	X			X	X
Florida	X		X		X
Hawaii	X			X	X†
Idaho		X		X	
Iowa		X		X	
Louisiana	X	X	X	X	X
Massachusetts		X	X		
Michigan	X		X		
Mississippi		X		X	X
Missouri	X		X		
Montana		X		X	
Nevada		X		X	X
New Jersey		X		X	
North Carolina		X		X	
Oklahoma	X			X	X
Oregon		X		X	X
Rhode Island	X			X	
South Carolina	X			X	
Tennessee	X			X	
Texas	X			X	
Utah		X		X	
Washington		X		X	
Total	17	13	7	23	11

Source: National Association of State Budget Officers 2002.

Note: Supermajority indicates a supermajority of votes in legislature required for any revenue increase.

*This applies only to taxes in existence in 1934 (not the sales tax).

†Two-thirds of elected members are required if the general fund expenditure ceiling is exceeded; otherwise a majority of elected members is required.

In more than half the states, the people play a key role in ratifying or proposing legislation. Eighteen states have an initiative process that offers voters the ability to propose constitutional amendments (constitutional initiatives) (table 5.4). In 21 states, voters can propose statutory initiatives—those that place the measure in law, not the state constitution. Fourteen states offer both constitutional and statutory initiatives. Twenty-four states use the popular referendum, whereby citizens can petition for a vote on statutes or ordinances that the legislature has passed and can, if they so vote, reject them. An example of the use of the popular referendum took place in November 2004 when California citizens petitioned to vote on a 2003 law setting up a pay-or-play type of health insurance system. Under the law, businesses with 50 or more employees would provide their workers with access to insurance (paying 80 percent of the premium) or pay into a state fund. The measure failed to get a majority vote (by 49-51 percent) and was not implemented. Eighteen states have a recall provision that allows voters to remove an elected state official from office. Together, the three mechanisms—initiative, referendum, and recall—are referred to as direct democracy.

Table 5.4
States with Constitutional and/or Statutory Initiative Processes

States with constitutional initiatives		
Arizona	Massachusetts*	Nevada
Arkansas	Michigan	North Dakota
California	Mississippi*	Ohio
Colorado	Missouri	Oklahoma
Florida	Montana	Oregon
Illinois	Nebraska	South Dakota
States with statutory initiatives		
Alaska*	Massachusetts*	Ohio*
Arizona	Michigan*	Oklahoma
Arkansas	Missouri	Oregon
California	Montana	South Dakota
Colorado	Nebraska	Utah*
Idaho	Nevada*	Washington*
Maine*	North Dakota	Wyoming*

Source: Initiative and Referendum Institute 2005.

*These states use an indirect method whereby, after the signatures are collected, the proposal goes to the legislature for consideration before the amendment can be placed on the ballot.

Direct democracy produces a type of accountability and responsiveness unmatched in Washington, D.C. It allows citizens to organize to support or fight an issue or person. Legislators and governors (and local officials) are aware of the latent power of the initiative, referendum, and recall and know they are accountable for individual decisions in a way a member of Congress is not. For example, in 1984, two Democratic members of the Michigan senate were recalled because they voted for a major tax increase (to balance a badly out-of-kilter, recession-affected state budget). Members of Congress might vote for a similar tax increase with the hope that two (or six) years hence voters will have forgotten the transgression or will wish to vote for them because of their positions on other issues.

Even if initiatives fail to garner the majority necessary for adoption, they may serve other purposes. The possibility of an initiative or referendum affects the kind of law proposed by the legislature. Unlike Congress, which has no public mechanism for citizens to express approval or disapproval of individual laws, a state legislator might see her long-sought law up for public approval, sometimes brought there by a petition-signing effort sponsored by interest groups defeated in the initial legislation. The possibility of such a reassessment, and of bringing up original bills, affects the design, strategy, and politics of state legislation, particularly in highly salient issue areas. Interest groups can send a message to legislators that the issue is important, and even if the initiative fails, it often lands on the legislative agenda following the election. Indeed, Elisabeth Gerber (1999) found that policies in states with initiatives more closely reflect voter preferences than do policies in states without and that this effect is greatest where access to the direct legislation process is easiest. It is also interesting to note that the initiative can be used to directly curb legislative behavior. Most term-limit provisions and TELs are put in place through initiatives, not legislation.

Direct democracy was the idea of populists at the end of the twentieth century who wanted to reduce corruption in legislatures by giving the people a direct voice. Ironically, some believe that this idealistic notion has led to what Gerber (1999) called a Populist Paradox, because it is special interests, particularly rich special interests, that benefit from the initiative process. However, Gerber found that economic interests do not necessarily benefit from initiating ballot measures (although they do better at stopping them). In contrast, citizens' groups do seem to benefit from having the initiative process available, much as the populists had thought. Citizens' groups are more successful than economic groups at getting new laws passed by initiative.

Initiatives are very popular in states and are increasingly used for major environmental and health issues. Toxic cleanup, nuclear waste, gun control, AIDS-related issues, medicinal marijuana, Medicaid spending for abortions, health insurance reforms (including a single-payer system), and right-to-die laws—all have appeared on the ballot in states across the country. Citizens' groups tend to initiate and support environmental measures, whereas health measures are often launched by economic and professional interests. One example was a California initiative in 2004 to establish a new state entity to conduct research on human embryonic stem cells, estimated to cost $6 billion over thirty years (Krane and Koenig 2005). Also in 2004, voters in 10 states enacted constitutional amendments to ban same-sex marriage, and Montana became the tenth state to legalize marijuana for medical purposes. In that same election, California voters expanded mental health services and programs by adding a 1 percent tax increase for those with incomes over $1 million.

State voters in 18 states also have the option to recall their governors, state legislators, and other statewide officers. In 2002, less than one year after reelecting Gray Davis to a second term, voters in California succeeded in recalling Davis and replacing him with former actor/bodybuilder Arnold Schwarzenegger. It was only the second time in U.S. history that a governor had been recalled.

The Press and the State Legislature

A major difference between most state legislatures and the U.S. Congress concerns media coverage. As discussed in chapter 1, members of Congress have become masters at manipulating the media by making clever pronounce-ments in 30-second sound bites and writing press releases and editorials that are often used verbatim in hometown newspapers. News coverage, especially local coverage, is widely available and highly useful to members of Congress. Press secretaries are important staffers, often highly influential in both for-mulating and packaging legislators' policy positions.

In states, the media coverage and press staffing are markedly different. Relatively few reporters cover the state capitol, and what coverage there is tends to be focused on the governor and a few legislative leaders and to high-light partisan bickering and embarrassing or ridiculous situations. Most state legislators do not have much access to public relations staffs, and even those who do are often unsuccessful in their efforts to make the six o'clock news. In "professional" state legislatures, press functions are often handled by party caucus staffs. Recently, however, several Michigan senators hired their own press secretaries—a movement noted with alarm by some observers. News directors and city editors often view state politics as dull and unappealing to viewers and readers. There are few exciting "photo opportunities," and the issues are often complex and not easily explained in a sound bite. Further, most state capitals are small towns relatively remote from the state's largest media centers. Thus, Albany, Sacramento, Lansing, Tallahassee, and Springfield may seem unimportant to the lives of the media—and the people they serve. Television coverage of state government is especially poor. Layton and Walton (1998, 45) called television reporters in state capitols "an endangered species, rarely glimpsed except for a major speech or press conference."

In 1998, 513 newspaper reporters and 113 wire service reporters were covering state capitols full time, ranging from 44 newspaper reporters in California to none in Alaska. Ironically, the number of reporters covering state government in a time of devolution has fallen. The Project on the State of the American Newspaper found that in 27 state capitols, there are fewer reporters today than in the early 1990s. In 7 of the 10 largest states, the number of reporters covering state government dropped over this period (Layton and Walton 1998). The simple fact is that state political coverage is considered dull, and it does not fare well in broadcasters' periodic "sweeps," which determine advertising rates and assess the popularity of shows and news coverage. As Karl Kurtz (1990, 10) put it, "Television doesn't cover legislatures because people are not interested in state government." But, he suggested, people are not interested in state government because television does not cover it well. One exception to the rather abysmal press coverage is that provided by public television. Several public television stations present regular legislative coverage, and some have gavel-to-gavel coverage similar to the popular C-Span coverage of Congress and other events in Washington, D.C. Other states now cover legislative proceedings on government cable channels.

This overall lack of media attention allows state policy making to take place in a setting without widespread public input and press coverage. The process is more closed and dominated more by those with special interests and concerns than in Washington, not because of any real intent or differences in state legislative rules or procedures but rather because of the media coverage, or lack thereof. As one North Carolina legislator put it, "One of the first things I was told when I came to Raleigh was, 'You can vote any way you want to up here because the folks back home will never know'" (Layton and Walton 1998, 54).

INTERSTATE DIFFERENCES

The similarities among the states are legion and unmistakable. A transplant from Rhode Island walking into the North Carolina state capitol would have little difficulty finding his way around or understanding the process, language, and operation of the legislative body. (Only in Nebraska would a visitor be confused: it has the country's only unicameral legislature.) Similarly, governors' offices, executive branch agencies, and lobbies operate in roughly the same manner across the 50 states. However, it would be a mistake to think that state legislatures are identical from Maine to New Mexico. They differ in many ways, especially in what is known as their "professionalism."

Every state in the country modernized to some extent in the 1970s, adding staff, increasing time in session, adopting procedures to expedite and streamline the legislative process, increasing salaries, and adding technology that links legislators to one another, to state agencies, and to the public. Many states reduced the size of their legislative institutions as a way to have more efficient organization and effective policy making. Reducing the size of the legislative body has an effect on the number of citizens represented per member, especially in large states. For example, the average member of the California assembly represents 423,396 constituents. At the other extreme, the average New Hampshire house member represents only 3,089 persons. The range in state senates is similar. A California senator represents, on average, 846,791 persons; a North Dakota senator must report to 13,106 (A. Rosenthal 2004). Is this fair? Certainly citizens of North Dakota and New Hampshire are more likely to know their representatives and participate more easily in the legislative process. For California and other large states trying to hold down the size of their legislative institutions so as to facilitate collective action decisions, there is a tradeoff between efficiency and representation.

Not every state made the same level of progress in modernization. Eight states can be referred to as professional—those with many specialized and personal staff, with relatively generous levels of compensation, and in session nearly full-time. At the other end of the spectrum are 17 nonprofessional, or citizen, legislatures, which have few staff, low pay, and limited sessions. Twenty-five states are hybrids, having some of the characteristics of each (K. Kurtz 1989).

Table 5.5 shows the range of professionalization of state legislatures, characterized by time in session, legislative salaries, and expenditures for staff services and operations. The level of professionalization reflects how closely each state legislature approximates Congress in the three areas. The measure used for each state is the mean of the percentage of the congressional standard the state achieves for each of the three areas (time, salaries, and staff spending). The table illustrates the enormous diversity of the states in their professionalization. California, the most professional state legislature, has a professionalization level of 90 percent (that is, 90 percent of that of Congress). At the other extreme, New Hampshire's legislature has a professionalization level of only 6 percent (King 2000). The mean level for all states is 26 percent. Also noteworthy is the big gap between the most professional state—California—and the other professional states (the professionalization

Table 5.5

State Levels of Professionalization (as percent) Compared with That of the U.S. Congress

>50 Percent		30–49 Percent		20–29 Percent		10–19 Percent		<10 Percent	
California	90	Alaska	45	Arizona	28	Delaware	19	New Mexico	9
New York	66	Ohio	43	North Carolina	28	Indiana	19	Wyoming	7
Michigan	50	Pennsylvania	40	Oklahoma	28	Rhode Island	19	New Hampshire	6
		Illinois	38	Vermont	28	Kansas	18		
		New Jersey	37	Colorado	27	Tennessee	18		
		Florida	35	Maryland	27	Idaho	17		
		Massachusetts	33	Minnesota	25	Kentucky	17		
		Wisconsin	33	Louisiana	25	Maine	16		
		Hawaii	32	Nebraska	25	West Virginia	16		
		Connecticut	32	Oregon	25	Arkansas	15		
		Missouri	30	Virginia	24	Montana	15		
		Washington	30	Iowa	24	Alabama	14		
				Texas	23	Georgia	14		
				Mississippi	22	South Dakota	11		
				South Carolina	21	North Dakota	10		
				Nevada	20	Utah	10		

Source: Data from King 2000.

level of the second-place state, New York, is only 66 percent). Clearly, state legislatures still retain their nonprofessional nature—at least compared with their national counterpart.

State legislatures also differ substantially in their levels of partisanship. Nebraska is the only state where legislators do not run on a party label. In other states, parties are important in identifying members to the electorate and in organizing legislative activities. The speaker or senate president is generally from the majority party, selected in caucus and then voted on by all members. But exceptions do occur—and more frequently than in the U.S. Congress. In 2005, a Democrat edged out a Republican for the top position (the speaker) in the Tennessee senate, even though Republicans held the majority of seats in the senate. The losing Republican candidate became majority leader in an unusual bipartisan leadership arrangement (Locker 2005).

Hawaii has long been one of the most Democratic legislatures, with only 5 of the 25 senators and 10 of the 51 house members Republicans in 2005. Massachusetts is also a strong Democratic stronghold, with only 6 of its 40 state senators in the Republican Party. At the other extreme, Idaho is highly Republican, with only 13 Democratic members in the 70-member house and 7 Democrats in the 35-member senate. In other states, parties are more competitive. The 2005 Colorado senate had 18 Democrats and 17 Republicans; the Tennessee senate had 16 Democrats and 17 Republicans. In many states, party control shifts with some regularity. In Michigan, for example, the lower house was controlled by the Democrats in 1991–92, was split evenly in 1993–94, was controlled by the Republicans in 1995–96, by the Democrats in 1997–98, and by Republicans again in 1999–2000. In contrast, some states have more stable party leadership. New York, for example, has had split party control for decades: the Republicans have controlled the senate for more than 35 years, and the Democrats have controlled the assembly for more than three decades (with one exception, in 1971–72).

In 2005, in 17 state legislatures, both houses were led by Democrats; in 21 states, both houses were led by Republicans. In 11 states, one house was controlled by one party and one by the other party (again, Nebraska has no political parties). When the party of the governor is factored in, only eight states had a full sweep of Democrats controlling the legislature and the governorship in 2005. Twelve states had Republican governors and Republican-controlled legislatures. The 2004 legislative elections produced ties in the lower house in Iowa and in the upper house in Montana.

A final difference among state legislatures, which has a large potential effect on state policy making, is term limits. Fifteen states now have term limits on their state legislators. Not all term limits are the same. The toughest provisions, in place in Arizona, California, and Michigan, limit service in the lower house to six years and in the senate to eight years, with a lifetime ban on further service. Nine states have consecutive-term limits, meaning a legislator could serve the limit of terms in the senate, stay out for a term, then return and start the term-limits clock again. Louisiana's term limits allow 12 years in the house and 12 years in the senate and are consecutive (National Conference of State Legislatures [NCSL] 2005c). In six states, term limits have been repealed, most often by the state supreme court.

Term limits are expected to change legislative composition, behavior, and power balance. Supporters clearly wanted to get fresher ideas and to turn out legislators who had, perhaps, become too ingrained in the system and not responsive to the electorate. Although the effects of term limits are only just becoming evident (they go into effect in Louisiana only in 2007 and Nevada in 2010), there is little evidence that legislative composition is greatly changed. The number of women and minorities elected to the legislature has not changed substantially, and legislators tend to be similar in occupation, education, income, religion, and ideology to those they replace. Hispanics in California are one exception to this. Their number has increased since term limits. Somewhat unexpectedly, legislators elected under term limits seem less inclined to be concerned about district needs and more concerned with statewide issues (perhaps because they are looking forward to their next race). They report spending less time keeping in touch with constituents than do non-term-limited legislators. But as yet there are no differences in the ability of the newly elected legislators to build coalitions or specialize in issues. The greatest impact seems to be on power. In term-limited legislatures, governors and state agency officials now seem to be more powerful, party leadership less powerful (J. Carey, Niemi, and Powell 2000). Though some argue that interest groups are more powerful in term-limited legislatures, others note that lobbyists have to work harder for their keep in these legislatures. In Michigan, for example, in 1998, lobbyists had to quickly acquaint themselves with 65 new members (in a 110-member house).

Gubernatorial power, too, varies across the 50 states. Term limits are more prevalent in states' chief executive offices than in legislatures. The majority of governors have some type of term limit imposed on them; most can serve only two terms. Governors' formal powers—those outlined specifically in state constitutions or statutes—include the length of the term, possibility of serving multiple terms, role in shaping the state's budget, ability to appoint cabinet members, and ability to reorganize state agencies. Some governors have relatively little formal power: limited to two terms, with few cabinet appointments and without the power to revamp the state bureaucracy unless they have legislative approval. For example, the governor of Texas does not present an executive budget to the legislature and cannot reorganize departments without legislative approvals. Other governors can serve many terms, have a large slate of possible appointments, and can make changes in state agencies with minimal legislative interference. Forty-three governors have the line-item veto, and 37 can reduce the budget without legislative approval. Fourteen governors can even veto selected words, and three can use a veto to change the meaning of words (NASBO 2002).

State judiciaries differ in how they are selected. States use three methods of choosing judges, and some states use a combination of methods (that is, one process for supreme court justices and another for lower trial judges). Many state judges are elected by the citizens, usually on nonpartisan tickets. In some states, judges are appointed by the legislature or the governor or both. Nearly half the states have adopted a modified merit approach, called the Missouri Plan, in which judges are initially appointed by the governor based on recommendations by a blue ribbon committee, then after a short period of time in service they must face the voters in an election.

State executive agencies also differ markedly, with some states having large professional bureaucracies dominated by civil service rules and others having fewer, more generalist officials who are not uniformly hired or protected by merit-based nonpartisan rules. State agencies in some states work closely with the legislature in drafting and producing legislation; agencies in other states might work in a more "arms-length" fashion, meeting only occasionally with legislative staff and others. Sparer (1996) found that differences in state agencies were key to understanding Medicaid programs in those states. In California, for example, officials implementing Medicaid enjoyed significant autonomy and were able to pursue the goal of cost containment. New York Medicaid officials, in contrast, operated in a fragmented, decentralized environment in which interest groups played an important role and agency goals played a secondary role.

Finally, the importance of lobbyists varies from state to state. Every state, like Washington, D.C., has seen the number of lobbyists increase over the past 20 years, and the style of lobbying and the effect of lobbying on the legislative product can vary considerably. In some states, interest groups are more influential than political parties in helping recruit and elect candidates as well as shape legislation. Especially in citizen legislatures, lobbyists serve to provide valuable information on both substance and political issues. Rules vary on who is considered a lobbyist and to what extent lobbyists must report their activities. In Iowa, lobbyists must register which bills they intend to support or oppose. In many states, multi-client lobby firms are the norm—a handful of lobbyists serve dozens of corporate and association clients (A. Rosenthal 1993). In every state, economic and professional health interests are important policy players.

The variations in state process and policy are, of course, not random but depend on large differences in citizens' wealth and education, the state's businesses and industries, and state residents' expectations, ideology, and views of government. A large body of political science research has considered the role of political and economic factors and measures of "need" in state policy choice and found that all are important, but with differences across policy areas. The variables that successfully predict why states are generous in welfare or Medicaid payments or eligibility criteria are not necessarily good predictors of which state policies will be enacted on water pollution or education or health professions education. Political variables, particularly, seem to weigh more heavily in some kinds of policy choices than in others (Lambert and McGuire 1990; Mueller 1992; C. Weissert, Knott, and Stieber 1994).

Also important is the presence of a policy entrepreneur who sells an idea and continues to push it through innumerable hurdles and who has the standing to make things happen. Governors are often very effective policy entrepreneurs: they can put issues on the agenda, work with legislative leaders and interest groups to shape the plan, and obtain the public's backing for the plan. Governors of Massachusetts, Florida, and Vermont played an important entrepreneurial role in health care reform. In each of these instances, the governor led the reform effort after much of the groundwork had been laid by the legislature or the private sector (Paul-Sheehan 1998).

FEDERAL-STATE HEALTH PROGRAMS

The state role in health goes back to long before the New Deal. Social legislation, particularly programs protecting the public's health and assisting persons who are poor or disabled, was initiated in many states in the early years of the twentieth century. States and localities were the traditional source of health care for poor people until World War II. States provided the money to build hospitals and adopted scores of public health measures. State regulation of health providers goes back to before the United States was established. The first law licensing physicians was enacted in 1639 in Virginia. State mental institutions trace their history to the early 1800s in Virginia and Kentucky; in the early 1950s, states began to establish departments of mental health. Following World War II, the federal role in health became more evident. Federal law permitted firms to deduct costs of employee health benefits, and in 1946 the Hill-Burton Act provided incentives for new hospitals and for care of the indigent (Rich and White 1996).

In the 1960s and 1970s, the federal government stepped up its spending in many health areas, including mental health, substance abuse, the environment, and public health. The biggest change in the national arena was the enactment of Medicare and Medicaid in 1965, which dramatically changed the nature of health care financing and services in the United States. Medicare and Medicaid put the federal government in the role of a major purchaser of health care and, as such, a shaper of the way in which care is delivered.

Medicaid

Medicaid is the premier federal-state health program. It is large, important, and controversial. In fiscal year 2005, Medicaid financed health care for 53 million low-income children, adults, seniors, and people with disabilities at a total cost of $329 billion. Medicaid is not one program but several, providing for different groups of recipients:

— low-income, uninsured children, some parents, and low-income pregnant women;

— persons who are disabled, including those with mental illness, and low-income elderly;

— people too poor to pay the premiums and co-pays required for Medicare, the federal program for elders; and

— safety-net hospitals and community health centers that serve the poor.

Medicaid accounts for nearly one-third (31 percent) of all federal outlays in health and well over two-thirds of state health expenditures. The most troubling aspect of Medicaid is not its size but its rate of growth. As table 5.6 illustrates, the program grew by more than $100 billion over the first years of the new millennium. No wonder Medicaid is viewed as an 800-pound gorilla or a monster by state and federal officials trying to control the program.

Several aspects of the Medicaid program entail policy choices that affect costs. The first is the number of persons eligible for the program—it is an entitlement program, which means that all eligible persons are provided

Table 5.6

Medicaid Spending (billions of dollars), 1970–2004

	Total	Federal	State
1970	5.3	2.9	2.5
1980	26.1	14.5	11.6
1985	41.3	22.8	18.4
1990	75.4	42.7	32.7
1995	156.0	89.1	66.9
2000	207.0	117.9	89.1
2004	309.0	176.2	132.8

Sources: OMB 2005; National Association of State Budget Officers 2004.

for under the program. Also important is the scope and level of recipients' benefits. A third important component is the level of payment to providers of the health care service. There is a substantial federal match in Medicaid, ranging from 50 percent for Connecticut, New Jersey, and 10 other states to 77 percent for Mississippi.

Federal law requires that certain groups of persons be covered and certain services provided to them. However, states can expand eligibility to include persons who are "medically needy." In the early 1990s, the federal government mandated expanding the Medicaid program to cover all children up to age 6 in families with incomes between 100 and 133 percent of the federal poverty level and children aged 6 to 15 in families earning up to 100 percent of the federal poverty level. All children on Medicaid get early and periodic screening, diagnosis, and treatment (EPSDT) services, and most Medicaid-eligible children also receive vision, hearing, and dental screening services. When states must reduce Medicaid, they can reduce eligibility for near-poor children and near-poor pregnant women and eliminate or reduce their programs for the medically needy.

Enrollments are cyclical and increase with a poor economy. In the early years of this century, enrollments of nondisabled adults and children in Medicaid rose by around 10 percent a year, while enrollments for people who are aged or disabled rose by around 3 percent a year. The larger increase in enrolled families likely reflects the national decline over that time in the number of individuals covered by employer-sponsored insurance (Kaiser Family Foundation 2005b).

It is also important to understand the distribution of enrollees and their relationship to costs in Medicaid. Children make up nearly 50 percent of those enrolled in Medicaid nationally but account for only 16 percent of Medicaid spending. In contrast, the elderly make up 11 percent of enrollees and account for nearly 30 percent of spending; people who are blind or disabled, 15 percent of enrollees and 40 percent of spending. Both the elderly and persons who are blind or disabled use long-term care services paid for by Medicaid. Nationally, Medicaid covers around 40 percent of all costs for long-term care and covers the care of more than half of all elderly nursing home residents. Demographic trends, including the aging of the baby boom generation, are troublesome to the Medicaid program. The CBO projects that long-term care expenditures for seniors could rise from $195 billion in 2000 (2.1 percent of GDP) to $760 billion in 2040 (about 3.3 percent of GDP) (Holtz-Eakin 2005).

Federal law requires that certain health services be provided to recipients, and states can offer a number of additional services from a list of optional services provided in federal law. During times of state fiscal stress, states limit these optional services, such as dental care, podiatry, chiropractic services, eyeglasses, hearing aids, hospice services, non-emergency use of emergency rooms, and prescription drugs.

States have flexibility in determining the reimbursement policies for most providers. Federal rules set forth administrative requirements in such areas as the designation of a state plan, provider certification, timeliness of provider payments, and quality control. States must also pay the Medicare co-payments of poor elderly who are dually eligible for both Medicare and Medicaid. Until recently, eligibility for Medicaid was tied to two welfare pro-grams: Aid to Families with Dependent Children and Supplemental Security Income. To be eligible, persons had to meet the requirements of cash assis-tance: age, blindness, disability, or membership in a family with dependent children. In 1996, the AFDC linkage was completely severed, with passage of the Personal Responsibility and Work Opportunity Reconciliation Act, which replaced the AFDC entitlement program with the TANF block grant. Under TANF, recipients are required to work, and TANF dollars often go into programs that help recipients find work, rather than providing direct subsidies. Former TANF recipients who find work are eligible for transition services under Medicaid.

A 1997 federal law (the Balanced Budget Act) gave states more flexibility in negotiating reimbursement rates for health providers; this was achieved by repeal of the Boren Amendment, which required states to reimburse hospitals and nursing homes at rates that were reasonable and adequate to meet the essential costs of efficiently and economically operated facilities. In a move typical of the give-and-take of federalism, the BBA also contained several mandates that "cost" the states more. The law restored Medicaid coverage for certain immigrants who lost their eligibility under PRWORA and increased the Medicare Part B premiums that states pay for low-income beneficiaries (Tannenwald 1998). In tight state budgets, states often freeze or cut reimbursement rates for physicians, pharmacies, hospitals, and managed care plans.

Medicaid not only provides funding for qualified individuals, it is also an important contributor to public hospitals that provide care to poor and near-poor persons. Medicaid is the largest source of support for both public hospitals and community health centers. In 2002, Medicaid accounted for 37 percent of revenues to public hospitals, which account for only about 4.3 percent of admissions nationwide but are responsible for 24 percent of uncompensated care provided by the hospital industry. State and local funding provides 15 percent of revenues for these hospitals. The Medicaid assistance comes primarily from Medicaid disproportionate share hospital (DSH) payments, designed to offset losses that hospitals experience from treating Medicaid and uninsured patients. Another source of funding is the Medicaid upper payment limit (UPL), which allows states to pay categories of providers as a group up to the "upper limit" of what Medicare would pay for those services. Both DSH and UPL have come under federal scrutiny and have been the object of Congressional action to curb their use by closing loopholes that allowed states to draw down extra federal funding with minimum state matching (Regenstein and Huang 2005).

Over the years, states have adopted a variety of innovations and administrative improvements in the Medicaid program, such as prior authorization (used primarily for prescription drugs—the physician does not have to obtain the state's permission to prescribe a particular drug), Medicaid Management Information Systems, provider profiles (the state examines physicians' practice patterns to identify any outliers on high-cost procedures such as surgeries), and computerized billing. Some states have established successful programs to control hospital costs, including rate setting based on prospective payment. In the 1990s, the states moved thousands of Medicaid recipients into full-risk managed care arrangements—far ahead of the progress in enrolling Medicare patients in these entities. States, led by Arizona, are also adopting managed care arrangements for the elderly. A provision in the Medicare Modernization Act supports creation of "special needs plans" or managed care plans for specific groups. Maryland has developed a special managed care plan for those who are dually eligible for Medicare and Medicaid, and other states are expected to develop other specialized plans (Foxhall 2005).

Medicaid Waivers

One way states have been able to innovate within the strictures of the federal guidelines on Medicaid is through Medicaid waivers. States can apply for a waiver for certain federal requirements to allow them to more efficiently operate the program. A key component of the waiver is a budget neutrality rule. Program spending under the waiver cannot exceed what it would have been before the waiver.

Several federal program waivers for Medicaid requirements are available to states:

— Section 1915(b) freedom-of-choice waivers allow states to waive statewide-ness, comparability of services, and freedom-of-choice provisions of the law. Many states have used this waiver to enroll beneficiaries in managed care programs, although a 1997 law allowed states to accomplish this via a state plan amendment. Others have used it to carve out a system for special populations or create programs that are not available statewide.

— Section 1915(c) home and community-based services waivers allow states to cover home and community-based services as an alternative to providing long-term care in institutional settings.

— Section 1115 research and demonstration waivers are more comprehensive, enabling states to deviate from standard Medicaid requirements to try out new approaches.

In the 1990s, states used these waivers, especially the broader Section 1115 waiver, to extend Medicaid coverage to previously uninsured groups, to expand the package of medical benefits available to program beneficiaries, and to mandate the enrollment of Medicaid recipients in managed care plans. The most famous pre-1990 waiver was the Arizona Health Care Cost Containment System (AHCCCS), a statewide managed care network, set up in 1982 to use the bidding process to select providers. For the first few years, AHCCCS delivered only acute care; in the early 1990s, it expanded to cover long-term care, home health care, and mental health care. In the mid-1990s, most Section 1115 waivers emphasized managed care.

Oregon used the Section 1115 waiver to provide a new system whereby all of its poor citizens would be provided with a set of health care benefits. Tennessee used the Section 1115 waiver to expand Medicaid to all poor persons in the state. In 2002, Utah used a 1115 waiver to launch its Primary Care Network. The state began to provide primary care to adults between the ages of 19 and 64, with or without children, who have not had health coverage for six months or more and who have annual family incomes of less than 150 percent of the federal poverty level. In order to expand coverage for this population, some services for Medicaid recipients were curtailed or eliminated, including hearing, vision, and dental services, non-emergency transportation, and mental health services. Newly covered recipients of Utah's program pay an annual enrollment fee as well as co-payments (AcademyHealth 2003).

A special subset of 1115 waivers is a pharmacy plus demonstration, which allows states to provide prescription coverage to individuals not eligible for Medicaid whose income is at or below 200 percent of the federal poverty level.

In 2002, a new type of waiver was launched to help reach uninsured populations. Health Insurance Flexibility and Accountability (HIFA) waivers enable states to access their unused S-CHIP allotments, increase cost sharing, and establish enrollment limits for S-CHIP and Medicaid. HIFA also has enhanced states' ability to build on employer-based coverage in programs designed to cover the uninsured. Early use of the HIFA waiver was hampered by states' fiscal difficulties. For example, California officials delayed implementation of an approved HIFA waiver that would have extended coverage to 30,000 uninsured parents of children receiving Medicaid or S-CHIP (AcademyHealth 2003). Other states have used the waiver simply to help reduce rising costs by increasing cost sharing and limiting enrollment. Nevertheless, the waiver has led to some innovations, including New Mexico's program that offers a "commercial-like" benefit package marketed by employers for newly eligible adults. Oregon, Idaho, and Illinois are offering some recipients the choice of usual coverage or premium assistance, in which Medicaid and S-CHIP funds can help subsidize private plans (Artiga and Mann 2005).

Although the purpose of HIFA was to increase the number of persons served under Medicaid and S-CHIP, states, as noted, can also use the waiver to help control rising costs through enrollment constriction and imposition of premiums. One analysis of the program found that little expansion had occurred by 2005, in large part due to states' fiscal problems and the budget neutrality rules (Artiga and Mann 2005). When state revenues are less problematic, HIFA may again be used as a source of program expansion as well as streamlining.

Medicaid's Growing Costs

In the past decade, increases in Medicaid spending were a major problem for states. From 1990 to 2001, Medicaid spending grew at an annual rate of 11 percent; in the first three years of the new century, the growth rate averaged even higher—13 percent (Kaiser Family Foundation 2005b). Partly in an effort to control costs, states enthusiastically adopted Medicaid managed care in the late 1990s. Growth in managed care coverage of Medicaid clients grew from 14 percent in 1994 to 61 percent in 2004 (CMS 2004). Also important to many state officials was the appeal of managed care as a "market solution" to dealing with health care delivery. For some states the change was accomplished swiftly. For example, Michigan's motto of "Fire, Ready, Aim" resulted in a program implemented statewide in only 18 months (C. Weissert and Goggin 2000). Other states, including Maryland, took the task more slowly. Still others, such as Kansas and West Virginia, had a difficult time launching any program given the dearth of managed care entities in those states.

Between 2002 and 2004, when many states were seeing greatly reduced revenues and tightened budgets, states tried to control Medicaid spending by raising eligibility standards, reducing benefits, and lowering provider payments. Many states also embraced disease management programs in Medicaid, whereby a state provides a case manager for those with specific chronic diseases such as asthma and diabetes. The idea is that a case manager will provide oversight and a treatment plan that will reduce expensive complications that require emergency care or hospital stays. Well over half of the states have adopted disease management as a component of their Medicaid program (AcademyHealth 2005).

Some states have targeted Medicaid spending for pharmaceutical drugs. Several have joined multistate purchasing cooperatives to increase their bargaining power for deeper discounts from pharmaceutical providers. States have set up preferred drugs lists, mandatory use of generic drugs, contracting with pharmacy benefit managers, quantity limitations, cost sharing, and prior authorization as mechanisms to hold down costs (W. Weissert and Miller 2005). A number of these states have been sued—often unsuccessfully—by PhRMA, the pharmaceutical industry's trade group, in an attempt to stop states' efforts to lower drug prices.

The huge program is a likely candidate for reform for states, given that it can consume as much as a quarter of the state budget. However, it is also important to remember that Medicaid spending is far from profligate. While Medicaid spending per enrollee grew at an annual rate of 6.1 percent between 2000 and 2003, after controlling for changes in demographics we find that this rate was lower than the annual rate of increase for Medicare (6.9 percent) and for private insurance (10.6 percent). During that period, premiums in private insurance rose by an average of 12.6 percent annually (Kaiser Family Foundation 2005b).

One study simulated the effects of covering privately insured individuals with Medicaid and covering Medicaid recipients with private insurance benefits. Hadley and Holahan (2003/2004) found that if low-income privately insured individuals were instead to receive Medicaid, their costs would be lower; and if Medicaid beneficiaries were instead covered by private insurance, their costs would be considerably higher. The researchers concluded that much of the difference in spending between Medicaid and private insurance is due to provider payment rates, which are much lower for Medicaid. Other studies have found that administrative costs are much lower for Medicaid than for HMOs and private insurance. Thus, Medicaid seems to be a good bargain—in spite of some political punditry that highlights its inefficiency and waste.

Florida has launched an effort to significantly reform Medicaid by turning it into a case-mix-adjusted vendor payment program, in which Medicaid recipients have allocations based on their health needs. Recipients can choose a plan from a "marketplace" of HMOs, preferred provider organizations, and new entities that offer clients a package of services that might differ significantly from one entity to another. One of the most interesting things about the Florida proposal is that it allows recipients to use their Medicaid payment to buy into their employer's health insurance. A federal waiver is required for the program.

In 2005, Medicaid was the target of federal cuts as well. The president's budget proposed establishing a new prescription drug price target for states and imposing penalties for individuals who transfer assets to become eligible for Medicaid long-term care. The president also called for $10 billion in Medicaid cuts over five years. The cuts were included in the final budget resolution, along with a new Medicaid commission to identify those cuts and assess the long-term prospects for the program. The NGA has offered its own set of recommendations to improve state flexibility and produce more efficiencies, including use of reverse mortgages; more ability to ask for recipient cost sharing and to establish differing levels of benefits; individual and employer tax credits for health insurance; state purchasing pools; reinsurance pools, in which employers and other payers would be reimbursed by the federal government for part of the cost of employees' catastrophic medical bills; and tax credits for long-term care insurance and long-term care partnerships, under which individuals who purchase private insurance and exhaust its coverage would be allowed to access Medicaid and still protect some of their assets. While states can come up with these innovations, it is difficult to put them in place without federal waivers, which can be a time-consuming and burdensome process (NGA 2005).

Medicaid is crucial to the country's health safety-net system. It provides care to the poorest and sickest citizens and props up the hospitals and clinics that serve those citizens. The states' role in Medicaid is pivotal—funding and, more importantly, defining the program and its parameters. The federalist nature of this program—its shared federal and state responsibilities—is both its strength and its weakness. It is a strength in that each state can meet the health needs of its poor population in the manner best suited to that state. It is also a strength in that states can innovate with the program in ways that can be replicated, if successful, by other states. The weakness is that states cannot spend beyond their means and thus must curtail the program when state revenues are reduced. This leads to a program that undergoes cycles of expansion and restructuring that result in uncertainty for recipients and providers alike. Ironically, program needs increase in times of national or regional economic difficulties—the very times when state coffers are also adversely affected.

Children's Health Insurance Program

A second important federal-state health program emerged as part of the BBA in 1997: the State Children's Health Insurance Program. Congress appropriated $24 billion over 5 fiscal years and $40 billion over 10 years to enable states to expand health insurance to children whose families earn too much to qualify for Medicaid but too little to afford private health insurance. S-CHIP is a block grant that allocates money to states based on the number of uninsured low-income children, adjusted for the state's average cost of health care. Since fiscal year 2001, the formula has also taken into account the number of all low-income children, covered or not, residing in the state. The program's matching-fund arrangement (the state's contribution) is more generous to states than is Medicaid's: 70 percent of the Medicaid matching rate.

States have considerable leeway in designing their S-CHIP programs. Under the federal law, states can establish a new children's program, can fold the new program into their existing Medicaid programs, or do both. Some 23 states elected to expand Medicaid, 15 set up a separate S-CHIP program, and 18 both expanded Medicaid and set up a new S-CHIP program (GAO 2000). States set eligibility standards limited only by federal ceilings of children living in families with incomes below 200 percent of the federal poverty level. However, states must deal with provisions in the federal law that stipulate minimum benefits, impose maintenance-of-effort requirements, limit use of premiums and co-payments, and prohibit states from enrolling in S-CHIP any children who qualify for Medicaid.

For Congress, S-CHIP was a popular issue for which both Republicans and Democrats could take credit. Democrats had long supported federally funded coverage for children. The Republicans also viewed S-CHIP, along with welfare reform, as part of an ideological plan to devolve more authority to states. For the president, S-CHIP represented a step toward dealing with one segment of the uninsured population and as such can be viewed as a "legacy of the Clinton administration's failed Health Security Act of 1993" (Hegner 1998, 2). Ironically, S-CHIP was of greatest benefit to states that had not acted on their own to provide health care for poor children. Three states in particular—Vermont, Minnesota, and Washington—already had programs in place for children in families living at or below 200 percent of poverty. Some additional federal dollars were available for these states to further expand their programs, but the amounts were small and the states were reluctant to participate in the program (Hegner 1998).

Enrollment of children in S-CHIP was slow. In the first 18 months of the program, states used less than 20 percent of the S-CHIP allocation. States were criticized in some quarters for being slow in developing the program infrastructure, including a potent marketing strategy, but other observers noted that many children referred to S-CHIP were actually eligible for Medicaid (Schram and C. Weissert 1999). In the third and fourth years of the program, enrollments increased. Further, states with the lowest level of coverage before S-CHIP expanded their income eligibility thresholds the most during the first two years of implementation, and states with the largest percentages of low-income uninsured children increased their income eligibility thresholds to a greater degree than states with smaller percentages of uninsured children (Ullman, Hill, and Almeida 1999). Some states used S-CHIP to expand coverage to parents. For example, Wisconsin's BadgerCare covers both children and parents with family incomes too high for Medicaid and without access to group heath insurance. By the end of the sixth year of the program, the national S-CHIP enrollment was four million children. Together with Medicaid, S-CHIP provides a critical safety net for poor and near-poor children.

Medicaid and S-CHIP, while important, are not the only health programs in states or the only area where innovations have occurred. In the 1980s, with rising concern for federal spending patterns and efforts to reduce federal grants and other program funding, states began to assume leadership in the area of public health, mental health, substance abuse, the environment, and health services delivery mechanisms and to offer innovative approaches to providing services while controlling costs. They continued that leadership into the new millennium.

Medicare Modernization Act

The 2003 Medicare Modernization Act contained some provisions that directly affect states. First and foremost, the law eliminated the federal provision that Medicaid is responsible for prescription drug coverage for dually eligible individuals—those who qualify for both Medicare and Medicaid—a group that uses drugs extensively. However, the law contains a "clawback" feature that requires states to repay the federal government 90 percent of what the state would have spent on drugs for this population if the state's program as it was in 2003 had remained in place. (After 10 years, the percentage falls to 75 percent.) The provision causes two problems. First, it puts in place a new federal grant feature in which states actually send monthly checks to Washington—what one observer called a reverse block grant (Adams 2005b). The second problem is that the provision is more costly to those innovative states that acted to cut prescription drug costs after the baseline year of 2003. California is one of those states. The state will send back 90 percent of higher pre-reform costs—a move that will cost the state $215 million more in 2007 than it would have cost without the MMA (Adams 2005b). Thus, ironically, states that were "pioneers" in reforming their Medicaid prescription drug costs might be punished the most, while states that had not acted will not be adversely affected (W. Weissert and Miller 2005). Some concerns have been raised about the constitutionality of the federal clawback, which might be viewed as "commandeering" state legislatures as revenue agents (Pear 2005a).

The law also requires states to help the federal government implement the new drug benefit, called Medicare Part D—a requirement without federal funding. States that operate state-only prescription drug programs must decide whether and how to coordinate their program with the new benefit. States worry that their negotiating power with drug companies for greater discounts will be harmed with the loss of the low-income dually eligible population from their program. States are also required under the MMA to work with the Social Security Administration to market to and recruit new participants in the federal program—an assignment not accompanied by special funding.

States benefited in the MMA from a new subsidy for employers (including states) that retain their current retiree drug benefits. Finally, the law created health savings accounts, which states may use as an option for covering state employees. Chapter 7 provides a more detailed analysis of this important new law.

Other Federal Assistance

The Health Resources and Services Administration offers state planning grants for states to launch programs to reduce their numbers of uninsured persons. The agency has provided both planning grants and pilot project grants to test new programs in one or more areas or for specific populations or to help implement a plan (AcademyHealth 2005, 18).

STATE INNOVATIONS IN HEALTH

Innovations in health and other key areas at the state level are very useful in that they can serve as test cases, working out problems and highlighting consequences before being implemented nationally. The use of the states as "laboratories of democracy" has a long history in the United States. The 1921 Sheppard-Towner Act, providing social and medical assistance to pregnant women and babies, was copied from a Connecticut law, and states provided models for the 1935 Social Security Act, the 1973 Supplemental Security Income programs, and dozens of health measures (Silver 1991). More recently, Medicare's DRG payment system was based on a program in New Jersey. S-CHIP was based on existing state programs, and federal patients' bill of rights legislation was patterned on state enactments. New York governor Nelson Rockefeller once noted that "those elements of the New Deal which failed were largely in areas *not* tested by prior experience at the state level" (Silver 1991, 445).

States have the resources, the infrastructure, and the desire to make health system changes that positively affect their citizens. Sometimes these changes are copied by other states and the policy "diffuses" throughout the nation. State efforts to regulate managed care organizations are one example. Over a period of three to five years, legislation on managed care was introduced in every state, and 40 states enacted new restrictions on managed care organizations (Hackey 2001).

A state can act to respond to issues and concerns in ways that might not be acceptable across all 50 states. Oregon's innovative Health Plan, which prioritized funding for health care by ranking medical services, is one example. Other examples are legalization of medical marijuana, legalization of assisted suicide, and laws requiring businesses to provide health insurance for their employees. While a handful of states adopted environmental standards in the direction of those proposed in the Kyoto Protocol, 16 states passed legislation or resolutions urging against adoption of the protocol in the U.S. Senate (Rabe 2004). The point is that states are composed of citizens with differing preferences for health care, taxation, and other issues. State policymakers recognize those preferences and produce legislation that serves their constituencies. In so doing, they often act before, and offer guidance to, other states and the national government.

States often act when political difficulties prevent national action. A good example is state action in the 1990s on genetically modified food. Minnesota was the first state to institute strict regulations on genetically modified food in 1992. New York petitioned the FDA to establish a formal review process and require the labeling of genetically modified foods in 1994. By 1997, Wisconsin, Maine, Vermont, and Minnesota had laws requiring the labeling of genetically modified milk.

Finally, states can often act quickly when issues arise that engage or outrage constituencies. For example, in 2005, when it became known that many new cars contained computer chips that store information on speed and seat belt use, Maryland and seven other states introduced legislation to inform consumers that their cars had the chip, and some prohibited use of data from the chip in court cases, unless there is a court order (Associated Press 2005b).

In recent years, states have launched innovative programs to provide coverage for the working poor, to reform small-group health insurance and establish risk pools for those who find insurance difficult to obtain, to mandate community rating, to develop new ways of delivering services to Medicaid recipients and state employees, and more (table 5.7). While some of these programs are funded with only state funds, many are jointly funded with federal funds and made possible through waivers or grant programs designed to encourage innovation.

Coverage for the Near Poor

In the 1990s, several states expanded coverage for near-poor people or provided a type of Medicaid buy-in. Connecticut, Florida, Maine, Minnesota, New York, and Vermont initiated health care coverage for children in the early 1990s. Washington State and Maine expanded Medicaid coverage to some low-income people (GAO 1992). New York adopted a state-funded children's health insurance program in 1991. The program subsidized health insurance for children up to age 13 in families with incomes up to 185 percent of the federal poverty level. Families with higher incomes could buy into the

Table 5.7

Some State Innovative Health Policies, 1965–2005

1965	New York adopts certificate of need
1974	Hawaii passes state-mandated employer-sponsored insurance
	Rhode Island enacts catastrophic health insurance plan
1975	Indiana enacts comprehensive medical malpractice act
	Connecticut establishes risk pool for uninsured
1976	Maryland establishes all-payer system for hospitals
1977	New Mexico adopts right-to-die act
	New York adopts "nursing home without walls" program
1978	New Jersey extends rate setting to all payers and hospitals
1981	Oregon receives Medicaid home care community-based care waiver
1982	California enables preferred provider organizations to do business in the state
	Arizona launches capitated program for Medicaid
	New York develops uncompensated care pool for sharing hospital revenues
1983	Virginia adopts natural death law
	Oregon contracts with providers on prepaid capitation basis for Medicaid patients
1984	Florida taxes hospitals to supplement state match for Medicaid expansion
	New Jersey reimburses hospitals using diagnosis-related groups
	New York enacts mandatory seat belt law
1987	Washington makes basic health services available for low-income residents in five areas of state
1988	Massachusetts passes first pay-or-play employer mandate
	Kansas enacts broad employee wellness program
1989	Oregon enacts legislation establishing rationing system
	Rhode Island passes "bare bones" insurance plans for small businesses
	Arizona launches capitated long-term care program for elderly
1990	Maine establishes practice guidelines to reduce medical liability
	Maine introduces Resource-Based Relative Value Scale into Medicaid
	Connecticut enacts small-group insurance market reform
1991	Connecticut receives clearance for state-endorsed long-term care insurance
	New York phases in requirement that 50 percent of Medicaid (AFDC) recipients be in managed care
	New York enacts state-funded children's health insurance program
1992	Minnesota attempts universal coverage through integrated service networks
	Minnesota institutes strict regulations on genetically modified foods
	Vermont requires community-rated health insurance

Table 5.7 *(cont.)*

1993	Washington and Florida adopt managed competition programs
	Tennessee expands Medicaid program to cover categorically ineligible people above poverty
	Missouri passes medical savings account law
	New Jersey guarantees issue of health coverage for individuals, requiring small-group insurers to either participate in the individual market or help cover the losses of insurers who do
1994	Mississippi and Florida sue to recover state dollars spent on tobacco-related illness
	Oregon voters adopt assisted suicide measure
	Kentucky establishes statewide alliance based on public employees
	California and Maryland adopt bans on smoking in any enclosed space that is also a place of employment
1995	Maryland passes anti-dumping law for nursing home residents
1996	Rhode Island requires all health plans in the state to provide subscribers with consumers' guide
	Massachusetts issues profiles of physicians, including disciplinary actions and settlements, on the Internet
	California, by approving a popular initiative, legalizes medical marijuana
1997	Texas permits patients to sue their health plan for damages if they are injured by the plan's decision to deny coverage for medical treatment
1999	Pennsylvania enacts patients' bill of rights calling for providers and health plans to use sound medical principles, not financial incentives, as the basis for patient care
2000	California requires hospitals to meet fixed nurse-to-patient ratios
2001	New York establishes Healthy NY, designed to assist small business owners to provide health insurance to employees
	Florida develops preferred drug list under Medicaid
2003	Maine enacts law setting special goals and timelines for greenhouse gas reductions
	Maine launches plan to achieve universal coverage in six years
2004	Minnesota launches reimportation program for drugs from Canada, Minnesota RxConnect
	California, by initiative, adopts $6 million stem cell research program
2005	Vermont files lawsuit against the FDA for failing to approve the state's proposal to establish a pilot program
	Florida launches major revamping of its Medicaid program by using health-adjusted vouchers

Sources: Data from *State Health Notes*, Intergovernmental Health Policy Project, various issues, updated with information from AcademyHealth 2003, 2005.

program. The New York program served as a model for the federal S-CHIP initiative (Brandon, Chaudry, and Sardell 2001).

One of the most daring and controversial attempts to cover the near poor was the establishment of TennCare, Tennessee's 1993 expansion of Medicaid to all uninsured residents of the state. The TennCare proposal is noteworthy for its genesis. It was put in place by the governor's executive order. Only minor changes, encompassing just one and a half pages of legislative language, were put into law. Though it dramatically increased access to health care in the state, covering 25 percent of the state's population, TennCare began as an effort to control Medicaid costs, which in 1993 accounted for more than 26 percent of the state budget. The choices, said the governor, were to raise taxes, slash medical benefits for poor people, or try something new. He proposed the third choice (Lemov 1994). The implementation of TennCare remained rocky and controversial for years. The state had to take over a large TennCare HMO and make major concessions to BlueCross BlueShield of Tennessee, which threatened to pull out of the program. The program was greatly underfunded. Finally, in 2005, the governor pulled the plug on most of the TennCare program, saying "TennCare was, and is, a wonderful dream" (AcademyHealth 2005, 10). The state dropped more than 300,000 adults from the program, transforming it from an innovative expansion to cover most of the state's uninsured to the more typical Medicaid program with eligibility tied to categories of illness or program qualification (Lemov 2005).

Other states have used Medicaid, S-CHIP, and state dollars to craft comprehensive programs. For example, in 2003 Maine adopted a comprehensive plan called Dirigo Health Reform (*dirigo* is Latin for "I lead"). Under Dirigo, the state increases access to health insurance for small-business employees, the self-employed, and individuals through expansion of S-CHIP and Medicaid and development of a public-private health plan for small businesses that encourages them to participate through lower rates. Individuals and the self-employed participate on a sliding-scale schedule (AcademyHealth 2005, 16). Funding comes from tobacco settlement funds, general revenues, and two new sources: contributions paid by employers and employees who enroll in the program, and an assessment on insurance revenues captured only when Dirigo's cost-containment efforts document reductions in health care costs. Its goal is to establish universal coverage in the state within six years.

Other states subsidize insurance for high-risk citizens, those working in small businesses, or those who are self-employed. Healthy New York provides standardized health insurance benefit packages, offered by all HMOs in the state. The packages are more affordable through state sponsorship so that more small employers and individuals can purchase health insurance coverage. West Virginia created a public-private partnership between the West Virginia Public Employees Insurance Agency and state insurance companies to provide subsidized health care coverage for small businesses (AcademyHealth 2005).

Some states have alleviated some of the mandates on health insurance sold in the state as a way to make health insurance more affordable. By allowing minimum benefit plans, 12 states have taken this route, although there is little evidence that such laws have been effective in increasing enrollment (AcademyHealth 2005, 31).

Managing Managed Care

Beginning in the mid-1990s, states began to regulate managed care entities. The first wave of laws dealt with providers, including many state laws that limited managed care entities' ability to exclude health professions. Dubbed "any willing provider laws," these laws were unpopular with HMOs trying to hold down costs but were promoted by health professionals of all stripes. By 2000, every state had passed some type of consumer protection in managed care, such as outlawing "gag clauses" that prevented physicians from advising patients about medically necessary treatment options, ensuring access to emergency care and using a "prudent layperson" definition of emergency, allowing women to see their obstetrician-gynecologist without first consulting a primary care practitioner, setting standards for length of hospital stay for maternity and mastectomy patients, providing continuing care after termination of a provider contract, and offering a range of new types of information to enrollees and prospective enrollees.

The spread of managed care led to calls for more consumer protection, such as the right to appeal adverse decisions or to sue the managed care organization. Although several states passed laws allowing patients to sue their HMOs for malpractice, in 2004 the U.S. Supreme Court ruled that ERISA preempts these laws (*Aetna Health, Inc. v. Davila*). Other states published performance reports for HMOs operating in the state and developed physicians' profile systems that make information on disciplinary actions and malpractice judgments available to the public. Meanwhile, there is no federal law regulating managed care.

Prescription Drugs: Access, Cost, and Quality Issues

States are working to improve access, control costs, and ensure the quality of prescription drugs for their citizenry. The access issue has revolved around the poor elderly who do not qualify for Medicaid. Almost two-thirds of the states have adopted pharmaceutical assistance programs for low-income persons who are elderly or disabled and do not qualify for Medicaid. Most of these use state dollars to assist in the purchase of prescription drugs. Well over a dozen states achieve price reductions through pharmaceutical discounts and manufacturer rebates. Other states provide assistance to this group through multistate purchasing cooperatives, in which states join together to negotiate lower prices for drugs (W. Weissert and Miller 2005).

States' efforts to hold down the costs of prescription drugs in the Medicaid program were discussed earlier in this chapter. In addition, some states established or joined purchasing pools for prescription drugs for state employees. One of the earliest such pools, the Minnesota Multi-State Contracting Alliance for Pharmacy (MMCAP), allows states and cities to negotiate for manufacturers' rebates with bulk purchases. A newer version of pools has both negotiated rates and a single pharmacy benefit manager who facilitates drug choices, makes recommendations based on research syntheses, and implements state pharmacy policies. One such arrangement is the RxIS Coalition, involving Ohio, Delaware, Missouri, New Mexico, and West Virginia, which negotiates prescription drug discounts for state employees using a single PBM. Georgia set up an intrastate pool including Medicaid, state employees' insurance, and its state Board of Regents that uses a PBM to negotiate manufacturers' discounts (Krause 2005).

Some states sought permission from the federal government to buy drugs from Canada and other countries at prices below U.S. prices (they must seek permission because federal law prohibits the reimportation of prescription drugs manufactured in the United States by anyone other than the original manufacturers). All state requests were rejected. An HHS-appointed task force on prescription drug reimportation also recommended maintaining the current policy, based on "safety concerns" (W. Weissert and Miller 2005, 131). Several states pursued their importation strategies without federal approval. Several local governments have also established reimportation programs. In a preemptive move, in August 2004, Vermont filed a lawsuit against the FDA for failing to approve its proposal to establish a pilot program (W. Weissert and Miller 2005). In 2004, five states—Illinois, Wisconsin, Kansas, Missouri, and Vermont—formed SaveRx, a program to purchase drugs from Canada,

Britain, and Ireland. When the Canadian minister of health announced plans in 2005 to limit prescription exports to the United States, the states added Australia and New Zealand to their medication sources (Ruethling 2005).

Finally, quality is the primary concern of a new multistate cooperative effort led by Oregon, which reviews published medical and scientific evidence on drugs in a particular class and makes the findings available to state officials in the program. When no differences are found between more expensive and much cheaper drugs, state officials can use the information in updating their drug formularies for Medicaid, and sometimes for state employees (Pear and Dao 2004).

Tobacco Settlement

The states' settlement with the nation's cigarette manufacturers in 1999 was one of the most interesting intergovernmental health policy stories of the decade and provided funding for numerous public health initiatives across the country. The story begins with a courageous attorney general from Mississippi who launched a lawsuit against cigarette manufacturers in 1994 to recoup state Medicaid dollars spent on diseases and disabilities caused by smoking. Attorneys general in Texas, Florida, and Minnesota soon followed suit. The tobacco industry decided to settle out of court rather than allow the cases to go to trial. By 1997, one cigarette manufacturer, Liggett, had decided to settle with the states—now numbering more than 40; the company agreed to accept liability in exchange for immunity from further suits by states or individuals. Later that year, the attorneys general reached agreement with the tobacco industry on the regulation of cigarettes by the FDA, on restrictions on advertising, and on payment of $369 billion over the next 25 years to compensate states for the costs of treating smoking-related illnesses, to finance antismoking campaigns, and to help finance health care for uninsured children. In exchange, the tobacco companies would be immune from future class-action suits and would not be liable for punitive damages for past misconduct. Because it involved a federal agency, the agreement had to be approved by Congress.

Congress proved to be a much more difficult battlefield for public health advocates. It simply could not come to closure on legislation implementing or modifying the initial agreement. In 1998, the attorneys general struck a new agreement with the tobacco industry—this time one that did not require congressional approval. Under this agreement, the 46 signatory states would get $206 billion over 25 years (4 states had settled out of court earlier). Also, the tobacco companies agreed to eliminate advertising on billboards and in sports arenas and to spend $1.5 billion on an antismoking ad campaign. In return, the states promised not to sue the cigarette companies again. Money began flowing to states in 2000. While some antismoking proponents had hoped settlement dollars would flow to health programs, and specifically to antismoking programs, this has not happened.

Very few states are spending anywhere near 20 to 25 percent of the settlement proceeds on smoking prevention programs. When states have fiscal difficulties, it is especially easy to reduce funding for these programs and spend the settlement money on Medicaid, education, or a myriad of other ongoing needs. In a report assessing states' use of the settlement funds, the Campaign for Tobacco-Free Kids (2005) noted that only three states—Maine, Delaware, and Mississippi—funded smoking prevention programs at or above the minimum levels recommended by the CDC. Thirty-seven states are funding programs at less than half of the suggested minimum.

Medical Malpractice

One of the most politically contentious issues that have dogged states for decades is medical malpractice. Malpractice insurance rates for some physician specialties have risen enormously—in at least eight states, 30 percent between 2001 and 2002 for internal medicine, general surgery, and obstetrics-gynecology (Jost 2003)—and when this happens, the call for action goes out to state capitols. While the situation early in the twenty-first century is less dire than in the 1970s, when private insurers were driven out of the market, any increases in malpractice premiums become more pertinent when the increases are difficult to pass on to patients in HMOs and fee-limited Medicare and Medicaid. The question is, what to do about it. While physicians and insurance companies are convinced that the costs are directly associated with court settlements, the evidence is not in their corner. A GAO study (2003) concluded that rising malpractice premiums were the result of a variety of factors, including poor returns on investments of insurance companies.

Nevertheless, a number of states have dealt with the issue by capping malpractice non-economic settlements. Many states copied the 1976 California law putting a $250,000 cap on non-economic damages, or those involving "pain and suffering." The law also limited attorneys' contingency fees, required large damage awards to be paid over time rather than immediately, and allowed defendants to introduce evidence of insurance benefits received by plaintiffs. Interestingly, states are still modeling their laws on the 1976 California law, even though a later (1988) California measure dealing with insurance reform actually reduced costs more significantly.

But caps are not the only component of malpractice reform. States have also enacted insurance reforms, mediation procedures, and underwriting programs. In 2001–2, three states—West Virginia, Pennsylvania, and Nevada—adopted comprehensive medical malpractice reforms that dealt with tort and insurance issues. Nineteen states enacted some legislation on malpractice in 2005 (NCSL 2005b). Among these innovative solutions were the following:

- state-established insurance funds from which doctors can purchase insurance if there is no other insurance carrier on the market (Nevada and West Virginia);
- state funds for paying a portion of settlements against a health care provider (Kansas, Pennsylvania, and Wisconsin);
- state-run medical malpractice insurance programs (West Virginia);
- voluntary arbitration programs (Michigan);
- requirements that hospitals report adverse incidents and that the aggregate hospital-specific data are made available to the public (New York);
- development of medical guidelines that physicians can use in defending against malpractice claims (Maine);
- creation of a data center to collect information on medical errors, to coordinate state agencies, and to develop innovative strategies to reduce errors and develop provider profiles and provide information to the public (Iowa); and
- strengthening of state medical boards' power to investigate and review physicians (Massachusetts and Pennsylvania) (NGA 2002).

In spite of the plethora of state actions, the president and the Republican House of Representatives wanted federal action—specifically, legislation to cap compensation for pain and suffering at $250,000 in successful malpractice suits. The national law was backed by interest groups representing insurance companies and physicians, who argued that national legislation would reduce the costs of court settlements and "defensive medicine," in which physicians prescribe excessive tests and procedures to avoid possible misdiagnosis (Stolberg 2002b). The calls for federal legislation in malpractice are nothing new. The same groups also lobbied the first President Bush, and he proposed legislation in 1991 to penalize states that did not enact a $250,000 cap on non-economic damages. The effort was unsuccessful (Jost 2003).

Mental Health

Mental health has long been a state and local responsibility. States serve as both third-party payers and direct providers of mental health services. States are the most important policy players in mental health, spending more than $13 billion to fund their state mental health agencies and match Medicaid mental health spending (Frank and McGuire 1996). States also influence mental health services through insurance regulation. Some states have adopted laws mandating a minimal mental health coverage for private insurance.

State mental hospitals were first established in the mid-1800s and soon became custodial institutions, to some extent mingling mental illness and indigence. The costs to the state were substantial. In the early 1950s, one-third of the New York State budget went to mental health care. Some relief came from the federal government with funding from Medicare, Medicaid, and the Community Mental Health Center program. With Medicaid, many elderly patients in state mental hospitals were transferred to nursing homes. In 1981, 10 federal categorical grants were consolidated into the alcohol, drug abuse, and mental health block grant (along with a 30 percent reduction in funding). Block-grant dollars make up only about 5 percent of state mental health budgets (Frank and McGuire 1996).

In the 1990s, states began to incorporate mental health services into Medicaid managed care, often through "carve-outs," or subcontracts to nonprofit or private entities. Some states use county or regional public or quasi-public bodies as the lead providers of mental health services to Medicaid patients. Mental health advocates, often well organized in states, have been active to ensure that contracts adequately protect the needs of patients. States continue to enact mental health parity laws, ensuring that mental health benefits are equivalent to those of other medical coverage, and to mandate insurers to provide mental health coverage.

Community Health

With the emphasis on devolution in the 1990s came a growing interest in the potential of community-based health. One could argue that community decisions have always been a major part of the nation's health policy, dating back to colonial poor laws. But the importance of communities in U.S. health policy increased during the 1960s with the development of community mental health and health centers, and this increasing community empowerment continued into the 1980s and 1990s with a strong business cast: local coalitions of health purchasers and other community-based efforts to hold down costs. In the 1990s, the emphasis was on more decision making at the community level. Several states set up mechanisms whereby local or regional health groups could make funding decisions and take the lead in prioritizing health care needs locally. The W. K. Kellogg and other foundations supported efforts to help communities organize to deal with health professions education and issues of health care for the uninsured. The task was not easy, in part because community was not an important theme in health care reform in Congress or among the citizenry. When health care reform is defined broadly to include long-term care and substance abuse, there is more support for community-based efforts (M. Schlesinger 1997).

At least 20 states have organized community-based systems of care for the uninsured, usually with counties as the primary focus (AcademyHealth 2005). Florida has long relied on counties to provide coverage for the uninsured and has several successful county programs that provide primary care to their uninsured residents. Michigan also has several county-based programs that provide coverage, commingling employer, individual, and county contributions.

Other Issues

In several policy areas, states are taking the lead where the federal government has refused to act. Two examples are greenhouse warming and stem cell research.

As noted earlier, several states have adopted laws on greenhouse warming, an area where the federal government has decided against meeting international guidelines set forth in the Kyoto Protocol. Rabe (2004) traces state activity back to the late 1990s when several states established carbon dioxide emission standards. Six New England states established regionwide standards for carbon dioxide emissions, along with Quebec and the four Maritime provinces of Canada. Since January 2000, new legislation and executive orders to reduce greenhouse gases were approved in more than one-third of the states (Rabe 2004). In 2003, Maine became the first state to pass a law establishing goals and timetables for greenhouse gas reductions (Scheberle 2005).

The federal government has also been reluctant to adopt far-reaching policy on stem cell research. Two states—New Jersey and California—have moved ahead on their own to provide funding for embryonic stem cell research. In addition, Virginia has funded research for sources other than embryos such as bone marrow or umbilical cord blood.

A third area is one where there is interest in Washington but little action: improving access to health records through information technology. A number of states are investigating or have launched statewide e-health networks to allow the sharing of patients' records among physicians, insurance companies, and pharmacies (M. Carey and Reichard 2005).

For residents with AIDS, states have purchased private health insurance, prohibited discriminatory practices, organized special facilities to provide targeted care, and provided their own funding for treatment. States have also taken measures to protect confidentiality in testing for HIV. Maine was the first state to expand Medicaid benefits to people living with HIV.

Long-term care, an area in which federal policy has floundered, has been the focus of several state efforts. States have led the way in providing home and community-based care programs in an effort to provide more choices for needy elderly persons. Washington State has authorized demonstration projects of social health maintenance organizations, HMOs that gather a full range of health and social services for elderly people under one organization. Connecticut was the first state to encourage the purchase of long-term care insurance.

States are launching programs to promote health and fitness among their own employees, offering a surcharge on insurance premiums for smokers (four states); reimbursing employees for health expenses, including exercise equipment and membership in fitness centers (South Dakota); sponsoring "weigh-ins" for state employees (Georgia); and establishing health savings accounts for state employees (Florida) (Cotterell 2005).

In sum, states have launched new programs in areas as broad as providing insurance to those who lack it and as specific as contracting with a vendor to monitor and pay for therapy for asthma or diabetes. States are concerned with efficiency but also effectiveness; they are trying to improve access to care while assuring that the care given is not redundant or excessive. They are using technology, research, and market-based approaches to achieve these goals. And they are learning from each other.

Diffusion of State Innovation

States learn and pick up ideas from other states. Sometimes policies go quickly from one state to another. For example, in May 1995, Maryland was the first state to adopt legislation to address what became known as "drive-through deliveries," mandating longer hospital stays for women after childbirth. Within

18 months, 24 more states had adopted this policy (DeClercq and Simmes 1997). Similarly, in 1992, when a U.S. Supreme Court decision gave state legislators more freedom to regulate abortion (*Casey v. Planned Parenthood of Southeastern Pennsylvania*), virtually no states had informed-consent abortion laws; eight years later, such laws were in effect in 27 states. In 2004, two states enacted legislation limiting cell-phone use for teen drivers; in 2005, eight more states acted (R. Tanner 2005). Similar diffusion occurred with bans or restrictions on late-term abortions and enforcement of parental involvement statutes (New 2005). In contrast, no other state adopted Oregon's Health Plan, which established a priority list of services available to Medicaid recipients, commonly referred to outside the state as "rationing" services. Thanks in part to federal insistence, Oregon was able to eliminate or "ration" only a few marginal services, saving little money. So states pick those policies they are interested in (often the "easy" ones) and perhaps ignore issues they do not like. And many states modify the proposals to their own needs.

States also learn from one another's mistakes. California was successful with its state-sponsored purchasing cooperatives, but other states—including Texas and Florida—had many problems. In 1999, the last carrier pulled out of the Texas Insurance Purchasing Alliance, leaving thousands of enrollees without coverage. Kentucky and Washington had difficulties with their innovative efforts at individual market reforms. In Kentucky, for example, most insurers left the state's individual insurance market in protest of the state law. Washington State had to abandon its efforts to move the SSI population into managed care in 1998. In 2000, just six weeks after it began operation, an innovative managed care mental health program for children in Arkansas was suddenly terminated. Each of these efforts was instructive to the state involved—and to others—in issues ranging from the importance of a strong base of providers to careful attention to adverse selection.

Many groups help states in their policy making. National interest groups with local affiliates often promote state legislation that they like. For example, the national organizations of nonprofit hospitals and other interests were active in promoting state legislation that prescribed how mergers and acquisitions of nonprofit hospitals were to be accomplished. Many national foundations fund states to deal with issues of concern to them. For example, the Robert Wood Johnson Foundation's Covering Kids initiative provides money to communities to improve health access initiatives for low-income uninsured children.

The diffusion of state policies has long been of interest to political scientists. Early research indicated that diffusion was largely regional, as states within a region looked to "leader" states for guidance in handling similar problems (J. Walker 1969). With improved technology and the expansion of sources of information and networking, states now tend to reach farther afield for their ideas, often to try out an idea of a state unlike their own in population, wealth, and ideology. Many state legislative staffs communicate with one another, and organizations such as the National Conference of State Legislatures and the National Governors Association provide opportunities for face-to-face meetings with counterparts across the country to obtain up-to-date information about what other states are doing, including legislative language and technical assessments.

Nevertheless, some states pride themselves on being more innovative than others. These are states with policy cultures or legacies that are conducive to major innovation. One observer of intergovernmental affairs, John Shannon of the Urban Institute, likened states to convoys. No state wants to be too far ahead of the pack, and no state wants to be in a vulnerable position in the rear. But some like to be among the first to try new programs. Maine, Vermont, Minnesota, and Oregon have often led the way in new approaches to dealing with problems in health, the environment, criminal justice, and other areas. Virginia, by contrast, is more comfortable letting other states try out ideas and work out the problems. There are some noteworthy exceptions, however. In 1993, Tennessee, generally comfortable in the middle of the convoy, launched its innovative TennCare program, which was examined and watched closely by states across the country. And innovative states are often not innovative in all areas. In one study of health professions education, for example, Maine, Massachusetts, and New Jersey, often innovative, were not among the innovators in this area (C. Weissert, Knott, and Stieber 1994).

Finally, the tendency of states to innovate can be traced to their political tradition or culture. In some states the populace believes government should be proactive, providing "good" to its citizens, who are actively involved in the political process. Other states have the opposite view: government should be avoided, the political process should be dominated by a few knowledgeable people, and citizens' roles should be limited. Elazar (1984) divided states into three political cultures. In the traditionalistic culture, government intervention is not generally desirable and citizens' participation is minimal; this culture is best exemplified by the southern states. In the moralistic culture, government is viewed as a positive instrument to advance the public interest, and citizens' participation is encouraged; Minnesota, Vermont, and Wisconsin are illustrative of this type. In the individualistic culture, the role of government is primarily to encourage private initiative, and citizens' involvement is encouraged only to the extent that it promotes economic concerns; examples are Illinois, Indiana, and Ohio. States with moralistic cultures are often the most innovative; those with traditionalistic cultures often do not value innovation involving government action (C. A. Johnson 1976; Sigelman, Roder, and Sigelman 1981; Sigelman and Smith 1980). Some states are a mixture, such as Florida (traditionalistic and individualistic) and California (moralistic and individualistic), making predictions based on political culture difficult. Nevertheless, the political culture does provide some explanation for state activities and policy choice.

Constraints on State Innovation

Despite some impressive innovations and reforms, states have political and economic constraints that limit their contributions. States must retain their businesses, companies, and citizens and are ever vigilant to avoid enacting policies that might drive out businesses from the state or attract poor citizens to take up residence. In one of the few examinations of the impact of state health reform on relocation of businesses, Kenyon (1996) concluded that some relocation of business activity is likely, particularly in states with metropolitan areas spanning state borders and in states with a relatively high level of current business taxation. Small and nonmanufacturing firms are most likely to be affected by health care reform. Because businesses are often prominent players in state politics, their concerns are major factors in states' health policy making.

In contrast, the evidence on the "race to the bottom," with poor citizens moving to a state where benefits are higher than in their home state, is more mixed and inconclusive. A migration of poor citizens to states with generous Medicaid benefits is unlikely. We should note, however, that politicians may be ignorant of, or may choose to ignore, research results. And if politicians believe that by raising benefit levels for welfare or Medicaid they will attract more poor people into their state, they may act on that perception by maintaining existing benefits or even reducing benefit levels—even without any evidence that such migration occurs.

There are also legal issues that greatly constrain state innovation, particularly in the health insurance area. The key one is ERISA, which preempts state regulation of health insurance provided by large companies that self-insure. State law cannot require these employers to cover certain procedures, insure high-risk groups, or make health coverage available to workers. Until recently, states could not impose taxes on self-insured companies to finance care for uninsured people in the state. Virtually every comprehensive health care reform law runs afoul of ERISA. In 1974, when the law was passed, a small number of health plans were self-insured; today, between 33 and 50 percent of the nation's employees are in self-insured plans (Butler 2000).

For years, the courts tended to strictly construe the language of the federal law to stymie state efforts at including self-insured companies in health care reform. For example, in 1992 a New Jersey court found that the state's surcharge on hospital bills to finance a trust fund for uncompensated care was a violation of ERISA, and struck it down. (A later court overturned the decision, but the state had already changed its financing scheme.) A 1994 court decision in Connecticut knocked down a tax on Connecticut hospitals to finance uncompensated care. However, in a 1995 case, *New York Conference of Blue Cross and Blue Shield Plans v. Travelers Insurance Company,* the U.S. Supreme Court held that ERISA did not preempt a state's hospital surcharges that had to be paid by self-insured plans. Subsequent Supreme Court decisions also began to set some limits on ERISA's reach, including decisions in 2002 and 2003 allowing states to require independent external review of coverage-denial decisions and upholding "any willing provider" laws.

Though states strongly support a change in ERISA to give them more leeway in health care reform, such a change has long been opposed by many business and labor interests that prefer uniformity in health insurance across the states. However, recent legislation may provide some hope for state officials. A 1996 ERISA amendment prescribes a minimum maternity hospital stay but allows specific types of state maternity length-of-stay laws. Federal laws enacted in 1996 and 1998 require insurers to provide both mental health parity (the same benefits for mental and physical health care) and breast reconstruction for women following mastectomy. In the case of mental health, the federal law preempts state laws; in the case of breast reconstruction, state laws are allowed that require at least the same coverage as the federal law. Generally speaking, these laws create a new relationship between state and federal governments by setting a federal floor for self-insured plans while also permitting states to enact stronger laws (Butler 2000).

Another problem related to self-insurance is the emergence of new health insurance arrangements and the blurring of government responsibility for accountability. For example, self-insured firms are now contracting directly with providers, and providers are forming joint ventures with insurance plans. As Holahan and Nichols (1996, 67) put it, "In general, financial risks are being shared in ways never envisioned by those who draft and enforce state insurance legislation."

In spite of ERISA, states moved forward rapidly in the 1990s to enact managed care regulation. Most states also acted quickly between 1996 and 2000 to establish grievance procedures, set up ombudsmen, ensure access to obstetrician-gynecologists, prohibit provider financial incentives, and establish "prudent layperson" standards for coverage of treatment in emergency rooms. Only laws establishing liability for HMOs were held unconstitutional by the U.S. Supreme Court (*Aetna Health Inc. v. Davila,* 2004).

STATE HEALTH AGENCIES

Every state has at least one agency that oversees health programs, but the scope and purpose of the agencies vary and, in many states, health responsibilities are shared by many agencies. A typical state health agency is responsible for quality control, including licensure and regulation of standards of practice for health care professionals; licensure and certification for Medicare and Medicaid reimbursement of hospitals, nursing homes, and other providers; and monitoring of laboratories, health-related services, and environmental and sanitation conditions. The agency collects and analyzes data, evaluates and assesses health services, conducts health-planning activities, coordinates with other agencies and providers, issues vital records, and sometimes provides services in underserved areas and regions. Around 40 percent of state health agencies administer the Medicaid program (see table 5.8). Many more agencies have mental health responsibilities (84 percent).

More than 30 percent of state spending in fiscal year 2003 was on health, but most (21.5 percent) went to Medicaid. Services most closely associated with public health—such as prevention of epidemics, protection against environmental hazards, injury prevention, prevention of chronic disease and promotion of healthy behavior, and disaster preparation—do not make up large percentages of state budgets. Across all states these programs represented less than 2 percent of total state expenditures, ranging from 0.2 percent in Wyoming to 4.6 percent in Hawaii. These public health services accounted for only 3 percent of state health expenditures in fiscal year 2003. Medicaid accounted for 71.3 percent of state health spending. The second largest category was health insurance for state employees, which made up 8.2 percent of state health spending (Milbank Memorial Fund et al. 2005).

In most states, other health services are administered by different agencies. These services include professional licensure and regulation (often carried out by independent boards), health insurance regulation (by insurance commissions or departments), mental disability programs (by mental

Table 5.8

State Health Agencies' Organization and Programmatic Responsibilities

Responsibility	Number of States
Part of larger umbrella agency	18
Decentralized public health system	51
Children with special health care needs	31
Health planning and development	38
Mental health	42
Environment	36
Alcohol abuse	45
Medicaid	18

Source: Data compiled from StatePublicHealth.org 2005.
Note: Data include the District of Columbia.

health and mental retardation departments), health personnel education (by higher education), health facilities construction (by direct appropriations and independent financing authorities), and cost-control activities (sometimes by independent commissions).

The 50 state health departments work closely with more than 3,000 local health departments charged with assessing the public health needs of their communities, developing policies to meet those needs, and ensuring that primary and preventive care are available to all. The systems have traditionally been very decentralized, with the state agency giving considerable discretion to local units. The state's lineage in public health is a strong one. In fact, the federal government is a recent entrant into the world of public health. Municipal and state public health departments were active in the nineteenth century and early twentieth century in improving housing, sanitation, nutrition, water quality, sewage, and inoculation in the nation's cities and rural areas. They were so successful, in fact, that there seemed to be little need for continuing such public health activity, and it declined in importance in states and localities, replaced by issues of chronic disease, unemployment, criminal justice and safety, transportation, and education. Many public health departments focused on health service delivery or personal health issues, including provision of health care for the uninsured, primary care, and teenaged pregnancies. But September 11, 2001, changed public health, as it did many things in the United States. The possibility of terrorists releasing pathogens into the air raised issues of prevention and possible action that made public health a key actor. "A lot of people who couldn't spell 'public health' now saw public health as the equivalent of the Department of Defense," said one state health director. And a conservative commentator observed, "The upheaval of September 11 poses a momentous opportunity for public health to reclaim its proper focus: to protect the population from disease" (both quoted in Markowitz and Rosner 2004, 8, 6).

Following the September 11 attacks, states and localities stepped up their efforts to deal with bioterrorism, particularly possible attempts to contaminate water supplies or launch air-based toxins. Federal legislation in 2003 provided $1.1 billion to help states strengthen their capacity to respond to bioterrorism and other public health emergencies. The money came from three sources. The CDC provided funding to support preparedness activities for bioterrorism, infectious disease outbreaks, and public health emergencies. The HRSA funding was targeted to create regional hospital plans to respond in the event of a bioterrorism attack. The third portion, supporting a Metropolitan Medical Response System, came from the HHS Office of Emergency Preparedness. The legislation was very specific and set forth critical benchmarks, including setting up advisory committees (with specific designation of what groups should be included), time lines, plans, assessments of capacity, and training needs.

The crisis—and the sudden attention focused on public health by the deaths of several postal workers from anthrax in October 2001—focused attention on public health in a way that public health officials generally welcomed. However, the federal government, the hand with the money, was also closely watching the states. For example, the CDC portion of the grant required states to submit semiannual progress reports (annual reports are more common), and the agency conducted site visits and assigned project officers to states. Even so, a GAO study two years after the law was passed indicated that 4 of the 14 critical requirements were completed by most states; 2 were met by few states, and the remainder were met by around half of the states (GAO 2004). This report and others critical of states' response led to some calls for federalization of public health, arguing that terrorism is a vivid reminder of the impacts of globalization and an indictment of state and local public health systems geared to local needs (Annas 2002). Other assessments were more positive, concluding that the funding had resulted in stronger relationships between law enforcement and health providers, greater epidemiological capacity, better training for response to possible bioterrorism activities, improved communications, enhanced laboratory capacity, and more and better-trained professionals working in the area (Markowitz and Rosner 2004).

The uneasy federalist alliance was tested again in December 2002 when HHS directed states to offer smallpox vaccinations to public health and health care workers, but without additional funds (funding was provided six months later, in May 2003). State departments of public health were thus hit with the task of massive smallpox inoculations, at the very time that many states were suffering fiscal difficulties and cutting their agency budgets, including those of public health.

In 2005, another $1.3 billion was provided to states to upgrade their abilities to respond not only to terrorism but also to other public health emergencies such as infectious disease outbreaks. Part of the money was targeted for an early-warning infectious disease surveillance program specifically for states bordering Canada and Mexico (HHS 2005a).

Even with public health now playing a major role in state policy on these timely and salient issues, some worry whether its time in the limelight will continue. Many states have used the federal dollars (and state dollars as well) to hire staff, purchase state-of-the-art technology and communications systems, and develop plans involving other state agencies, local governments, and the private sector. "Yo-yo funding has been the history of public health," said one state public health director who fears public health may see reduced funding in future years (Markowitz and Rosner 2004, 17).

CONCLUSION

Few would question the role of state governments as key actors in health care in the United States. They serve as the providers, financiers, administrators, initiators, and regulators of health care delivery. Their reach cuts across traditional health providers, insurers, businesses, educational institutions, and, of course, citizens. State governments are capable of adequately performing all their roles and representing all the groups and citizens they serve. They are the innovators and creators of many of the most promising ideas considered in the nation's capital and elsewhere. They are probably the most pivotal government actor in health care, since they implement and help define federal policies, define and implement their own policies, and define and oversee local health-related activities.

States and their local governments were the primary makers of health policy for the first 150 years or so of this country's history. States made laws dealing with public health, provided services for the mentally ill and the elderly, and even considered comprehensive health insurance.

Before World War I, there was intense interest in many states in adopting a compulsory health insurance program funded by employers, employees, and the public. At least 16 states introduced health insurance bills based on a model bill prepared by the American Association for Labor Legislation, a group that had led the successful drive for workers' compensation (O. Anderson 1990). In the 1930s through the 1960s, the states provided essential health services but were generally not leaders in innovation or responsiveness to the public. A key turning point was the adoption of the Medicare and Medicaid programs, which developed into the major public health safety net for the elderly and poor.

The 1970s and 1980s witnessed a spurt of innovation and activity in the states. In health care, innovations in financing, new forms of delivery, and systems allowing citizens to make tough "rationing" choices were developed at the state level, and in the early 1990s the states developed the ideas of managed competition, global budgets, and major insurance reforms—ideas only talked about in Washington, D.C. In the rest of the decade, states led the way in the use of managed care in Medicaid programs and in regulation on behalf of citizens in public and private managed care systems, in providing prescription drugs to those unable to pay, and in controlling costs for public programs. States dealt with legal protections, accountability, and health access and quality—issues that stymied congressional attempts to enact national laws. In the early years of the twenty-first century, the states saw renewed interest in universal health coverage—a response, perhaps, to frustration with the lack of interest in Washington, D.C., in increased domestic spending coupled with frustration with rising premiums and health care costs. Bills to set up a statewide single-payer system were introduced in 18 states in 2005 (Leingang 2005).

Nevertheless, state actions are stymied by fiscal constraints such as federal law (ERISA), balanced budgets, and limits on revenues and expenditures that are not in place at the national level. States that enact broad health care reforms (Tennessee, Minnesota, and Washington State) can be forced to abandon the reforms when the needs of citizens swamp the resources of the state to deal with them. States that lead the way in controversial areas such as medical marijuana and assisted suicide may see their actions nullified in federal court. States that enact incremental reforms are often criticized for being cautious and masking the failures of the private market (Beamer 2004). These reforms also illustrate what Paul Peterson (1995) calls the "price" of federalism—inequity. For citizens in a progressive state, eligibility for and benefit from health services differ from those for citizens in another state. Critics argue that only the federal government can successfully reform the many faults of the current health care system. But the truth is that it hasn't.

The failure of the national government to deal with comprehensive health care reform brings to the fore both the strengths and the weaknesses of a health care system led by state innovations. The system cannot be dominated by states, which simply lack the resources and constitutional scope to run a national health care system. Some commentators continue to bemoan the lack of a national system and the impossibility of a decentralized health care system. However, states can and do dominate in designing effective policy for their own citizens. States recognize what Craig (1996) called "taste differences," and they operate in different "specialized political markets" (Oliver and Paul-Shaheen 1997) and in different health policy regimes (Hackey 1998). The products of these various tastes, markets, and regimes will be different from those emanating from Washington, D.C. They may not "travel" to other states or to the capital and may not be viewed as optimal by outside observers. Yet they serve the needs and desires of citizens of the state.

Examples in the environmental area—particularly related to greenhouse gas effects—highlight both the strengths and weaknesses of federalism in public policy. The fact that some states are acting when Washington, D.C., does not is important and relevant. Equally important and relevant are the large majority of states that are not acting. The policies are not national—the question is whether they should be.

The U.S. health system is neither a decentralized health market nor a centralized health system. Rather, health is a combined federal-state responsibility with substantial federal oversight and funding, imbued with state innovation and implementation. The system may be confused and confusing, but it seems to work.

Part II

Health and the Policy Process

6

The Policy Process

ONE SISTER, Rosa, moved a few years ago to a beach town halfway down the long eastern coast of Florida, making her and her husband two of that day's approximately 1,000-person net increase in the state's burgeoning population. Unaccustomed to managed care and aware of its bad reputation among older people, Rosa initially opted to continue her fee-for-service Medicare coverage. After some persuasion from a friend in her bridge club, she and her husband agreed to call one of the local Medicare managed care firms and hear its pitch. They were amazed to find that the plan would charge no monthly premium, cover drug costs of up to $800 a month, and cover stays at either of the two nearby hospitals in their beach community. Clearly, coverage in the same federal program differed between fee-for-service and managed care, and it might be still different at a managed care firm other than the one Rosa and her husband chose.

When she had a small stroke a few days after joining the managed care plan, Rosa was very pleasantly surprised at the range of specialists who were quickly assigned to her case: a neurologist, a neurosurgeon, internists, and a physical therapist. After her first night in the hospital, she was visited by the managed care firm's medical director, who was taking a special interest in management of her potentially high-cost case. Had she remained in her fee-for-service plan, or had her stroke occurred a week earlier, before she'd made the switch, Rosa would have been worse off in several ways. She would have faced a one-day cost-of-hospital-care deductible, a daily co-payment, a 25 percent co-payment for drugs, a major gap in her drug coverage once she'd spent the limits of her coverage a few months after her stroke, and substantial co-payments for ambulatory care visits to her physicians after leaving the hospital.

Meanwhile, across the state, her sister Mae, not yet 65 and working for one of the thousands of service industry firms in Florida, needed back surgery—or at least was told she did, despite government warnings (based on government-sponsored research studies) that back surgery is often not very effective. With no health insurance and an income not close enough to poverty to qualify for Medicaid, Mae and her husband would not be able to pay for her hospital care or for the doctors who would do the surgery.

Were she to collapse at work, Mae might be able to claim workers' compensation coverage. If she were in a car accident and further injured her back, she might be able to get some of her medical expenses covered by the mandatory medical injury coverage that many states, including Florida, require auto insurance companies to include in their policies. Or if she were rushed to a hospital emergency department after such an accident, the federal EMTALA (Emergency Medical Treatment and Active Labor Act) law would require that her condition be diagnosed and stabilized by physicians and staff before they could send her home, with no plans for follow-up.

Of course, that would not stop the hospital from turning over the bill to a collection agency, which would dun Mae repeatedly and quite likely try to garnishee her wages to force her to pay the bill. In fact, Medicare and Medicaid agreements signed by the hospital would require it to go after her for payment—unless hospital management wanted to adopt a policy of going after nobody who owed them money, since Medicare and Medicaid want to be assured that their patients are not singled out for extra charges.

U.S. Representative Jones heard about the problem of the bad-debt collection policies of hospitals and was concerned that poor people were getting worse care than the nonpoor. She asked the administrator of the Centers for Medicare and Medicaid Services to testify before her house committee to explain how Medicare and Medicaid policies affected bad-debt collection by hospitals. The CMS administrator answered the committee's questions, many of which were written for the committee members by congressional staff who had read a report on the subject—most likely prepared by the Government

Accountability Office, Congressional Budget Office, or Medicare Payment Advisory Commission (MedPAC).

For their research in preparing a report of this type, any or all of these agencies or individuals quite likely made use of the extensive Medicare and Medicaid data on use and cost provided by the hospitals, as well as cost reports covering all patients and all expenses and bad debt that hospitals must file regularly if they want to participate in Medicare or Medicaid. Or the researchers might have made use of one of the many surveys of hospital admissions, discharges, payment sources, and other features paid for with public funds.

If Rosa, the sister with Medicare coverage, were discharged to a nursing home, Medicare might pay for a few days' stay. A longer stay would have to be paid for out of her own pocket, until she was poor enough to qualify for Medicaid to cover that portion of the bill that her Social Security and other funds could not pay each month. If either sister died during her hospital stay, state law would dictate whether the case had to be counted in some kind of published hospital mortality index, since the federal mandatory hospital death index was repealed some years ago and replaced in only a few cases, including Florida, by state law. The federal Centers for Disease Control and Prevention would, of course, want to know about the death from a death certificate, so that mortality rates by cause of death and by state and county could be reported. The death might not result in an autopsy, since state laws vary on whether an autopsy is required in routine cases. Florida leaves the decision to the discretion of the state attorney, if he or she thinks a crime may have been committed.

But the hospital might do an autopsy anyway, if it had the permission of the family, because the Joint Commission on Accreditation of Healthcare Organizations (JCAHO), a private group operated by hospitals, is a strong proponent of autopsies, and the hospital would not want to risk its state and local licenses to operate as a hospital, or lose its Medicare and Medicaid certification, by becoming careless and losing its JCAHO accreditation. Licensure and certification often require accreditation as one condition among many others. Furthermore, some states might require, as Florida does, that the deceased be transported from the hospital to a burial site under the direction of a funeral director, since the funeral industry has been successful in some states in lobbying the legislature to make it illegal to transport a corpse without involvement of a funeral director.

If neither sister died, after recovering at home they might go out and celebrate, vowing to give up smoking and go on a diet, especially after reading the antismoking, diet, exercise, and other health promotion materials prepared by the CDC and state public health agencies that their husbands had picked up for them in the hospital cafeteria. Driving home from the celebration, whoever was driving would want to be quite sober to avoid violating state driving laws aimed at preventing motor vehicle–related morbidity and mortality.

This is health care policy in the United States: who is and is not eligible to receive subsidized care; what share the individual pays; which types of health care and which services and procedures are covered; who can render care and get paid for rendering it; what government does and does not do when a person needs care but does not have the money to pay for it; who gets financial help with medical care training; what nurses can and cannot do for patients; how wide the doorways of hospital bathrooms should be; what data must be supplied to the federal and state governments; how federal tax policy and workers' protection laws interact with various health care laws; how federal agencies translate congressional intent into regulations affecting health care providers and patients; what records must be kept, how they must be kept, whom they can be shared with, and whom they must be shared with; what kinds of educational materials about healthy living are distributed and which behaviors are restricted or encouraged in the interests of improved health status—and much, much more.

Health care policies are not unique to government. Hospitals have their own private policies: some will not perform abortions; many operate as not-for-profits while others operate for profit, many of them part of a chain of hospitals owned by investors; some have data system firewalls that protect medical records from unauthorized access; bad debts are absorbed graciously or collected aggressively; infants under a certain weight at birth must be kept in the hospital until they gain weight; the hospital does or does not operate a drug detoxification center. Insurance companies, in the interest of reducing liability, may require of their nursing home clients that all residents be accompanied to the bathroom whether they need help or not. These private policies share many characteristics with public policies. They differ in that they do not usually have an explicit public purpose and are not compelled by public authority. People do not go to jail for violating a corporate policy (but they may be fired—for example, for violating corporate policy that forbids one worker to tell another worker his pay rate). The real difference, however, is that government policies are made by government and, as such, are the product of a political process in which public elections are a key determinant of who gets to make policy.

THE AMBIGUITY OF PUBLIC POLICY

It would be naive to think that the purpose of health care or other public policy is always obvious (box 6.1). Policy is formed by compromise. In chapter 1 we described how Congress forms an enacting coalition—a specific group of members willing to vote for a specific proposal at a specific time—with a majority large enough to pass a proposal, sometimes just barely. Things are left deliberately vague so that many people with different perspectives can see their views represented in the same ambiguity. More detail might lose a vote. For this reason (and also because of incompetence, uncertainty, time pressures, and bad writing), even though policy always has a purpose, that purpose may not always be easy to figure out. Indeed, the members of Congress who voted for it may have many different purposes in mind. Program evaluators find this out early, for health care and every other type of program. Asked to evaluate how well a program is achieving its goals, more often than not the evaluators discover the program does not seem to have any goals. Sometimes it has too many, often conflicting, goals. That a program has been running for several months or years on some vaguely worded rationale may be

---

Box 6.1
Defining Public Policy

   Public policy has been defined as "what government does." But J. E. Anderson (1994) and others ask, who is government? (A member of Congress? the president? the chair of the Physician Payment Review Commission?) And what does *does* mean? (Making a law? a proposal? a speech? a proposed regulation? a ruling? a conference report recommendation? Writing of a Medicare check to pay a hospital?) Simon (1960) called check writing and similar activities "programmed" decisions, because they are repetitive, routine, and based on standard operating procedure. He said that policy involves discretion: making choices that are novel, unstructured, and consequential.
   According to Dye (1984, 1), public policy is "whatever government chooses to do or not to do." That captures the kind of power lobbyists are best at: keeping unwanted proposals from being adopted or even debated. But not addressed by these definitions is the difference between nominal policy and actual policy. Medicaid law requires "statewideness" (no urban-rural differences in access to Medicaid-subsidized services). But who would argue that there are no differences? Nonetheless, the law gives rural dwellers a legitimate claim that efforts should be made on their behalf to try to mitigate these differences. Sometimes nominal policy is the goal, while actual policy is the route being followed toward that goal.

disturbing to evaluators, but this rarely seems to get in the way of the actors. So an evaluator quickly learns that goals must often be deduced by translating from something implicit in the actions taken by the actors.

At other times, ambiguity can be quite troubling. Laboratory administrators serving doctors or hospitals in different states complain about the contradictions and administrative burden of interstate variations. The same firm must adopt different procedures for different states and, in some cases, for counties or regions within a state.

The (Unintended) Consequences of Public Policy

Policy action in health care and other fields often differs, sometimes painfully, from intention. As we noted in chapter 1, policymakers vote only on policies, not on outcomes. Their committee specialists tell them what is likely to work, but they may not be right. When health care policy makers wrote new standards for participation in the Medicaid program in the late 1980s and 1990s, they intended to improve the quality of nursing home care for publicly subsidized patients. Though that purpose was accomplished for many patients, for others—low-income, privately paying patients living in facilities too poor to meet the new standards—life was probably made worse when nursing homes dropped out of Medicaid because they could not afford to comply with the new standards. Similar dilemmas face those who wish to upgrade fire and sanitation standards for poor inner-city apartment buildings and hotels (flop houses) and for assisted living facilities serving people who are elderly and disabled. Tenants too poor to pay the higher rent that accompanies the improvements demanded by new regulations have to move to settings worse than those they inhabited before the government decided to help them. Indeed, in health care policy, much of the problem lies in trying to resolve the inherent tension between reform efforts aimed at improving quality and their unintended consequences for poor people's access to care, or between cost-containment strategies and reduced quality or access. Every time premiums rise, some people drop their insurance.

The Evolution of Public Policy and Policy Legacies

Policies evolve. Ask any nursing home operator about Medicaid's policy on the quality of care in general, or on the prevention and treatment of decubitus ulcers in particular, and you will most likely get a puzzled look followed by a long-winded answer. By the end, the operator will probably have worked herself into a bit of a pique and may finish by saying, "You tell me" or "Do you mean this week or next?" Policy is not written in stone. It is dynamic, a potpourri of laws (often vague), regulations (often late, ambiguous, changing), government officials' interpretations (often conflicting, sometimes wrong), court decisions (sometimes bizarre), and, in the final analysis, the level of compliance by providers, fiscal intermediaries, and patients themselves—who sometimes find ways to systematically alter policy by, for example, giving away their assets instead of spending them for care in lieu of public subsidy. Policies evolve and change because they reflect the negotiated preferences of many parties over differing periods of time. They change because the world changes and the policies must reflect the private sector and the everyday activities of consumers. They change and evolve because they must, so as to be effective and reflect changing demands.

The evolution of public policies builds in part on what is called policy legacies or path dependence. Initial decisions, particularly those affecting institutional choice, become self-reinforcing and develop networks of individuals and groups that benefit from the status quo. As Pierson (2000) put it, earlier actions may "lock in" options that actors would not now choose to initiate. Thus future decisions are path-dependent on past policy decisions. In health policy, the current system of employer-based health care, which flows from a decision of a half-century ago, tends to curtail the reform options that are considered. While the system could be drastically changed (through a single-payer system, for example), in fact, most policy options to improve access in the intervening years—and there have been many—have built on this employer-based system.

DEMANDS FOR HEALTH CARE POLICY CHANGE

In health care, as in every other field, policies come from demands for action or for deliberate inaction. Poor people want access to care. Physicians want a new procedure paid for by Medicare. Hospitals want a place to send discharged patients who cannot find a bed in a Medicaid nursing home, or they want relief from antitrust enforcement, which makes it risky to talk about mergers with other providers. Nursing homes want fewer visits from federal quality-of-care surveyors; the Citizens Coalition for Better Long-Term Care, a patient advocacy group, wants more such visits. Demands may be general or specific: demand that something be done or that something very specific be done. The demand may inspire new health care policy or give existing policy content, direction, or interpretation. The form of the policy may be a new law, a change in an existing law, a regulation, a court decision, or a supervisor's memo interpreting policy to the field staff.

Whatever the genesis, the demand is important to the success of any public policy. Who participates, what resources that person or group possesses, and how that group translates its resources into influence are all important elements of policy development (Hayes 1992). In addition to the important role of interest groups (see chapter 3), informal groupings of experts in academia, think tanks, and agencies can also play an important role in helping policymakers understand issues and come up with reasonable solutions. These actors, part of what Kingdon (1995) called the policy community, constitute their own attentive public, which can actively aid the progress of an idea. When this community is integrated and in agreement on the nature of the problem and its optimal solution, it can play a major role in policy development. If it is fragmented, or if multiple groups claim community standing, its influence is diminished and the likelihood of successful comprehensive policies is lessened.

An important distinction in public policy is that it reflects the public's concerns. Members of Congress and the president (and their counterparts in the 50 states) do not make policy in a vacuum. They listen to their constituents, interest groups, and colleagues and (increasingly) rely on polls and focus groups for policy guidance in answering crucial questions. Are the prescription drug costs of Medicare patients too high? Should guns be more tightly controlled? Is food safety a real concern? Experts in think tanks, universities, and the bureaucracy can help answer these questions, but expert advice alone is not the key to policy initiation. The public must perceive a crisis—and for health care coverage, for a while in 1993, it did.

The pattern of public support for health care reform closely follows what Downs (1972) called the issue attention cycle: the public becomes interested in an issue (or problem) and, for a while, its attention grows as the issue gains salience, is covered by the media, and is the focus of congressional hearings and presidential speeches. At some point, however, it becomes clear that the problem cannot easily be solved, that it will likely involve great expense, and that some groups will be hurt by proposed solutions. The public may now begin to lose interest, and policymakers may lose support for making tough decisions to solve the problem. The public, fickle in its attention, may switch its concerns to another issue. So Congress moves on as well. The 1993–94 debate on national health care reform seemed to fit this pattern. In the spring of 1994, health was the top concern of the public; a few months later, it had been replaced by crime. One thing that pushed health care reform off the agenda was widespread concern that it would raise the insurance premiums of the middle class. In 2005, health care reform was again a focus for several national foundations and a new coalition of business groups and nonprofits interested in alleviating the growing numbers of uninsured while holding down health care costs.

Downs's model, then, is pessimistic about the possibility of major reforms. But others believe that actions can be taken within the attention cycle to perpetuate the interest and promote long-term reform. Baumgartner and Jones (1993, 87) argued that "even [a] short-lived spurt of [public] interest may leave an institutional legacy" such as an office, group, or staff committed to the issue.

The public is very susceptible to symbolism, and politicians are often successful at manipulating such value-laden issues as patriotism or universal health care coverage to seek public support. When President Clinton promoted national health care reform as "health security" for everybody—ensuring portability from job to job and coverage of existing conditions—rather than focusing on the problem of the uninsured, he was, in Schattschneider's term (1960), trying to "widen the scope of conflict." He wanted to make average Americans feel they had something to lose if health care policy was not reformed. The public likes symbols that oversimplify and often finds comfort in their use (Edelman 1964). A more recent explanation of public opinion and health policy deals with the idea of policy metaphors, or the combination of norms, practices, and organizational arrangements that shape the public's interpretation of a given policy. M. Schlesinger and Lau (2000) argued that public opinion is based on policy metaphors rather than details of policy or the workings of U.S. politics. In health, they identified five policy metaphors: health care can be viewed as a community obligation, marketable commodity, societal right, employer responsibility, or an issue under professional control.

CATEGORIES OF PUBLIC POLICY

Policies can be categorized in a variety of ways. They can be grouped by issue (say, the health care workforce) or target audience (Medicare beneficiaries or vulnerable populations or people with disabilities). Policies change over time and so may also be categorized by period: as New Deal policies, or

Clinton-era policy, or current policy. Some policies emanate from the states, others from the federal government, others from the 82,000 or more local jurisdictions making policy on everything from screening for HIV to water quality. Campbell (1992), writing about health policy making in Japan, classified policies in a matrix: big or small, old or new. Old, small policy ideas, he noted, are easiest to pass.

Policies are either substantive or procedural. Substantive policies do things like improve health care, protect the environment, or regulate employment practices. Procedural policies are concerned with *how* the government is doing things. The Administrative Procedures Act of 1946 is the quintessence of a procedural policy, or set of procedural policies. It requires that government regulatory and administrative actions be taken only after notice of proposed rulemaking, opportunity for comment, publication before becoming effective, explicit procedures for relief and appeal, and more. The National Environmental Policy Act requires environmental impact statements before government agencies can act. Title XIX of the Social Security Act (Medicaid) requires states to adopt a state plan for Medicaid participation and seek approval of any changes in its plan from the CMS (formerly, Health Care Financing Administration), which manages the Medicaid program for the federal government and pays states the federal share of costs.

Of course, procedural policies may have profound substantive effects. Oregon's request for a waiver of federal rules so that it could explicitly introduce the notion of rationing into its Medicaid plan was initially turned down by the HCFA on grounds that were later regarded as both substantive and political (too close to the election to endorse rationing), though initially the focus was on procedural inadequacies. Environmental policy is fraught with opportunities for both sides to call in their attorneys to argue that proper procedures were not followed. Often the effect (and the intent) is to slow things down, delay, and wait for a better deal or make time for negotiation. Cynics have called the Administrative Procedures Act the "Lawyers Relief Act," but every day this act protects many citizens from arbitrary action by a civil servant. Changes in abortion policy are often sought through procedural requirements. Michigan pro-choice supporters argued that a state legislative proposal requiring that women seeking an abortion must be advised of the risks of abortion was a substantive policy masquerading as a procedure. They were particularly outraged by the requirement that the information be provided only by state officials.

Politics shapes policies, but policies also determine politics. Policies can be viewed as distributive, regulatory, or redistributive (Lowi 1969). James Wilson

(1989) noted that distributive policies often concentrate benefits on hospital corporations, medical schools, or other such beneficiaries, whereas costs are diffused among taxpayers at large and concentrated on no one specific group. So the winners have a big stake in the policy and actively support its passage, while the losers do not lose much and pay little attention. A typical distributive program would be one that sets up federal scholarships for nurse-practitioners who agree to practice in medically underserved areas of the state. The witnesses before Congress would likely be nurse-practitioner groups, nursing school deans, and spokespersons from hospitals in rural areas that would benefit from the program. There would be few, if any, witnesses speaking against the program. The only possible opposition might come from physicians' assistants or other providers who might think they should have similar programs. Overall, it would be a "love fest," to be repeated in the other house and passed with little fanfare some weeks later. Office of Management and Budget representatives or the Congressional Budget Office might point out that the program would be expensive and ask how it was going to be funded. To the extent that the nurse-practitioner program would be in competition with programs for physicians, pharmacists, or community housing advocates, the politics of distributive programs can become more turbulent and sometimes downright nasty. (The impact of the federal budgetary constraint on policy making is described in chapter 1.)

Regulatory policies restrict the behavior of private and government actors. In health policy this includes hospitals, physicians, nurses, and graduates of foreign medical schools who want to practice in the United States; drug manufacturers, medical laboratories, and home health agencies; hospital janitors in charge of disposing of medical waste; dentists, who must wash their hands, change gloves, and wear masks to prevent transmission of infections; nuclear power plants, auto manufacturers, farmers, food processors, restaurateurs, and hospital CEOs who want to take over the competition. Continuing the nurse-practitioner example, regulatory policies would be state laws requiring that nurse-practitioners practice only under the guidance of physicians. There are clear winners and losers in regulatory policies, and though the losses may be limited (nobody gets killed), they can also be substantial—the opportunity to earn millions or even billions of dollars. Generally speaking, regulatory policies are more controversial than distributive policies, and they are often fought out on the congressional floor and in committee markup sessions. Many are salient and can easily arouse the ire of the group to be regulated. Sometimes the group is state or federal government, as in the case of federal restrictions on state regulation of self-insured managed care firms under the federal Employee Retirement Income Security Act of 1974 or more recent laws to prohibit liability suits against gun makers.

Some regulatory policies—a substantial number in the health care field—are "self-regulatory." Physicians set the standards of practice for physicians, hospitals accredit themselves based on standards set by their own organization (the JCAHO), and schools of public health decide what courses will be required of graduating students in order for them to receive their association's (Council on Education for Public Health's) imprimatur. Government often devolves authority to these self-regulating bodies, taking their seal of approval as evidence that minimal standards have been met and removing some of the political heat—and the cost of enforcement—from government actors.

Redistributive policies take money or power from some and give it to others. In health care policy, redistribution translates to taxing those with higher incomes to pay for health services for those with lower incomes. The U.S. income tax system is progressive, taking taxes at a higher rate as income rises, because those who have the ability to pay are believed to be the ones who should pay. Economists argue that extra or marginal units of almost any good are of less value to the recipient than the first units. Following that logic, a little money to a poor person has a lot more social utility than a little more money to a rich person. Religious teachings make a similar point in parables: for example, the New Testament story of the poor widow whose small gift was valued more highly than the larger gift of the rich man.

Medicaid is a redistributive program, taking tax dollars from the middle and upper classes to pay for health care for the very poor and near poor. Minority hiring policies redistribute job opportunities from white middle-class men to women, persons of color, and members of other minority groups. Many expensive public programs are not very redistributive, and many of those that are redistributive are rather small. Medicaid is an exception. Once tiny, this program, which spends nearly three of every four dollars on people too poor to get care by any other means, has grown larger than Medicare in size.

Redistributive policies produce fierce politics. These policies are combative, controversial, constantly under attack, hard to obtain, and hard to retain. When the Reagan administration ushered in its program of government spending cuts, which health care program was the first to be cut? Was it Medicare, the (then) nearly $100 billion program serving all elderly Americans, a group that is mainly middle class and has a poverty rate lower than that of the population in general and roughly half that of children? Or was it Medicaid, a program for the very poor or needy and those who must "spend down" everything they own to a few dollars per month of personal money before they can qualify for benefits? Of course, it was the latter. Because many people wrongly think that Medicaid is more or less exclusively a welfare program aimed at unwed mothers and their children, many of whom are members of a minority group, this is never a popular program with the majority of voters. President George W. Bush's fiscal year 2007 budget cut both Medicare and Medicaid spending (Pear 2006).

Most policies are economic in nature: someone or some group wins, another loses. Someone pays—although the payment may be spread over so many individuals that little notice is taken. Some scholars have focused on policies with clearly identified losers. The loss might be experienced by a group (dropping those who are medically needy from Medicaid), a geographic area (allowing oil drilling off the Florida Gulf Coast), or a business (cuts in hospital reimbursement in Medicare). What is interesting in this line of inquiry is the strategies available to policymakers who must act but who do not want to offend any potential voters. Pal and Weaver (2003) noted the several available choices:

— manipulate procedures: delegate responsibilities to bureaucrats or advisory bodies, bury the policy choice in a reconciliation bill or omnibus bill where it might "get lost," or shift venue to the states or the courts;

— manipulate perceptions: use technical language or changes to lower visibility and find a scapegoat (globalization, for example); or

— manipulate payoffs: delay or phase in implementation of the policy or provide some benefits along with the pain.

A nonmonetary loss can also be incurred, something Pal and Weaver (2003) categorize as a symbolic loss. This loss is often in the area dubbed "morality" policies, a subset of non-economic public policies. Several health issues fall into this category, including abortion, the "morning-after" pill, the right to die, and gun control. These issues address social relationships and are associated with "values" rather than facts. Morality issues tend to be highly salient and very controversial in a way that sets their development and implementation apart from other issues. Morality issues tend to be seen as absolutes by those who care about them, making it difficult for politicians to take a middle ground or for compromise to occur (Mooney 2001). Morality policies are generally technically simpler than most other types of policy; everyone can be reasonably well informed on an issue and have an opinion. In abortion policy, for example, the issue is well understood and individuals have staked out a position. In one national survey, only five respondents—0.3 percent of the sample—had no opinion on the abortion question (Norrander and Wilcox

2001). Finally, morality issues generally involve grassroots organization and mobilization. Given the political difficulty with morality issues, legislative bodies often avoid making decisions in these areas—frequently leading to judicial action (McFarlane and Meier 2001).

THE EXTENT OF POLICY CHANGE

Not all policy changes are equal in their scope, range, and depth. Some changes are clearly monumental, generally reflecting a value change in society, often leading to institutional changes and pointing policy in a new direction. One example was the enactment of Medicare in 1965, the first major federal health program guaranteeing health care for a large targeted population. But most public policies are not comprehensive. Rather, they are incremental: they build on earlier policies, are implemented by existing agencies and departments, and generally follow the policy direction of earlier policies. The Children's Health Insurance Program, passed as part of the 1997 Balanced Budget Act, was more incremental than comprehensive, even though it was in many respects a new program. It built on Medicaid, left many choices to the states, and started as a 10-year block grant that would have to be renewed.

The politics of the two types of policies—comprehensive and incremental—are quite different. Comprehensive policies flow from major changes in public attitudes, often expressed through election results. Hayes (1992) argued that these nonincremental policies can be adopted only when values are agreed upon and when there is an adequate knowledge base. Even with these two criteria in place, the environment must be right for change—usually a turbulent environment characterized by a dramatic shift in the political world or public opinion. Public support is crucial to successful adoption of nonincremental change. Support by "elites," those who are influential in the thinking of policymakers and the president, is important as well. Leaders willing to take a chance and opponents unable to defend their position can also help. But as Hayes noted, nonincremental change is simply impossible for many issues. Incremental policies are most likely to emerge from situations in which there is not much information and no national agreement on values. Incremental policies pit interests against interests in a situation where public attention is low and interest groups, federal agencies, congressional committees, and other interested parties grapple with the problems and their possible solution quietly and without public fanfare.

Some argue that the distinction between incremental and nonincremental change is extremely vague and may reside in the eye of the beholder. And, in fact, a series of what one sees as incremental changes can have the combined power of major change, and seemingly nonincremental change may be simply an amalgamation of incremental steps. For example, changes in federal reimbursement systems encompassed in the Medicare Prospective Payment System in the 1980s led to a redefinition of health care delivery by hospitals and other providers. Yet the changes were accomplished across several years and several decisions and are hard to view as a single comprehensive change. The Medicare Modernization Act of 2003 was a major change in Medicare—offering for the first time selective coverage of prescription drugs. But other aspects of the law, such as expansion of health savings accounts, were clearly incremental.

Those authors who initially described the policy process as incremental wrote before the field had focused on the role of uncertainty in public policy. Were they writing now, they might have characterized what they saw as a response to the great uncertainty that faces policymakers trying to address a new problem. For example, these early writers noted that nonincremental change sometimes starts with an incremental step that provides knowledge to policymakers and mobilizes public or group support. In a second stage, the changes converge toward noncomprehensive reform (Hayes 1992). Kingdon (1995, 83) quoted one of his sources as saying, "These things proceed in small, incremental steps. Something is enacted, everybody concludes that it's not so bad, and that gets people ready for the next bite." Aware of the higher likelihood of success with incremental rather than nonincremental approaches, national health reformers have battled for 40 years over which approach would produce more success: going for broke when the opportunity arose, trying, as did President Clinton, to cover everything and everybody, or being satisfied with accomplishing a little bit each year.

Despite the failures of most past presidents who sought major change in health policy, President Clinton rejected a narrowly focused plan addressing only catastrophic care costs in favor of a broad plan that covered everyone, expanded benefits, reduced co-payments, and mandated businesses to pay three-quarters of the cost of premiums. Political and health policy advisors urged him to focus on the vision of major change that he had promised in the campaign and that, they argued, the American people demanded and expected. Economic advisors, sensing Clinton's preference for this visionary approach and swallowing their reservations, couched their support in conditional language that took advantage of the fact that the choice between broad and narrow reform was being made without the benefit of cost projections (Woodward 1994).

The post mortems would suggest that in addition to ignoring and then badly underestimating the costs, the boosters of comprehensive change had misread the voters. What the voters meant by major change was a guarantee of portability—an assurance that insurance would not be lost or priced out of their reach when workers changed jobs or lost employment. But to the Clinton administration and its potentially most ardent supporters—the AARP, labor, and other beneficiary group lobbies—this type of paltry change was the worst kind of incrementalism. Two years after delivering a crushing defeat to Clinton's nonincremental approach, Congress passed legislation guaranteeing portability of health care coverage for up to 18 months after job loss or change, suggesting that it was indeed an incremental change that voters wanted.

Clinton was not the only president to succumb to the sirens' song of comprehensive change. President Jimmy Carter ridiculed incremental efforts, saying that "most of the controversial issues that are not routinely well-addressed can only respond to a comprehensive approach" (Wildavsky 1979, 242). He thought incremental efforts were doomed because of interest groups' opposition and that, with strong public support, comprehensive change could be implemented. Carter, like Clinton after him, found mobilizing and maintaining such public support difficult indeed.

Incrementalism is often an easier sell to the voting public and Congress because most people are averse to risk. They are reluctant to make large and risky changes because the consequences and costs are hard to predict and unintended consequences can be costly. Many have observed that savvy politicians use this understanding of the policy process to select a strategy for creating policy change. No one was a greater master of this incrementalist strategy than the very liberal Henry Waxman (D-CA), former House health and environment subcommittee chair. "He sets such ambitious policy aims that colleagues might consider him a pie-in-the-sky fool if they were not by now so familiar with his technique of taking a small slice at a time until years later he is holding the whole pie—even in the face of spending retrenchment. Persistence and patience are his strengths" (Duncan 1993, 188). Others call this strategy "the nose of the camel under the tent." Once the nose is in, it is hard to keep the rest of the camel out.

THE POLICY PROCESS FRAMEWORK

The public policy process is too complicated, mutable, and variable for easy understanding, much less predictions. There are simply too many variables, and many of them are contingent on other variables and contexts. Institutions, rules, policy legacies, temporal conditions, electoral preferences, catastrophes, economic conditions, technology—all play a role in policy making. Individual behavior is also key: lawmakers' preferences are contingent on many of the aforementioned factors plus their own personal views on the issue, their perceptions of voters and groups in their district, their relationship to party leaders, their electoral popularity, and on and on. And these are only the variables predicting policy adoption. There is an entire other aspect of policy, related to implementation, involving a different, although sometimes overlapping, cast of characters and incentives.

Then there are the theoretical mechanisms for understanding the process. Elinor Ostrom (1999) has helped us by categorizing the levels of analysis into frameworks, theories, and models. Frameworks are the most general and help us identify the elements and relationships among the variables that should be considered. Theories go a step further to include specification of which elements in the framework are particularly relevant to which questions and to make assumptions about the relationship. Models are the most specific and set forth precise assumptions leading to outcomes in ways that can be tested.

Using the framework approach, we can talk about the components that make up the policy process. One elementary, yet instructive, framework is the progression that public policies follow: (1) a problem is recognized and defined, (2) a public policy is developed to deal with the problem, (3) the public policy becomes law or is otherwise put in place, and (4) the public policy is implemented. The story does not end with policy implementation, however. During implementation, the lessons learned are applied to revising or improving the policy in an important feedback mechanism. But here we concentrate on the definition of the problem, the formulation of policy, its legitimization, and its implementation.

Problem Definition

One point on which all models and most students of the policy process agree is the importance of defining the problem. It is certainly true that policies sometimes begin with someone pushing a favorite solution, but these must ultimately be coupled to a problem or they do not become law. Problems are essential. Loomis (1995) asserted that "successfully defining conditions as problems (smog, learning disabilities, global warming, etc.) is perhaps the most important single step in obtaining policy change." According to Baumgartner and Jones (1993), problem definition is the very engine of change because it is the essence of power. Problems are inherently political, because they are not simply "out there waiting to be solved"; they must be formulated and defined, using political skill to mobilize support for the desired position.

Definitions of problems are chosen strategically, "designed to call in reinforcements for one's own side in a conflict" (D. Stone 1988, 122). Is it more accurate to describe a procedure to terminate a pregnancy as dilation and extraction or as partial birth abortion, and which will be more effective in rousing the ire of antiabortion groups? Is requiring an HMO physician to use one brand of medication rather than another interference with medical decision making by faceless bureaucrats, or is it cost control? Should the focus be placed on medical errors or patient safety? Is smoking a choice made by adults or an addiction perpetrated on children by tobacco company advertising? The definition of a problem sets the parameters for discussion and lends legitimacy to an issue. The definition flows from the choice of values (Dery 1984) and can also determine whether the problem demands public policy action. Not all problems are candidates for public policy. Some may be viewed as either intractable or not in the government domain. Eyestone (1978) provided three prerequisites for governments' recognition of a policy problem: governments must correctly identify a social problem or issue, governments must have the capacity to respond, and politicians must be persuaded that they should respond.

There is a strong pragmatic streak in problem definition. Policymakers tend to select for consideration those problems that can be solved. As Wildavsky (1979, 42) put it, "A difficulty is a problem only if something can be done about it." Problems that tend to defy solution, according to Downs (1972), are those for which one or more of the following conditions hold:

— A numerical minority (not necessarily ethnic) is suffering from the problem.

— Suffering is caused by social arrangements that provide benefits to the majority or a powerful minority of the population.

— The problem has no exciting qualities (or is no longer seen as exciting).

These qualities seem to fit the plight of the uninsured pretty well.

Consumed as entertainment, the news must stay lively to keep its readers and viewers. If the problem is of national scope and is, objectively, a major concern, it may sporadically recapture interest or attach itself to another problem taking center stage. When it does so, it will usually receive a higher level of attention, effort, and concern than problems still in the prediscovery stage. As Schon (1971, 42) put it, "Old questions are not answered—they only go out of fashion." The uninsured are a sad example: important in 1965; back on the agenda and even more important in the early 1980s and again in the 1990s; rarely mentioned in the early 2000s, despite their growing numbers.

In health, the definition of a problem is crucial. Is the problem an unequal system of health care delivery, costs that are rising too rapidly, or the quality of the care provided? Is the problem excessive paperwork or waste, profiteering insurance companies, greedy doctors, or a third-party payer system that encourages inefficiencies? Or is it all these things, as President Clinton proclaimed in his health address before Congress in September 1993? Part of Clinton's task, as defined by Eyestone (1978), was accomplished: identifying the problem. But his harder task, convincing politicians and the country to respond, was only beginning. President George W. Bush decided that the problem was costs, proposing consumer-driven, high-deductible health savings accounts in his 2006 state of the union address (Lee 2006).

Where Problems Come From

Problems do not just emerge. Citizens, leaders, organizations, interest groups, and government agencies create them in the minds of their fellow citizens. Problems come to what Cobb and Elder (1972) called the systemic or public agenda. Problems originate from people perceiving bias, groups seeking advancement or assistance, or groups seeking (their view of) the public good. Triggering devices for a problem can be a natural catastrophe, an unanticipated human event, ecological change, or technological change. If sufficiently affecting many people, a problem can enter the formal or institutional agenda, where policymakers will recognize and consider the matter. Problems can also reach the institutional agenda through interest-group lobbying, congressional staffers, bureaucrats, constituents, or members of Congress themselves who discover a problem and wish to "solve" it with government action.

Measuring and Framing Problems

Problems are usually ill defined and, more often than not, exaggerated. Advocates often approximate prevalence and severity in congressional testimony and press reports. Their goal is to dramatize the problem and create a sense of urgency. They want to make people feel the problem is so widespread that they could be its next victims. Advocates must "oversell" their positions to avoid losing their audience, Kingdon (1995) contended. Some recent examples make his point.

Estimates of the prevalence of battered women offered by the National

Coalition against Domestic Violence were so large as to include half of all married women. One-third of these women, the group said, are battered multiple times each year. When pressed for the source of the estimates by the *Washington Post* (Brott 1994), the coalition revealed that the numbers were actually "guesstimates." On a major investigative news show the estimate was raised to 60 million women—a number that, as the *Post* pointed out, exceeds the number of women living with men in the United States. Somewhat more disciplined in her estimates was the secretary of HHS, who said that women were battered by their mates about as frequently as they bore children: an event occurring for 4 million women a year. A more accurate estimate is probably one from the National Institute of Mental Health's National Family Violence Survey. It found violence in 16 percent of all American families, most of it slapping, shoving, and grabbing. More violent abuse is limited to 3 or 4 percent of families, about 1.8 million families, and fewer than 200,000 women are harmed to the point that they require medical attention—far too many, but far fewer than advocates' guesstimates. The problem needed to be addressed, and supporters thought this was more likely to happen if half of or all married women were battered rather than fewer than 5 percent (Brott 1994).

Another form of exaggeration is mischaracterization of the group suffering a salient problem. When homeless people began to make news, the aging lobbies described the homeless as "bag ladies," drawing attention to the needs of elderly women. Only on closer examination of the homeless population did it become clear that most homeless people were nonelderly and most were men, many of them Vietnam veterans and other middle-aged and younger men (Rosenheck, Gallup, and Leda 1991). Heterosexuals who contracted AIDS during its first decade were mostly intravenous drug users. Yet to garner middle-class support, public education campaigns focused on heterosexuals in general and children in particular. Even pupils in middle-class elementary schools were taught how to avoid AIDS (Fineberg 1988; Goodman 1988). Near hysteria ensued when newspapers and the evening television news headlined the story that a small-town Texas high school had "discovered" six cases of AIDS in young men with no homosexual experience (Suro 1992). The embarrassing follow-up story two weeks later, revealing that the results could not be verified and the school nurse who had released the story could not be located, was given barely two inches near the bottom of an inside page in the *New York Times* (Associated Press 1992). Most newspapers simply ignored the follow-up.

Another example of mischaracterization of victims is the kidnapping of children. Pictures of missing children began arriving through the mail and appearing on milk cartons. Only later did it emerge that most of these claims of kidnapping involved divorces and child custody disputes (Best 1988; Gelles 1984). And a decade after this, a more systematic definition of kidnapping excluded 350,000 family custody cases, leaving 4,600 incidents involving a stranger and 200 to 300 per year defined by researchers as long distance and long term or ending in a fatality—again, far too many, but far fewer than initial estimates (P. Davis 1990; Greif 1993).

Advocates for elderly people, kidnapped children, and even hospitals like to present their group as disadvantaged if this serves their policy interests. Many hospitals in the 1980s complained that they were losing money on patients they wanted to discharge but could not do so because there were not enough nursing home beds. Hospitals said that states should pay for the wasted hospital days (Dubay, Kenney, and Holahan 1989; Welch and Dubay 1989). In reality, as the researchers showed, in many states the problem barely existed. And there seemed to be other explanations for the delays that did occur, such as slow Medicaid eligibility determination, a problem that could be solved by more caseworkers or a presumptive payment system. Instead, the hospitals went to state legislatures for more money. The point is that hospitals have a major stake in defining the problem, estimating its magnitude, and attributing its causes. It is in their best interest, so they believe, to present themselves as the victims, seeking legislative relief in the form of extra compensation for any unnecessarily long stays. Is this because hospitals are run by dishonest people always seeking a public handout? No; it is because hospitals are highly complex organizations facing urgent demands from many constituents. If they can solve one of their problems by shifting the load to public policy, they are likely to do so. The policy-making process must sort out the validity of the demands and decide whether a public policy solution is warranted or hospitals should be left to solve their own problems.

Finally, problems can be "framed" in ways that lead to very different solutions. This framing of problems can also be crucial in engendering public support for the problem—and its subsequent solution. One example of the importance of framing in understanding policy is in the area of assisted suicide. Proponents of assisted suicide framed the issue as one of individual rights and personal empowerment, emphasizing patients' dignity, individual rights, and autonomy. Opponents of assisted suicide framed the issue as contrary to the healing mission of physicians. A Michigan physician, Dr. Kevorkian, helped personify this notion of a physician gone amok (Glick and Hutchinson 2001).

Attributing Causes

For years, airplane crashes were invariably attributed to pilot error. Manufacturers did not take kindly to having their aircraft designs and construction blamed, and flight controllers were not willing to accept blame when a plane missed the runway or two planes had a close encounter. Mechanical failures or accepting bad landing instructions became the pilot's fault: he was blamed for not doing a better job of inspecting his aircraft before takeoff or not figuring out that another plane was already using the runway to which he had been directed. As the aircraft industry improved, as air traffic controllers realized they were unlikely to get better pay and lighter workloads unless they admitted mistakes and reported near misses, as terrorism became a competing cause of aircraft downings, and as National Transportation Safety Board bureaucrats got better at their jobs, we began to hear more candid representations of the facts—though still typically couched in the most careful, caveat-ridden technical language, because powerful interests have a stake in the causes to which bad outcomes are attributed.

So, too, in health care: much of framing the problem involves linking the problem to its root cause. And different causes lead to different solutions. For the first half of the twentieth century, tobacco companies claimed that smoking did not cause health problems. When the data had mounted to the point of undeniability, the companies' lawyers worked to put the blame on the smokers themselves, who should have known better. Finally, by the late 1990s, blame for smokers' deaths had shifted from individual smokers to cigarette manufacturers and their advertising and marketing campaigns, especially those targeted at children. Policy shifted with each new perspective on the problem: from the federal government's including cigarettes in military box lunches until as late as the mid-1960s, to government warnings about adverse health effects printed on cigarette packs from the late 1960s, to restrictions on tobacco companies' marketing techniques, especially those directed at youngsters, in the 1990s. When bartenders selling drinks to obviously intoxicated customers began to be seen as part of the problem of drunk driving, dram laws were passed in state after state.

The linkage between cause and effect is crucial to policy choice. In fact, Deborah Stone (1989) claimed that people choose causal linkages not only to shift blame but also to create the idea that they can remedy the problem. The focus on "deadbeat dads," for example, is ideal for a quick and popular legislative initiative: track them down, garnishee their wages, or throw them in jail for nonpayment of child support. Fair enough, but this is hardly a solution to the intractable and complex problem of out-of-wedlock teen pregnancies.

Formulating Public Policy Options

Not all problems are public problems; many can be solved in the private sector or simply will not be solved at all. Determining what is a public problem—to be solved by government—is, not surprisingly, not always easy. And it varies from generation to generation. In recent years, what once might have been public problems have been more and more relegated to the market. Other issues are also important in this formulation stage, including equity issues and the cost of the endeavor.

Is It a Public Problem?

American culture is built around core beliefs of individual liberty—defined as freedom from government constraints—in a way that has a powerful effect on how people perceive the meaning of *public problems* (Bosso 1994). In health care, as in other areas, the criterion for defining public involvement is this: is the problem better settled by the public than by the private sector? Policies on issues as disparate as airline industry regulation, sexual harassment, job training, international trade, and needle-exchange programs have all had to meet this "public role" criterion before government intervention could be justified (Rochefort and Cobb 1994).

The meaning of *public,* however, is in the eye—or rather the ideology—of the beholder. People (including policymakers) differ in their views on the proper role of government. One recent issue illustrating this point is obesity. Many people in public health think the increasing incidence of obesity in the United States, particularly among children, is a public problem, but most of the public does not agree. For example, a 2003 survey of Michigan residents found that only 28 percent thought being overweight was a public concern (Ford, Olson, and Baumer 2004). While much attention has been focused on this issue, several barriers need to be overcome before it can be justified as a public problem, including broad-based social disapproval, definitive research linking obesity with adverse health effects, emergence of a self-help movement, the "demonizing" of the relevant industry, organization of a mass movement, and interest-group action (Kersh and Morone 2002). One step in that direction is *The Botany of Desire: A Plant's-Eye View of the World,* by Michael Pollan (2002). In this book the author attributes much of America's obesity problem to federal farm subsidies that make corn cheap, encouraging the oversupply and overconsumption of corn syrup, a high-calorie substance found in most fast food and soft drink products. It quickly became a best-seller.

For many, markets are the preferred solution: government should be limited to instances of market failure. But does this simplify things? Not really, because claims of market failure do little more than open a debate about whether the market has failed. Is health care a well-functioning market? Or is it plagued by market failures because of several distinctive characteristics, including, for example, information asymmetry: patients as buyers and health care professionals as sellers are not equal players? Professionals use enormous amounts of technical knowledge to judge whether their patients need the care they prescribe. Most patients are completely or almost completely ignorant of the science underlying clinical decision making. This information asymmetry distorts the principle of consumer sovereignty and, to many, justifies public action to at least license professionals so as to weed out unqualified providers. Others would go farther. Given that the physician has the power to influence the patient's decisions about how much of a product to buy (McCall and Rice 1983), they advocate regulating physicians' fees and reviewing the appropriateness of prescribed care.

Externalities—costs or benefits falling on others—are also a concern in health care policy. Some health care problems affect more than the individual; infectious diseases are the principal case in point. Because of the risks involved in the spread of diseases, government must take responsibility for ensuring that everyone is vaccinated and, under some circumstances, evaluated for the presence of disease. Public health and sanitation laws and enforcement are justified on this principle. "Free riders" are another problem sometimes necessitating public action. Young healthy workers who decline to buy insurance are counting on the rest of us to pay for emergency rooms to care for them if they get sick or have an accident. They are free riders on an expensive health care system maintained by the insurance premiums paid by the rest of society.

These rationales for government involvement are intended to bypass issues of ideology and justify a limited role for government: correct the market failures, then get out; disrupt the private sector as little as possible. Following this economic orthodoxy, Rice (1998) argued that there is no reason to assume that a competitive marketplace will result in superior outcomes in the health area. Rather than putting the burden of proof on those who believe that government intervention is justified, we should consider alternative policies equally and judge them using the same criteria.

In health care, ideology plays an important role in determining what gets defined as a problem and what gets on the agenda for policy making. Ideological differences about the role of government action help policymakers pick sides in the debate over whether government action is needed. Party affiliation helps people make up their minds. While Republicans are often quite willing to use government to restrict behavior related to moral issues, they tend to favor minimal government for solving domestic problems. They want the market to solve such problems, unless there is strong evidence that this approach is not working and cannot be fixed. As chapter 7 illustrates, ideology played a role in the development of the Medicare Modernization Act in 2003. Republicans strongly supported market-based approaches, including improving competition between Medicare fee-for-service and managed care, imposing substantial co-payments, prohibiting the government from setting national drug prices, and instead setting up health savings accounts to encourage consumers to pay their own health care bills. Democrats, particularly liberal Democrats, are quicker to give up on the market and seek government intervention, and more of it. The high cost of prescription drugs is a good example. Democrats were the first to call attention to the problem and to offer a proposal for extensive coverage. Republicans quickly focused on the concern that most elderly people already had private drug coverage, which Republicans were loath to replace with public coverage. When President George W. Bush asked Republicans to support Medicare drug coverage, even a bill with great gaps in coverage barely passed Congress.

This tension between the parties over the role of government is predictable for many issues, as pointed out by Eyestone (1978). He noted that most social questions are not neutral with respect to the issue of government involvement. For any two competing issues, he said, one will almost certainly call for more government involvement than the other, and the contrast will invoke the government role to some degree. Further, he noted, the appeal against bloated government is often a conscious political strategy—a charge also made by Democrats when Republicans criticized President Clinton's proposed health insurance purchasing alliances.

The public, too, is often skeptical about government intervention and evaluates a proposal by whether or not its extension of government power will directly affect the public (Eyestone 1978). Public skepticism has a long history in health policy and has played a major role in stymieing the development of national health insurance. The arguments used in 1964 and 1994 on freedom to choose a physician, quality of treatment, and the possibility of bureaucratic medicine were nearly identical. And both were effective. When a poll asked people to choose between reliance on a government or a private-oriented approach, a majority chose the private approach (Jacobs 1993b). Further, though Democrats are more likely than Republicans to support a tax-financed national health plan, even liberal support is "tempered by concern over the problems of bureaucracy and the practical limits to what government can accomplish" (Jacobs 1993b, 634).

Appropriateness of the government role is an equally critical standard of acceptability for health care policies—that is, for solutions. This criterion is easier to meet at some times than at others. During more liberal times, a significant block of voters moves from serious distrust of government's ability to solve problems to a willingness to suspend disbelief long enough to try out a new set of reforms. The Great Depression was a time when the private market had clearly failed many Americans and they were willing to turn to government for help. Again, during the Johnson years, Americans seemed willing to experiment with public approaches to meeting a pent-up demand for solutions to a host of social concerns. Values seem to oscillate between relatively more liberal and relatively more conservative positions; these cycles are difficult to predict but at times seem to span three decades or so. In the current decade, pharmaceutical companies were greatly concerned that Medicare price setting would stifle innovation and discourage new cures. Congress responded by passing a law that essentially guarantees that drug makers will have their prices set by the market rather than by government, even though government was already a large purchaser of drugs, and through Medicare is becoming much larger.

Even in more liberal times, a high level of distrust remains, making some proposals unacceptable. One such proposal is mandatory participation in government health insurance programs. To many liberals, mandatory participation is the only effective solution to the free-rider problem—people at low risk avoid insurance, producing adverse selection as the sick seek insurance and premium costs increase, thus inducing more drop-outs, more uninsured individuals, more adverse selection, and so forth, sometimes called a "death spiral." Yet little seems to more enrage conservatives than mandatory participation in a public program they do not support. This is particularly true when the problem is, as Downs (1972) suggested, one that does not affect most members of society. National health insurance proposals involve significant dislocations and costs for all those who feel they are already well served in the private market. With premiums for nonelderly people substantially paid by employers and care for the elderly and many people with disabilities paid for by Medicare and Medicaid, most people fall into this category. Either they have insurance or think they do not need it. The exceptions are the poor and the near poor: they need it, want it, but cannot afford it.

Over time, for some kinds of solutions, attitudes soften and ideas that were once anathemas gain support and can be adopted. Mandatory use of seat belts, initially strongly opposed as government intrusion into private lives, was later grudgingly tolerated and eventually welcomed as a necessary safety device effective against real harm. By 2000, some 30 years after the use of seat belts was first required and resisted, laws were being passed (with little opposition) allowing police to stop drivers for seat belt violations alone.

Requisites for changes in attitudes are the passage of time and accumulation of overwhelming evidence that benefits justify government intrusion. Kingdon (1995) noted that softening up occurs while time is passing. Promoters talk about their proposal and make people more familiar with it. They may also change it enough to make it more acceptable. As a result, ideas that failed the appropriateness test when first introduced tend to be introduced time and again, becoming better understood, more familiar, and easier to accept as time goes by. Prospective payments to hospitals are a case in point. Unfortunately, the time required for softening up is unpredictable. For some proposals in some places, more than a half-century has not been sufficient. For example, the fluoridation of drinking water was still an issue in Arkansas, Massachusetts, Oregon, and Washington State in 2005. Even though there is substantial evidence that fluoridation reduces cavities, the state legislatures in those states continue to discuss whether to impose it statewide—succumbing to citizens' concerns about government intrusion in their lives. Ironically, while the American Dental Association celebrated 60 years of water fluoridation, in 2005, research findings emerged that indicated a possible link between fluoridated tap water and bone cancer in adolescent boys (Eilperin 2005).

There may be an interaction between the quality of an idea and its increasing likelihood of passage with time and familiarity. Kingdon (1995) conceded that there seems to be a compelling power to an idea whose time has come. Explicit rationing of health care to control costs is still unacceptable to most Americans, but the idea began creeping into public policy discourse in the 1990s (Lamm 1990) and was explicitly adopted for Oregon's poor residents early in the decade—though in response to fierce objections, its most controversial provisions were watered down. Conversely, some solutions grow less acceptable with time. Forced screening for various infectious or inherited diseases, particularly those that uniquely affect a minority group, is not a publicly acceptable method of disease control or cost control and shows little sign of becoming acceptable, though quarantine for infection was once more or less routine.

Equity

The reliability of government as a problem solver is not all that is at stake in the debate over the government's role. Often lurking behind the symbols is the real point of departure between conservatives and liberals: income equality, or redistribution. Liberals typically want to use government intervention as a means of redistributing power and wealth to the poor and disenfranchised. Deborah Stone (1993) even pushed for such an outcome from the private sector on the issue of pooling health insurance risk. Arguing that the nation is a community, she rejected an insurance company's definition of actuarial fairness: "the lower your risk, the lower your premium" (288). On the contrary, she argued, each person paying for his own risk, when taken to its extreme, would mean every person having his own premium based on a perfect prediction of health care costs. The result would be the end of insurance, since all who could afford to would simply put the money in the bank to avoid insurance company profits and administrative costs. She called actuarial fairness "anti-redistributive ideology" (294). In contrast, she argued, "Social insurance operates by the logic of 'solidarity.' Its purpose is to guarantee that certain agreed-upon individual needs will be paid for by a community or group . . . In the health area, the argument for financing medical care through social insurance rests on the prior assumption that medical care should be distributed according to medical need or the ability of the individual to benefit from medical care" (290).

Harvard philosopher John Rawls (1971) would most probably agree. Most people are risk averse; in situations in which their future status is unpredictable (they wear a "veil of ignorance"), they tend to adopt policies that raise the position of the least advantaged. Fearing that they could become part of the minority, they adopt redistributive policies that lead to greater equality of outcomes.

In voluntary insurance plans, the sickest people buy insurance, well people (especially young people) wait until they get sick, and premiums rise over time, exacerbating the problem. Insurance companies find it in their interest to sell insurance only to people who are not likely to use it, excluding in any way they can those who are likely to get sick: through physical exams, exclusion of preexisting conditions, long waiting periods, and high and rising premiums for those who present an elevated risk, especially when "experience" shows that an individual has a tendency to use substantial care. Information about risk indicators and health care utilization is often accessed at the time an individual applies for a new job that includes health insurance. The result is that people with elevated risk may be unable to change jobs without becoming uninsurable or facing prohibitive premiums. Sometimes the policies of an entire small firm face cancellation owing to the risks or costs of one unlucky individual.

Mandatory national health insurance covering the young and old, sick and well, and those who have no health problems today but may have them tomorrow is offered as one way to increase the size of the risk pool and distribute the costs of high-risk individuals among all policy holders. This raises the premiums of well people above what they would pay in an experience-rated plan and lowers the premiums of sick people. It may also require an expansion of the benefits package to meet the needs of enrollees with special problems, including high limits on prescription drugs and coverage of experimental treatments, adaptive housing, transportation, special communications aids, and personal care for chronically ill patients. Because these are typically limited in the benefits packages and premium calculations of private plans, they may further increase premiums above those for private, experience-rated plans. The result tends to be premiums that redistribute wealth from some premium payers to others and expansion of the role of government into new sectors of the economy as it referees disputes among beneficiary subgroups over what services should be covered. The side one chooses in this perennial debate reflects one's values and typically involves a trade-off between greater efficiency and greater fairness in solving problems.

Reliance on the market to distribute income, wealth, and equity of access to health care may produce particular problems for minority groups. Even a quick review of the data shows that the market has not worked very well to remove differences in health status between minority and nonminority Americans. Members of minorities live sicker and die sooner from a wide variety of acute and chronic conditions. African Americans experience the poorest health outcomes of any racial or ethnic group in the United States. Minorities account for half of all the uninsured in the United States. Even when they are insured, minorities are less likely to receive adequate care (Kennedy 2005). African Americans and other minorities also confront significant treatment disparities. Socioeconomic status is a powerful determinant of both health and mortality (Fiscella 2003).

Nevertheless, advocates of market-oriented solutions to health care problems, such as Winn (1987), simply do not see racial barriers as a problem. Free-market advocates do not regard African Americans as a special group, ignoring "the fact that blacks experience shorter life spans, a higher rate of chronic and debilitating illnesses, and lower protection against infectious diseases" (Winn 1987, 240). Failure to confront the reality that poverty is highly correlated with minority racial status in the United States means that the special needs of minorities will not be met. Racially neutral policy thus perpetuates the effects of racial discrimination and enhances its persistence. Likewise, policies that require poor individuals to pass through invasive and demeaning eligibility screenings to prove they are poor enough to receive benefits, as well as requiring them to accept care from providers willing to work for the invariably lower prices paid by government, are an affront to many advocates for the poor: these policies produce "two-tiered" care, the lower tier disproportionately provided to minority-group members. Recent efforts have highlighted the need for an infrastructure for monitoring and tracking disparities, including a new, congressionally mandated National Healthcare Disparities Report, which has developed consistent definitions and is tracking changes in quality of care over time (Moy, Dayton, and Clancy 2005).

Means Testing and Redistribution

Liberals and conservatives often part company over means testing as a way of limiting public subsidies and the scope of the public role. The two major political parties subscribe to different philosophies of how best to improve the lot of the poor. Conservatives fear creating dependency among those given free care, and they worry that further taxing the well-off will stifle investment and that the inevitable standards that accompany subsidies will discourage innovation. They prefer to restrict free care to the poorest of the poor and count on a growing and innovative economy to provide more income for everyone and more efficient production than a highly regulated economy can offer. Physicians tend to side with the conservatives on this issue, because they prefer to earn their incomes from middle-class, privately paying patients, restricting government health care programs to those who cannot pay on their own. Their fear is that with government subsidies will come fee schedules and other controls, eroding their income and freedom. Liberals prefer to use progressive taxation to raise revenues and provide the health care benefit free to all, removing the stigma attached to "charity" care and mitigating the temptation to render poor care to poor people (though this is hard to avoid if the poor and the middle class use different providers). Means testing is an approach to limiting government's role and making proposals more affordable. Even some liberal U.S. senators supported it, based on cost concerns, when Republicans made it a part of the MMA (see chapter 7).

These differences in perspective between what are loosely referred to as liberal and conservative views reflect fundamental differences in social priorities and views about the efficacy of government as a solution to social problems. For these reasons, merely pointing out that a problem exists in no way ensures a consensus on the need for government action. In defining health care problems for public policy intervention, technical arguments must take shape within an ideological context. Values are often at least as important as data.

Who Will Pay the Costs?

When policy analysts think of costs, they think in terms of efficiency: the amount of output for each unit of input. Often they are concerned with cost-effectiveness or cost-benefit ratios: the marginal benefit for a marginal expenditure. Politicians make a similar but slightly different calculation. They are worried about how to pay the political costs—dollars, disruption, administrative burden—and whether the juice is worth the squeeze. Proposals that are very costly and of dubious effectiveness are dead letters.

National health insurance is a case in point. In most proposals, costs typically fall on one of two groups: businesses (through a government mandate or another form of taxation) or taxpayers in general (usually through a payroll tax such as Medicare supplemented by "sin taxes" or through taxation of employer-provided health insurance premiums). In an important if ill-fated variation in the 1980s, a catastrophic health insurance plan for elderly people tried a third approach: it taxed wealthy beneficiaries of the program to pay some of the costs for poorer beneficiaries. The law was repealed the following year as those who were targeted to pay complained about the cost for the value received. A more recent variation proposes to charge wealthy beneficiaries higher co-payments for home health visits, and the 2003 MMA limits premium subsidies based on income.

Taxation of health insurance premiums provided by employers, either in full or over some threshold premium value, is appealing economically because, in addition to raising money, it can make consumers more aware of their health care costs in a way that might help restrain spending or at least ensure value for price. But, of course, it has one very great drawback. The benefits are diffused among the entire beneficiary population, many of whom are poor and most of whom are not well organized around the health insurance issue, but the costs are heavily concentrated on employers. Proposals that concentrate costs on powerful interests such as business are sure to be met by well-financed, well-organized resistance. Even though many economists have argued that costs of health insurance are shifted ultimately to employees, employers tend to see themselves as paying the bill. Hence, from their perspective, employer mandates put the burden on business, especially small businesses not now offering coverage; firms make the point that a person employed in a business not offering insurance often can get coverage through a spouse's employer. All these strategies involve major political problems. This creates incentives for employers to organize and spend resources to oppose the plan, while most beneficiaries individually have little to gain and cannot be inspired to act collectively.

Costs, no matter where they fall, have become much more important than they used to be, especially in health care policy and regardless of whether the budget is in deficit or surplus. For decades, costs were a secondary consideration at best, and even then only for large, expensive projects costing billions of dollars, and they were of no concern at all for smaller projects of only a few million dollars. Mere thousands have long been rounded off in federal budgets. Debate challenging the feasibility of Medicare in 1965 did address the cost issue, and even President Johnson's staff was concerned about the higher than expected rate at which health care costs were rising after its passage, but those concerns were not given the weight that they are today. Nor were there so many sources of competing cost estimates. Few politicians want to raise taxes, so they must find other programs to cut or must claim that their program will actually save money. An important aspect of the CBO staff's job is validating—or, more likely, rejecting—claims of expected savings. Nevertheless, in one recent example—the Medicare Modernization Act—the costs were grossly underestimated by the CBO to meet a ceiling that was set by the White House and enforced by conservative Republicans. Only a few months after the measure was signed, the cost estimates shot up and continued to increase in the ensuing years.

Complexity

Calling a proposal "bureaucratic" is another rallying cry. Fear of bureaucratic red tape can bring a proposal under deep suspicion if opponents are successful in making a plausible case (often laced with exaggeration) that it is likely to spawn bureaucratic growth and replace private decision making with decisions made by bureaucrats. This concern is paramount in health care. It puts proponents on the defensive and can greatly diminish the likelihood of adoption. Proposals that seem to replace physicians' clinical judgment with bureaucratic rules are strongly resisted, as are efforts to direct middle-class patients to specific providers. Likewise, much of the so-called managed care backlash of the late 1990s and early 2000s arose from the requirement for patients to jump through administrative hoops to see a specialist. Ironically, it was principally Republican members of Congress who designed and passed the MMA, one of the more complicated expansions of health care coverage ever adopted, including income-adjusted premiums that change each year, gaps in coverage, availability through managed care firms or competing local pharmacy benefit management plans, penalties for late sign-up, and the authority of various plan administrators to change the drugs they cover from time to time (see chapter 7). If further proof was needed, the MMA showed that it is difficult to write a law and not be "bureaucratic" when it tries to strike a balance between public and private responsibilities, includes incentives for prudence, accommodates regional variations and individual preferences for care delivery, and holds down costs.

Even when restrictions on freedom are minimized, paperwork burdens by themselves cause fierce resistance. Business, particularly small business, is viscerally fearful that any government-mandated compliance, however innocent at first, will eventually prove to be the nose of the camel under the tent, as Congress, bureaucratic regulators, and the courts reinterpret the scope of their authority, the degree of compliance, and, most especially, the scope of reporting required. This fear of paperwork has made businesses unwilling to accept federal subsidies intended to get them started on employee health insurance coverage, even companies that could clearly benefit from the subsidies.

Political Action or Legitimization

A proposal that seems appealing on an analyst's slide presentation software may have no chance of passage, or even consideration, in the real political world. Thus, political action—passage into law, adoption as an executive order or regulation or, increasingly, an issuance of the court—is far from a given. Many factors come into play: besides elements of the issue itself, these include saliency and timing and institutional factors.

Saliency and Timing

Public opinion plays an important role in political feasibility. If the public is engaged with an issue, it will be supportive; if the public is in strong opposition, the issue will fade quickly from the agenda.

The saliency of an issue dictates the kind of politics that accompanies it. Salient issues draw heavy press attention and thus provide legislators with the opportunity for credit taking, which encourages individual grandstanding and partisanship. Compromise around a majority position becomes harder. Party discipline tends to break down, because members of Congress know that voters will hold them accountable and may punish them for not protecting district interests. For the president, salient issues involve big stakes, making him vulnerable to demands for concessions by lawmakers willing to bargain for their vote. But if the issue is nonsalient, private interests and lawmakers' attentive voters are likely to call the shots. An actual or perceived emergency—such as the Medicare trust fund going broke—can help proposals, giving legislators political cover from interest-group pressure and allowing program or budget cuts that would otherwise be impossible.

President George W. Bush found out that even a popular, engaged president cannot necessarily control public opinion. In 2005, Bush introduced and strongly endorsed the idea of private accounts as a substitute for part of the nation's Social Security system. In spite of an all-out personal effort and tireless support from his cabinet, the idea gained little popularity with the American public and therefore met with fierce resistance in Congress.

Timing can easily kill an issue, either because another issue pushes it off the agenda (foreign affairs events, for example) or because the issue has not been resolved as election time approaches. The policy debate becomes grist for campaign debate. Issues that have been the subject of negotiation and compromise become campaign slogans and sound bites, widening rather than narrowing the gap between the parties. Compromise becomes even harder if one party believes it may gain enough seats in the election to change the lineup supporting or opposing a particular proposal. Kingdon (1995) made the point that the policy window opens only briefly. Proposals that are ready to go when the opportunity arises have a better chance of being adopted than ones that still have to be worked out. Downs's issue attention cycle (1972) characterizes the tenuous hold that problems have on the national agenda, especially if they are costly to solve. They enjoy saliency only so long as they are not replaced by another, more interesting problem.

Timing has generally been unkind to national health insurance proposals. They tend to be proposed early in the legislative session, but because of their complexity, serious battles over the most important features—the role of government and financing—often are delayed until well into the first year or early in the second year. By then, the congressional midterm elections are looming. Differences in opinion about policy issues become the focus of ideological tirades. Members begin looking to the election and thinking about how to use the health care debate to embarrass the other party or how to delay a vote on the legislation. If things go as hoped, the party will come back with additional seats, thereby improving their bargaining power on the health bill. This political maneuvering has been the death knell of health care reform proposals for decades.

Yet, electoral maneuvering had a great deal to do with the success of the MMA of 2003. The Republican White House and Republican Congress thought passage of a prescription drug bill could take away a pivotal campaign issue for Democrats in the 2004 congressional election. The strategy may have worked—the Republicans maintained control of both houses. Cleverly, they postponed program implementation—which proved to be problem prone—until after the election but then had to worry that elders might still be having problems as the 2006 election neared.

Institutional Factors

Implied in various authors' notions of political feasibility is a set of issues related to the role of institutions in the policy process. Proposals are much more likely to succeed if backed by a president with substantial political capital, including a large majority of his party controlling both houses. In its absence, with two houses and two parties to get through, along with interest-group opposition, a general distrust of government, affordability concerns, and issues as complex as health care policy, the default is policy failure. Any remaining hope must come from a policy entrepreneur, someone—often a member of Congress—pushing the solution forward, bargaining, and making persistent demands for progress (Kingdon 1995). The possibility for success depends on this individual's legislative and policy prowess, placement on key committees, and level of expertise and determination. If the president is the policy entrepreneur, success is more likely if the proposal is one that helps fulfill campaign promises or helps establish his legacy. Prospects rise further if he is a savvy master of the congressional process and is clever enough to court rather than offend powerful interests that wield influence with congressional leaders or delegations. Legislators must be able to see how the proposal will benefit their reelection prospects, either by giving them an opportunity to claim credit for serving the interests of their attentive constituents or by allowing them to trade their vote on this issue for another that is important to them.

Big plans require big majorities and a powerful policy entrepreneur. Again, for national health insurance this means a president who is popular and whose party commands a large majority in both houses. Medicare slipped through because of the lopsided Democratic victory in 1964. Votes can be lost through the traditional disagreements between the parties but also through the inevitable tension between groups of liberals: those who favor comprehensive change and those who want something more scaled down with a better chance to win. In the Carter years, Democrats split their support for national health care reform over the issue of comprehensive cradle-to-grave versus catastrophic-only coverage: President Carter versus Sen. Edward Kennedy (D-MA) and Big Labor, then Carter versus labor. Then, in the Clinton years, single-payer advocates versus managed care advocates did the same thing during debates on the health care proposal. Presidents with small majorities are simply not able to muster the votes for large comprehensive proposals. As criticism of their proposal heats up, it tends to cost them support in the polls as well, further depleting their reserve of capital.

A large number of factors impinge on the willingness of members of Congress to provide the votes the president needs. Chief among them are district concerns. Proposals that require members to set aside the interests of their districts are often doomed to failure. So-called sin taxes fall on a small number of industries, usually represented by a block of important legislators such as those representing wineries in California and New York or tobacco interests in the South. Especially ill advised are proposals that offend an industry concentrated in the district of one or more key committee chairs (as did a graduate medical education reform proposal when the Senate Finance Committee was chaired by a senator from New York, a state with many teaching hospitals). Conversely, proposals are likely to succeed by wide margins if they serve the interests of many legislators' districts and allow them to take credit for bringing projects and services to their districts, such as subsidies for hospitals.

Not all these criteria of political feasibility carry equal weight. For some criteria the weight changes with the issue; others are always heavily weighted. Effectiveness is likely to be a less important consideration in a debate on subsidies than a debate on mandates. Timing and comprehensiveness are less important if the issue is less salient. Concentrated costs and benefits are always important, however, because members of Congress place service to their districts at the top of their priority lists, and members from districts chosen to bear concentrated costs are by definition well financed and likely to use their resources to fight the proposal. The public's support is crucial, especially for salient policies.

For many issues, the criteria for political feasibility are both additive and interactive in their effect on the probability of success. Appropriateness of the government role is especially debatable if the costs of the proposal are high. Comprehensiveness tends to raise costs, which are likely to be concentrated somewhere. Effectiveness becomes more uncertain with each additional complexity, and complexity means more time and debate—and the proposal is most likely still under debate as election time approaches and the parties are looking for issues useful for defining themselves. These additive and interactive effects highlight the difficulty of getting the planets in the right alignment for successful enactment of comprehensive policy change.

Implementation

Once a policy is put in place, it is rarely self-executing. Rather, federal agencies must issue regulations, write checks, set up oversight committees or boards, and collect data on the process and impact of the new law (see chapter 4). In many instances, states and localities are the implementers, and they must designate or hire staff, develop procedures, select recipients, send checks, and collect data—among many other tasks. Implementation is not the end product of public policy but rather the beginning of feedback to policymakers about the progress of the program, its successes and failures and any unintended consequences. In the United States, implementation also has a special value in that the 50 states can implement differently—even the most stringent program—thanks to differences in institutional arrangements and in the demographic and social makeup of the states. By studying the implementation process and effects across the states, policy analysts and political scientists can gather information that is helpful both to Congress and to frameworks and models of the policy process.

ANOTHER APPROACH TO UNDERSTANDING THE POLICY PROCESS

The policy process can also be understood through a focus on components of the policy environment, rather than on the more linear notion of activity. David Baron (2000) summarized the policy process by focusing on four components: issues, institutions, interests, and information.

Issues may include the environment (noise, water, air pollution or land use constraints); externalities, such as the impact on local wages or tax revenues; health and safety concerns, such as lack of employee health insurance or worksite safety; public policy toward new technologies, such as bans on imports or exports or on genetic modification, or advertising, or age or gender constraints on research, or price and patent barriers to needed drugs; or moral issues.

Institutions include the city council, which may grant a license or tax relief or a construction variance; the hospital board, which may close its emergency room; the state legislature, which may demand discounts for poor or near-poor patients or ban certain marketing techniques; the courts, which may grant standing to parties not thought to have a stake in a dispute; or the European Union, which may decide that your trade practices violate antitrust rules. Each is characterized by a set of rules, by a constituency, and often by professional values or disciplinary standards or conflicts.

Interests are, for political scientists, the usual suspects, ranging from business coalitions to street marchers, to unions, to consumer groups, to pet lovers who mount a boycott against your product, to advocates for medically disenfranchised refugees on another continent.

Information is also key: how the public or stakeholders react to information may be wholly a function of how effectively the issue is framed. Information may be good or bad, right or wrong, science or myth, urban legend or ideology, complete or incomplete, preliminary or final. It may be reported by researchers at major universities, or it may be a malicious rumor or a misleading campaign advertisement; it may be a warranted or unwarranted investigation, lawsuit, or indictment; or it may be medical error or a patient satisfaction survey or a leaked memo. Gun makers have been masterful at framing gun sales as a Second Amendment right, shifting the debate away from their products' enhanced killing power. Physicians have had some success in framing medical errors as broader patient safety issues, and malpractice lawsuits as the excesses of greedy lawyers.

According to Baron (2000), issues come up because technology has changed, an interest group has become active, new research has uncovered the adverse effects of a drug or procedure, a prominent figure has been caught in a compromising situation, or a law or regulation has been issued or reinterpreted or grossly broken. Typically, issues follow a lifecycle that moves from early recognition by experts to broad demands for action, to realization of costs, difficulties, and opposition, to loss of interest and replacement by something new and more interesting. Stages often, but not always, include issue identification, interest-group formation, legislation, administration, and enforcement. The concerns over managed care abuses in the mid- and late 1990s, leading to demands for a national patients' bill of rights, certainly followed this cycle, from topping the news, conversation, and the national agenda to a forgotten issue.

THEORIES OF POLICY CHANGE

The policy process framework is important in understanding the process of policy making, but it fails to answer questions such as why some policies pass and others don't and why policy change does occur. Numerous explanations have been posited as to why policy changes. We briefly summarize three of these theories: the garbage can model, the policy advocacy model, and the punctuated model.

Kingdon's Revised Garbage Can Model

John Kingdon (1995) argued that policy change occurs in unpredictable ways as separate elements of the policy process intersect, as in a garbage can collecting trash. Three streams—problems, policies, and politics—merge. These streams develop and operate largely independently. Problems are defined and moved to the government agenda; policy solutions are developed, whether or not they respond to a problem; the politics may change suddenly with the election of a new administration, whether or not the policy community is ready or the problems facing the country have changed. The separate streams come together at critical times: a problem is recognized; a solution is available; the political climate makes the time right for change. This critical time, or opening of the policy window, is an opportunity for advocates to push their pet proposals.

A policy window is open but a short time. Precipitating events may be enabling legislation that comes up for renewal or the influx of new members of Congress. The item suddenly becomes "hot" because things come together at the same time: problems, solutions, policymakers' attention, and the desire to act. Kingdon (1995), like Cohen, March, and Olsen (1972), called this process coupling. Typically this comes at the hands of a policy entrepreneur: a cabinet secretary, senator or representative, lobbyist, academic, lawyer, journalist, or career bureaucrat—inside or outside the formal policy circle—who does the brokering to make things happen. "No one type of participant dominates the pool of entrepreneurs" (Kingdon 1995, 204). The entrepreneur's job is to push, shape, negotiate, disseminate, and couple the problem to a solution or a pet solution to a problem. "As to problems, entrepreneurs try to highlight the indicators that so importantly dramatize their problems. They push for one kind of problem definition rather than another . . . As to proposals, entrepreneurs are central to the softening-up process. They write papers, give testimony, hold hearings, try to get press coverage, and meet endlessly with important and not-so-important people . . . The process takes years of effort" (205). An important contribution of this model is the recognition that solutions sometimes precede problems. The process is anything but well ordered.

Advocacy Coalition Framework

A model that recognizes the long-term nature of policy change is the work of Sabatier and Jenkins-Smith (1988, 1993), who argued that policy change should be viewed over a long time-horizon—at least a decade. Problems are not "solved" and taken off the policy map. Rather, as Wildavsky (1979) noted, once a solution is carried out it creates new sets of issues, ensuring that no public problem ever really dies.

The framework developed by Sabatier and Jenkins-Smith, called the advocacy coalition framework, suggests that analysis of policy change requires a time perspective of a decade or more and should focus on policy subsystems, or what they call advocacy coalitions. Policy change, they posit, occurs as a result of competition within the subsystem and events outside the subsystem. This approach differs in that it focuses on *coalitions* of interests composed of actors including Congress, the president, interest groups, and the press, rather than on the actors themselves. Advocacy coalitions are composed of people who share a particular belief system and who are committed to working toward a policy over time. These coalitions spend time "venue shopping," or trying to find government entities that might be most amenable to their cause. Policy change occurs following an external shock or intervention or when very solid empirical evidence leads to policy-oriented learning across belief systems.

Punctuated Equilibrium

Baumgartner and Jones (1993) argued that policy making is generally characterized by long periods of relative stability (equilibrium) punctuated by the occasional major change. Significant policy shifts occur when the balance of forces that generally promote the status quo is disrupted such that the forces protecting the current situation are overwhelmed. One way this can occur is by fashioning a new policy image and exploiting multiple policy venues. Change is most likely when a positive feedback system forms and even those who previously objected to the change conclude that it is inevitable and participate in the change process. The Medicare Modernization Act of 2003 fits this model in that several major interest groups that had previously opposed versions of the bill (particularly PhRMA and the AARP), and even a staunch Democratic proponent, Senator Kennedy, supported a measure that included components they had earlier opposed and was not as comprehensive as they might desire.

CONCLUSION

Taken together, the various understandings of the policy process framework suggest that problems and solution options must meet certain criteria if they are to reach the political agenda and survive the political process of policy making. Those who are suffering as a result of the problem must have interesting or attractive features. The problem must be (viewed as) appropriate for government action, not usurping state sovereignty or replacing market solutions with government interference. Its solution must seem to be technically feasible and effective and must reflect a general consensus among experts. Policy solutions must be equitable in both who gets benefits and who pays for them. Costs must not be concentrated on powerful interests and must not be budget busting, nor should they involve too much redistribution from the haves to the have-nots.

Means testing can be invoked to attract conservative supporters, but may (or may not) offend liberals. Proposed solutions must not involve (or imply for the future) excessive reporting or other administrative burdens or transaction costs, especially if the burden will fall on states or small business. The district interests of powerful congressional committee chairs must not be transgressed. Someone who can speak for others, someone who has great political skill, institutional endowments, political capital, and great persistence, must shoulder the duties of policy entrepreneur. The other party's turf must not be encroached upon. Members of Congress must be able to claim credit for bringing home the pork or good policy. Supporters must not be balkanized or uncompromising; opponents must not be well organized, concentrated, moneyed, prestigious, or otherwise well positioned to mount a well-financed and well-orchestrated fight. Public support is key.

Health policy is typically, but not always, complex. The exceptions are areas, such as abortion and sexual abstinence education, that are best characterized as morality policies. The health policy domain has long been characterized by incremental change, but as the Medicare Modernization Act of 2003 aptly illustrates, nonincremental policies can be adopted, especially if the issues—and solutions—have been considered in the legislative world and thus have been shaped and brokered, and if legislators have been softened up and made familiar with its provisions. In the next chapter we apply these lessons to see how helpful the models are in understanding why, in one particular case—the MMA—some problems won a place on the agenda and the solutions to which they were attached became law.

7

Problem to Policy

Politics of the Medicare Prescription Drug Law

MOST PROBLEMS become issues for politicians when they can be used to win elections. Not that politicians are crass opportunists. Rather, they are pragmatists. Solving problems that no one cares about would mean neglecting problems they do care about, and it is these issues that bring people to the voting booths and inspire supporters to volunteer for campaigns and make campaign contributions. Prescription drug prices and restricted access to life-saving and pain-relieving drugs are ideal issues for candidates and parties to run on because they represent real problems and attentive voters care a lot about them.

On December 8, 2003, President George W. Bush signed into law the largest addition to Medicare, the health insurance program for people who are elderly or disabled, since the program was initially enacted in 1965. The new plan was designed with a two-year implementation delay for its major features, coming into full effect in January 2006. It provides full drug coverage with no premiums or co-payments for poor people, income-adjusted small to modest premiums and co-pays for people who are near poor and have few assets, and coverage for spending up to a certain level with a 25 percent co-payment, annual deductible, and monthly premiums. That certain level will rise each year, based on all Medicare beneficiaries' drug spending; it was $2,250 in 2006. Everyone in the program gets catastrophic coverage for costs exceeding just over $5,000, and that level too will rise yearly. A large gap in coverage (commonly dubbed the "donut hole") is left in the middle range of spending, to keep program costs down and ensure that market forces are setting prices. The gap, requiring out-of-pocket spending, started at about $3,600 in 2006, and the level will rise yearly.

The new program, which added a new Part D to the Medicare law and modified Part C (in the managed care portion of the law), can be accessed as a traditional fee-for-service option or through managed care entities, including some new forms of managed care voluntarily combining various types of providers and vendors. In either case, enrollees must go through a regional pharmacy benefit manager; PBMs will compete for enrollees' business, decide which specific drugs to carry within classes of drugs, and negotiate drug prices with the pharmaceutical companies. In the MMA, the federal government is expressly forbidden to set prices. Other provisions cap the percentage of drug and other ambulatory costs that the government will pay, expand access to health savings accounts, and establish future demonstration projects.

Supporters of the new law call it a historic improvement in the program. Critics say it is a first step toward privatizing Medicare. Many agree that it is a complex program full of uncertainties as to how it will affect many aspects of the world of prescription drugs. Medicare's share of overall drug spending was expected to rise from about 2 percent in 2005 to about 25 percent in 2006 (Heffler et al. 2005).

In this chapter we chronicle the 108th Congress's process of crafting, debating, and passing this historic bill, the Medicare Prescription Drug, Improvement and Modernization Act of 2003 (the MMA), which became Public Law 108-173. Drawing on the theory perspectives discussed in earlier chapters, this chronicle highlights the role of the president, key congressional committees, and House and Senate leaderships; the powerful contributions and rather unorthodox process of the conference committee that reconciled differences in the House and Senate bills; the role of think tanks and commissions; and the overweening presence and influence of key lobby groups.

THE PROBLEM AND THE AGENDA

By the turn of the new century, prescription drug prices had been a problem for at least two decades as new therapies became available and more care shifted from hospitals, where Medicare paid drug costs, to ambulatory settings, where it did not. For winning policy agenda space, a problem's having been around for a few years can be helpful. Brand new issues don't typically garner much attention from candidates, because too few voters care passionately about them yet, and no one knows how long a new issue's political legs will be. Congress had been working on the problem of drug prices for at least 20 years.

THE HATCH-WAXMAN ACT OF 1984

Drug companies had long complained that they lost years of revenues while they waited for an overburdened FDA staff to review their drug approval requests and accompanying clinical trial evidence. Those delays also cut into the period during which the company would enjoy patent protection—that is, protection from generics. Consumers and the generics industry, however, complained that the makers of name-brand drugs used a variety of legal maneuvers to prevent generic versions of major drugs reaching the market. Congress, led by the bipartisan efforts of the House Commerce Committee's Health and Environment Subcommittee chair Henry Waxman (D-CA) and Senate Health and Welfare Committee chair Orrin Hatch (R-UT), wrote the bill that permitted pharmaceutical companies to pay fees to the FDA that allowed the government to hire more staff and thus speed up the approval process. The bill passed Congress on September 12, 1984, and became PL 98-369, the Drug Price Competition and Patent Restoration Act, often called the Hatch-Waxman Act (*CQ Weekly* 1984). In exchange, generic drugs could be brought to market without retesting of the same compounds used in patented versions (Wehr 1984).

This solution struck a delicate and controversial compromise between the powerful brand-name manufacturers and their generics counterparts. The law included provisions that ultimately allowed some brand-name drug patents to be extended at the whim of the manufacturer by filing an allegation of patent infringement, changing drug packaging, or other tricks. Critics said the law made the problem worse, and, indeed, both Congress and the president intervened many years later to correct some of those problems. But the new law's defenders nonetheless argued that it accomplished the major goal sought by its congressional sponsors: the share of generics rose from about 19 percent of the prescription drug market in 1984 to 43 percent in 1996 (CBO 1998, 27), largely as a result of the new law and cost-conscious purchasing policies by managed care firms, Medicaid, and others. According to a CBO report (1998,

27), "The Hatch-Waxman Act greatly increased the probability that a generic copy would become available once the patent on a brand-name drug expired. It also contributed to a dramatic rise in generic market share. In addition, the act reduced the delay between patent expiration and generic entry, but that acceleration was roughly offset by patent-term extensions and exclusivity provisions [of Hatch-Waxman] that postpone generic entry."

By the spring of 2005, the share of generics versus brand names had risen to more than half (53 percent) of the U.S. prescription drug market, though in the rest of the world the generics share exceeds three-quarters of the market (*Medical News Today* 2005). Nonetheless, despite the growing availability of generics, from 1990 to 2000 drug spending rose at alarming rates, and in subsequent years rose even more dramatically from less than $300 billion in 1990 to more than $600 billion in 2003 (Express Scripts 2004), faster in many years than most of the rest of health care (which typically well exceeds general inflation). In 2003, the year in which the MMA would be voted on, drug spending accounted for 11 percent of all health care spending.

In 1988, in the Medicare Catastrophic Coverage Act, Congress amended the original Medicare statute to provide (among other things) limited coverage of prescription drugs. Congress repealed the reform a year later when Medicare recipients revolted against the income-based, sliding-scale higher premiums that accompanied the expanded coverage (of drugs, nursing home care, mammograms, and other benefits). In fact, many of those who led the revolt would have been net beneficiaries; only high-income seniors would have paid more (Kollman 1998).

AN EXPERT'S PERSPECTIVES ON THE PROBLEM

In the spring of 1994, *Health Affairs,* a journal read by policy analysts, policymakers, academics, researchers, and others with an interest in following health policy issues, featured an article by a respected health economist from the RAND Corporation (S. Long 1994). (By coincidence, 1994 was the death-knell year for both the Clinton health security proposal [which included prescription drug coverage] and the Democrats' four-decade control of the House of Representatives.) The author of the *Health Affairs* article, Steven Long, made the case for prescription drug coverage under Medicare. His interest in this issue dated back to at least his work managing health issues at the Congressional Budget Office and, more directly, to his brief stint in 1989 as executive director of the Prescription Drug Payment Review Commission, created by

Congress in the Medicare Catastrophic Coverage Act of 1988. The commission had died aborning with the repeal of the act, repealed in part because of the impression that the drug coverage provisions were expensive and unneeded given that about three-fourths of seniors already had drug coverage through Medicaid, their current or former employers, Medicare managed care plans, or their supplemental insurance policies.

Using an analysis from the National Health Accounts compiled by the HCFA (later CMS), supplemented with analysis from the 1987 National Medical Expenditure Survey (produced by another HHS agency—the Agency for Healthcare Research and Quality), Long showed that drug spending was highly skewed: a few elderly people were the big drug spenders—11 percent accounted for nearly half of all drug spending, and more than half of that spending was out-of-pocket. Most seniors spent little on drugs and had some form of coverage.

To those who think about such issues, this is the classic profile of an insurable event: a low probability of large losses—a point that Long made early in his article. Yet he was also quick to make the case that this skewness in drug spending and the conditions that produced it created a poor situation for the purchase of drug insurance, because those who expected to have big drug costs would be most likely to buy the insurance—if the companies would sell it to them. The big drug spenders were most likely to be treating chronic illnesses—long-term conditions that were already known to them, had known drug costs, and were not likely to go away. In short, from the insurance provider's perspective this was the worst situation for selling insurance: asymmetric information between the insured and insurer. Unless the government mandated that everybody, sick or well, must buy insurance against the possibility that they might someday need it, the drug insurance market would fail due to adverse selection. Long also showed that the Medigap policies offering drug coverage were likely to be so stingy in their coverage that most would pay little. The people with good insurance tended to be the younger, healthier, employed population, least likely to need the insurance.

Long's article, supported by a grant from the AARP's public policy institute, identified the problem, quantified it (using data from bureaucratic agencies), legitimized it, talked about the burden on a sympathetic group of elders, and made the case for government intervention—all necessary steps in the policy process, and all outlined in the first few paragraphs and tables of a report in a widely read journal. The article went on to consider various policy options, ranging from comprehensive coverage to limited coverage intended to inspire cost-awareness. Long's analysis reminded would-be advocates about the legacy of the Medicare Catastrophic Coverage Act, which provided benefits to few and costs to all, and he suggested that a principal concern must be how to deal with the fact that some seniors already had drug coverage and would not want to see their tax dollars go to providing public coverage for what they already had. He also raised the matter of cost controls, noting that some analysts would come to the issue with a penchant for price controls, while others would loathe that idea and instead favor some sort of market discipline. Finally, in his list of proposal options, Long suggested that one approach might be to cover only the financially neediest population, while noting that this would leave many near-poor beneficiaries without coverage and no effective means of getting it. Long's article presaged what would become the major sticking points of the policy debate as it reached its peak in Congress nearly a decade later.

Meanwhile prescription drug prices were rising, research showed that some Medicare recipients were doing without drugs or skipping doses, other studies showed the adverse consequences of not taking needed medications, and some drug companies seemed to be abusing their patent privileges by gaining patent extensions (blocking generic drugs) for such minimal improvements to their patented drug as changing the color of the package.

1999 National Bipartisan Commission on the Future of Medicare

Problems with prescription drugs were but one aspect of Medicare's shortcomings, however. There was not enough money even for the services already included in Medicare. By 1997, the Medicare Trust Fund, which pays for hospital inpatient and some skilled nursing services, had, several times over, been projected to go broke in future years. The day of reckoning had been put off a few times but was almost at hand, with the prospect of millions of baby boomers retiring and enrolling in Medicare in 2010. This was not an attractive election issue (as deficits typically are not) and so had not gotten much attention from the press or the general public. Congress liked it that way, and rather than put the problem on the evening news by debating it, the members quietly created a commission to come up with a solution. Commissions are a favorite way Congress has of addressing, while not getting too close to, hot potato problems. The National Bipartisan Commission on the Future of Medicare (1999) was created as part of the 1997 Balanced Budget Act (PL 105-33) to make recommendations for strengthening the Medicare program ahead of the baby boomers' retirement. It was chaired jointly by Sen. John

Breaux (D-LA) and House Ways and Means Committee chair Bill Thomas (R-CA), both conservative members of Congress despite their bipartisanship. The commission membership, nearly evenly split between Republicans and Democrats, was a mixture of congressional party and presidential appointees, and it was charged with adopting recommendations only if they could muster an 11-vote majority, two-thirds of the 17 members. Nominally, this requirement could foster bipartisanship and improve the chances of drafting something that could pass muster with the then Republican-controlled House of Representatives and Democratic-controlled Senate, and President Bill Clinton. Functionally, it could promise failure to reach a consensus among the commission's politically diverse membership.

Senator Breaux, aided by his co-chair, Representative Thomas, crafted a plan for the commission that strongly favored a broad role for private insurance firms in Medicare service delivery and the use of managed care and would provide an ambulatory care prescription drug benefit. The two legislators also favored a "defined contributions" subsidy to replace Medicare's existing "defined benefits" plan. In a defined benefits plan, the insurer—in this case the government—essentially promises to increase its payments if the costs of a defined set of benefits should rise in the future. In a defined contributions plan, the government implicitly limits its payments to a fixed amount, or a fixed rate of increase, regardless of what benefits ultimately cost.

This "restructuring of Medicare" through the use of managed care was intended to save more than $350 billion over the coming decade. Other features of the Breaux-Thomas plan included a gradual increase in the Medicare eligibility age to 67 years, higher premiums for higher-income beneficiaries, payment for medical education through a trust fund, full subsidy for those whose incomes were below 135 percent of the federal poverty level, and other features not directly related to the drug issue. Some commission members, including some Democrats, supported the approach. Others saw the plan as dismantling the Medicare program, replacing it with a "premium support," or defined contributions plan (as opposed to its current defined benefits plan), and radically reducing the role of government in program management (M. Carey and Adams 1999). Breaux and Thomas's critics also wanted benefits available through fee-for-service, not just managed care, plans, and they wanted the defined benefits approach retained.

President Clinton's appointees to the council were among those opposing the proposal. The president was accused of instructing his appointees to block the Breaux-Thomas plan by refusing to work toward a compromise. But the Clinton appointees themselves, Laura Tyson, former chair of the President's

Council of Economic Advisers, and Stuart Altman, well-known Brandeis University professor and former Republican White House adviser—no shrinking violets and fully capable of strong policy convictions—unequivocally denied even having met with the president or in any way following his bidding on the commission (M. Carey and Adams, 1999).

At a February 24, 1999, meeting of the panel, 10 members supported the Breaux-Thomas approach, short of the 11 members needed to adopt it as the commission's position. When the commission briefed the president on its progress to date—perhaps noting members' fractionated positions, including opposition by his appointees—he let them know he wasn't interested and that he would introduce his own proposal. This message probably hurt the commission's already limited likelihood of finding sufficient support for their Breaux-Thomas plan to muster the two-thirds majority needed to adopt it. The commission disbanded in March.

The president introduced his own plan on June 28, 1999. It differed from the Breaux-Thomas plan in several respects, while sharing some similarities. Both plans would strive to restructure Medicare and add prescription drug coverage. While the Breaux-Thomas plan would provide only stop-loss coverage—that is, catastrophic coverage so that Medicare patients would be covered only above a certain level, though that level was not specified in the plan—the Clinton plan would cover half of drug costs, but only up to a certain level. The level below which coverage would be provided would be phased in. During the first year, the Clinton plan would cover half of up to $2,000. After eight years, coverage would rise to half of up to $5,000. Beneficiaries would pay premiums of $24 per month under the president's plan, rising to twice that amount with the increasing stop-loss level. While beneficiaries would be entitled to spend more than $5,000 on drugs, those extra costs would be fully borne by the beneficiary. Low-income beneficiaries, those making less than 135 percent of the poverty level, would not pay premiums or a share of drug costs. Those with incomes between 135 and 150 percent of poverty would pay costs adjusted to their income level.

This plan would turn out to be less generous than the plan the Republicans eventually adopted, which would then be widely criticized for both stinginess and costliness. Critics said the president's plan would do little good for the two-thirds of beneficiaries who already had drug coverage, while it would be too limited in scope to help those without coverage who were sick enough to need much higher levels of spending. They also worried that the plan would encourage employers to drop the drug coverage provisions of their retiree health coverage plans. Clinton responded that he would also provide subsidies to employers to encourage them to keep up their coverage. The plan would cost an estimated $118 billion over a decade (Adams 1999).

Key common elements in the two plans were limits on total coverage and the reintroduction of means testing—different subsidy rates based on income—into Medicare. That these ideas were introduced by a Democratic president may well have surprised many Democrats, since most had fought against them for more than three decades. These ideas would become part of the policy legacy of the developmental phase of the MMA of 2003 and would be revisited when later bill drafters sat down to devise their own plans. Nonetheless, they were not exactly radical. Medicare already had limits on hospital and nursing home coverage, as well as limits on various ambulatory care services.

The Search for Solutions

Meanwhile, employers, insurers, and state Medicaid programs had begun to look for ways to reduce their drug costs. With many minds working on the problem, the range of responses was richly variegated. Some firms and later many states sought ways to get bulk purchasing discounts. Other firms and payers decided instead to pass on some of their costs to consumers through increased co-payments. Often the co-payments were directed at trying to drive the consumer toward choosing a generic alternative to a brand-name drug. But consumers often have little choice about what drug they select, because their physician makes the choice when she writes the prescription.

Managed care plans came up with one answer: adopt a policy that all prescriptions must automatically be filled by a generic when one is available, unless the physician notes on the prescription that it may be filled only as written. To counter the influences of drug company representatives—who are typically allowed to walk past the receptionist and into the physicians' offices, where they talk up their newest and most expensive drugs with physicians and staff—some hospitals either adopted policies barring these so-called drug detailers from direct contact with physicians or hired and trained their own "counter detailers," whose job it was to tell physicians and their staffs about generic or cheaper brand options. (It is worth noting that drug company representatives are allowed into physicians' back office because many physicians and staff welcome the information provided by these friendly, knowledgeable, quick-to-pick-up-the-lunch-tab reps.)

Many self-insured firms took a combined approach. They contracted with

PBMs to select and manage the drugs their plans would cover, those they would not cover, and those they would cover only with prior authorization by a managed care authority before a physician could write the prescription. Others took a surer, simpler approach to controlling their drug costs: they stopped, or didn't start, offering health insurance to their employees.

Some individuals—especially older individuals with no drug insurance coverage—discovered they could buy drugs from abroad at greatly discounted prices (unlike in the United States, prices are set by government in most countries). Many seniors began traveling to Canada to buy drugs. Later, Internet-based Canadian pharmacies filled millions of prescriptions for U.S. consumers, and still later a few enterprising firms opened U.S. outlets of Canadian pharmacies and helped consumers buy abroad. Many of these firms were quickly closed by the FDA or by other agencies' actions at the FDA's instigation.

State Medicaid programs adopted all of these strategies and a few others, including limiting the number of brand-name prescriptions they would pay for on behalf of a patient in a given month. This wide variety of strategies had taken many years to develop. Interestingly, the pace of solution development seemed to follow closely the increasing awareness of the problem, as more and more consumers and employers grew irritated by high drug prices and sought solutions.

By the mid-1990s, the problem had reached a tipping point and solutions were broadly sought. The range of options being used to battle rising drug prices diffused quickly across the country, throughout the public and the private sector, demonstrating the importance of state innovation and diffusion (see chapter 5).

Congress got back into the issue in the early 1990s when Medicaid programs sought federal legislation to compel the companies that sold them drugs to give bulk purchasing discounts. Congress included this requirement in the 1990 Omnibus Reconciliation Act. It mandated that firms selling to Medicaid programs must sell at the lowest price at which that drug was sold in the United States. By some calculations, this resulted in rebates equal to about 20 percent of manufacturers' average prices (CBO 2005b).

Congress acted again two years later in the Veterans Health Care Act to demand even larger discounts for its own federal purchasers: the Department of Veterans Affairs, the Defense Department, the U.S. Coast Guard, and the Public Health Service, including federal health clinics around the country. As the piecemeal, ad hoc, and widely differing solutions spread throughout the 1980s and 1990s, they eased some aspects of the problem of high costs and restricted access, but they sometimes caused new problems or shifted the burden to others. Restriction on coverage of specific brands caused problems for some Medicaid recipients doing well on an old drug but unable to tolerate its cheaper equivalent. Loss of employer health insurance coverage swelled the ranks of the uninsured. Purchase of prescription drugs in Canada and import for consumption in the United States by private individuals continued to be illegal, eventually leading to periodic law enforcement crackdowns and pharmaceutical manufacturers' reprisals against the offending Canadian vendors. Customs agents had to decide whether to look the other way when they found drugs intended for personal use in travelers' luggage. Members of Congress, especially those whose constituents lived in states near Canada or Mexico, had to decide how they were going to respond to growing hordes of silver-haired fugitives boldly flouting U.S. laws. Several legislators decided to join them, sometimes renting a bus to take groups of constituents across the border for drug-buying runs.

Welfare advocates were troubled by the state-to-state inequity in Medicaid coverage of prescription drugs. Maryland and Massachusetts, for example, were generous, while West Virginia baldly restricted coverage.

2000: ELECTION YEAR POLITICS

Presidential candidate Al Gore seized on the prescription drug issue. His message was essentially, "If you want prescription drugs covered under Medicare and PhRMA's pricing power controlled, elect me." He proposed a comprehensive plan that would cover all 15.2 million Medicare beneficiaries. For a time, Republican candidate George W. Bush was silent on the issue. But by the first presidential debate, he had a proposal and a promise to address the prescription drug issue if elected. His plan was much more limited than Gore's. Bush would cover only about 5 percent of Medicare beneficiaries, about 600,000 people, and would spend only about $158 billion over 10 years on the plan (Thorpe 2000). Meanwhile, House Republicans, concerned that seniors might punish them for not acting on prescription drug coverage, were determined to pass something well before the November 2000 elections.

Just in time for the spring recess, Republican legislators responded to Democratic attacks that they had done nothing on prescription drugs by introducing a set of principles, with few specifics other than a determination to rely on private insurance companies to offer the plan (M. Carey 2000a). This plan, introduced by House Ways and Means Health Subcommittee chair Nancy Johnson (R-CT), would provide subsidized coverage for poor and near-poor beneficiaries, much like President Clinton's 1999 plan, with the level of coverage dropping as incomes rose above poverty. But it would provide no coverage at all between near-poor subsidies and a catastrophic, stop-loss level, above which insurance would pay all or most of additional spending. The rationale for this approach was that two-thirds of beneficiaries already had coverage, mostly from private sources or Medicaid, and covering the near poor would target those lacking coverage.

Congressional Democrats were unimpressed, saying the plan neglected the middle class. They also objected to the basic notion of giving up on universality (M. Carey 2000d). Two weeks later, House Democrats announced their own plan, essentially mirroring President Clinton's 1999 plan: it would pay half the costs between near-poor level and a stop-loss level to be specified, but perhaps as low as $3,000. But the 50 percent cost sharing would again be phased in—that is, to keep public spending down, the full 50 percent subsidy would not be available for several years (M. Carey 2000a).

Meanwhile the Senate worked on other plans, including a revised version of the earlier Breaux-Thomas bill, now becoming the Beaux-Frist plan. Bill Frist (R-TN), the only physician in the Senate, was viewed as an expert on health care issues. (Before much longer he would, unexpectedly, become Senate majority leader when the current majority leader, Trent Lott (R-MS), was forced to resign his leadership after making racially insensitive remarks.) The Breaux-Frist plan emphasized managed care, coverage of poor and near-poor beneficiaries, and catastrophic coverage above some stop-loss level. Subsidies would range from full coverage for poor beneficiaries to one-quarter of high-income earners' costs (M. Carey 2000b). It was essentially the National Bipartisan Commission on the Future of Medicare plan.

Given the House and Senate differences, fundamental differences in approaches between the parties, and the election-year atmosphere, few observers expected any bill to pass. But House Speaker Dennis Hastert (R-IL) was determined not to have his party go back home to campaign without a response to the Democratic claim that House Republicans were ignoring older Americans' need for drug coverage. Emphasizing party loyalty (and with zero likelihood of passage in the Senate), on June 28, 2000, the House voted 217-214 to pass HR 4680, the House prescription drug bill. Democrats did their best to defeat it, meeting in "war council" in a "war room" to pump themselves up for battle by watching scenes from the popular movies *Gladiator* and *Apollo 13*. From the latter film they watched the clip in which the key sentiment delivered is "failure is not an option" (M. Carey 2000c).

107TH CONGRESS

First Session, 2001

The new president, George W. Bush, began his first year in office with a bang—or, at least, economists thought the economy started that way. Most projected a continued growth of the GDP at 2.4 percent. (Not until November would they declare that a recession had actually started back in March, only to be made significantly worse by the events of September 11.) Given the rosy outlook as the year began, much seemed affordable.

The GOP, which now controlled both houses of Congress and the presidency, spoke of a new approach to health care that would rely on the marketplace (M. Carey 2001c). Yet their new president gave Republicans little direction in his 2001 state of the union address on January 20. "We will reform Social Security and Medicare," the president said, "sparing our children from struggles we have the power to prevent. And we will reduce taxes, to recover the momentum of our economy and reward the effort and enterprise of working Americans" (*CQ Weekly* 2001).

Some commentators on the 2000 election would speculate that Bush's decision to put forward a prescription drug proposal to counter the one offered by his opponent, as well as his suggested education reforms and other domestic improvements, had helped him characterize himself as a "compassionate conservative" and might have helped him win votes in key swing-vote states (T. Patterson 2003). Polls showed widespread support for such a drug program aimed at seniors. A January 25, 2001, poll released by the Kaiser Family Foundation, a strong promoter of Medicare prescription drug coverage, showed that 56 percent of Americans supported such an expansion of Medicare, with support by two-thirds of self-identifying Democrats and 43 percent of self-identifying Republicans (*Congressional Quarterly Almanac* 2001).

On January 29, 2001, the president quietly released his initial drug plan, an interim approach intended as a stop-gap measure while awaiting congressional action on a broader plan. His proposal was called an Immediate Helping Hand. It would give $48 million in block-grant money to states to provide free drugs to low-income seniors, 50 percent subsidies for near-poor seniors, and catastrophic coverage for drug expenses above $6,000 by any beneficiary. Critics charged that the president's helping hand would be extended to only about 5 percent of those eligible for Medicare (*Congressional Quarterly Almanac* 2001). According to Consumers Union (2001), the measure would not curb prices or cover most beneficiaries. Nearly full coverage would end at the eligibility standard of 135 percent of poverty (below which beneficiaries would pay no premiums and only small co-payments). From 135 to 175 percent of poverty, beneficiaries would pay 50 percent of premiums plus co-payments. Above 175 percent of poverty there would be no coverage. The president's plan, the group noted, would rely on states for administration, a problem because the states had enjoyed only limited success with their own programs in reaching many Medicare-eligible seniors, and this program was more complex. Introduction of the plan with little more than a press release, no public fanfare, and few details was taken to mean that the president was leaving to Congress the task of writing a drug bill. Few took this particular proposal seriously (M. Carey 2001b).

On July 12, 2001, at a Rose Garden ceremony, the president tried again to fend off critics and send a signal that he was moving forward on prescription drugs, although in fact he was waiting for Congress to get on with the task of designing a drug plan while he was principally occupied with other issues (M. Carey 2001a). Flanked by representatives from several PBMs, whose business is to buy drugs in bulk for various health plans and manage their drug coverage, the president announced that these and other firms would sponsor private drug discount cards on behalf of the Medicare program. The cards would be used to obtain volume discounts at pharmacies. Discounts of 20 percent were anticipated. The cards would cost beneficiaries $25.

But the AARP and several other organizations already offered such cards, some of them claiming larger discounts than the government was expecting, and some of them free. Democrats charged that the idea was of little value. But the president announced that he had been advised that the plan could be adopted on his own authority and would not require congressional approval. The National Association of Chain Drug Stores saw it differently. They feared that the savings would come from store profits and would do nothing to arrest manufacturers' price increases. The association sued in federal court to stop the program, charging that the president had exceeded his authority, essentially altering the Medicare program by introducing a new benefit not enacted by Congress. Two months later, a federal judge agreed with the association's argument and ordered the program halted.

Two other drug coverage plans were also competing for attention. One was the plan that the House had passed in 2000, now sponsored by Ways and Means Committee chair Bill Thomas, which was similar to the Breaux-Frist plan but would cover only costs above a catastrophic level. The leading Democratic plan was offered by Sen. Bob Graham (D-FL) on July 13, 2001, with nine cosponsors, as an amendment to an appropriations bill. It would pay half of drug costs up to $3,500, after an annual deductible of $250. The Democrats were forced to tack their drug bills onto various other bills in order to get them considered by the Republican-controlled Congress.

The CBO put a damper on everything with its budget pencil. The CBO director Dan Crippen, testifying on March 22, 2001, before the Senate Finance Committee, said that any drug plan would be enormously expensive. Coverage for all enrollees could cost $1.5 trillion over the coming decade. Covering even half their costs over that period would cost $728 billion. And covering everything above $1,000 per beneficiary would cost $1.1 trillion.

Senate Finance Committee chair Charles Grassley (R-IA) quickly noted the implications for drafting of the drug plan: "In light of the enormity of the potential costs of prescription drug coverage and Medicare's worsening financial condition, we must be fiscally responsible in adding any new benefits" (*Congressional Quarterly Almanac* 2001, 12-8). (He did not mention the looming budget deficit or the president's proposed tax cut, though others did.)

Second Session, 2002

Much of the health debate in 2002 was focused on providers' demands for givebacks of the phased-in cuts coming pell-mell, year upon year, as provisions of the 1997 BBA kicked in. With the Senate controlled by Democrats, following loss of the Republican majority when Sen. James Jeffords of Vermont switched to independent, there was little chance it would pass the House Medicare prescription drug bill. But neither party wanted to go into the November 2002 elections without responding to the providers who were complaining that hospitals and physicians would be forced to leave Medicare if they did not get relief. Knowing that provider-relief questions would come up when members went home for the Memorial Day recess, the House Ways and Means Committee circulated a summary of their giveback proposal: $1.6 million for nursing homes; rollback of a planned 15 percent cut in home health payments; $3.5 billion to Medicare+Choice managed care firms; 2 percent increase for physicians every year for three years, totaling $20 billion; and $9 billion for hospitals over the coming decade. These givebacks would be important lures for providers' support should a Republican prescription drug and Medicare reform bill eventually emerge. The Ways and Means Committee summary assured members that the provider givebacks, totaling $30 million, would fit within the House version of the budget resolution target for Medicare reform for 2003, now set at $350 billion.

Republicans also wanted to show the electorate that they were responding to the demand for coverage of prescription drugs. "It is more important to communicate that you have a plan than it is to communicate what is in the plan," a GOP pollster told the party (M. Carey 2002a). By adding $30 billion in provider givebacks to their prescription drug bill, HR 4954, Republicans hoped to make it easier to win sufficient support for the bill to get it through the House, even if it was sure to be ignored by the Senate. Reforms in the bill were intended to make Medicare a financially viable program that could serve the baby boomers, but also to make sure it did not break the bank. This could be assured by keeping its costs within $350 billion over 10 years. This budget target thus became a key design parameter for the bill. To stay within it, the plan simply could not afford to provide government coverage to all of the two-thirds of Medicare beneficiaries who already had some sort of coverage, many of them through a retiree health plan. A gap in coverage would accomplish this goal, meaning that beneficiaries would have to pay drug costs between $2,000 and $3,800, a burden for beneficiaries, yet a more generous plan than the version passed by the House in 2000. The bill would also rely on private providers to deliver the drug benefit and would pay them quite generously. Other provisions revealed later would also be attractive to one or more interest groups.

Mary Agnes Carey (2002a) of *CQ Weekly* observed, "The decision to include billions in additional funding for Medicare providers has brought in support from well-known medical groups, such as the American Medical Association and the American Hospital Association. But it also has subjected the bill-drafting process to immense pressure from lobbyists, who sent out scores of e-mail and advocacy letters urging members to include more money or a specific policy change to benefit their group." "It appears as though you are all concerned about subsidizing . . . the insurance companies rather than subsidizing the cost of prescription drugs," said Charles B. Rangel (D-NY), ranking member of the House Ways and Means Committee (M. Carey 2002a).

Democrats offered a substitute plan during a Ways and Means debate on June 18. Their bill would be much more generous to seniors, offering universal, nearly comprehensive coverage (80 percent of costs over a yearly deductible of $250, then 50 percent of costs above $1,000). But it would cost $800 billion. It lost that day in the Ways and Means Committee by a party-line vote of 16-23, and on June 20 in the House Commerce Committee by a 24-30 vote, also along party lines. Democrats ridiculed Commerce Committee members for adjourning early to attend a drug maker–sponsored party during the markup process (M. Carey 2002a).

On June 29, 2002, the House Republican drug bill, HR 4954, passed the

House on a vote of 221-208. Eight members of each party broke partisan ranks. Several features of the bill, which was a revised version of the House-passed bill of 2000, reflected Republican convictions that private market forces were needed to keep prices down, including private plan administration with considerable flexibility to tweak coverage and premiums; extra payments to managed care firms, as well as the other provider givebacks negotiated earlier; a major drug coverage gap, now excluding from coverage all costs between $2,000 and $3,700; benefits varying from insurer to insurer and region to region; and varying beneficiary premiums. Democrats, angry at the nature of the bill, were not allowed by the majority to offer their own, much more expensive bill. Their party's revenge would come in the Senate, where majority leader Tom Daschle (D-SD) said the House bill would not be taken up and that it was a "terrible bill." He aimed to consider the Democratic bill offered by Senator Graham and others, estimated to cost between $400 billion and $500 billion over several years (M. Carey 2002b). But Daschle predicted that if the bill was not taken up by September, it was not likely to emerge during this election year. His fears proved correct.

GETTING SERIOUS: THE BUDGET RESOLUTION IN 2003

With both Houses controlled by Republicans following the election, the drug bill debate for the new 108th Congress in 2003 began with the annual task of formulating a budget and passing a budget resolution that would provide spending targets for the ensuing session. President Bush started the process with his 2003 state of the union address in which he called for Medicare reform, including improved access for seniors to prescription drug coverage. He followed up with his proposed budget for the coming fiscal year, 2004, due to start in September 2003 and continue through the following August. The president's priorities for the 108th Congress would be expensive: $400 billion for defense, up 2 percent over the prior year; and $38 billion for homeland security. But the biggest new spending would be an additional round of tax cuts, extending those made in 2001 that were due to expire. The price tag: $758 billion in the coming fiscal year; $1.57 trillion over 10 years. To pay for these tax cuts, nondefense spending ranging from international affairs to farm subsidies, operations of the Justice and other departments, the District of Columbia's annual federal subsidy, and many other aspects of domestic government were cut by 2 percent. The expected cost of the drug benefit was now set at $400 billion.

With assumptions of a faster growth in the economy and accompanying increases in revenues despite tax cuts, the Bush budget estimated that revenues would total $1.922 trillion in the 2004 fiscal year, expenditures would total a bit over $2.229 trillion, and the deficit would reach $307.4 billion.

Budget hawks objected to the larger deficit, but because revenues were not as high as expected, by the time Congress finished with its budget resolution, modifying the Bush proposal, the tax cuts themselves were reduced, the Medicare drug bill reserve was $400 billion over 10 years, and the deficit was estimated at $385 billion for fiscal year 2004. Looked at over the period 2004 through 2013, these shortfalls in annual budget estimates would reach $1.4 trillion, even after being offset by the Social Security surplus being held in anticipation of the baby boom beginning to retire in 2010. The *Congressional Quarterly Almanac* (2003) reported that if Social Security's temporary (earmarked) surplus were not counted as offsetting the deficit, federal spending would exceed federal revenues by $4 trillion during the next 10 years, and the public debt, estimated at $7.4 trillion in 2004, would be approaching $10 trillion by the end of 2013.

Given these impressive shortfall numbers, Republicans were convinced that they needed to hold new prescription drug costs to their $400 billion target for the decade and, indeed, would agree to that amount only if some of it were offset by close to $28 billion in Medicare cuts from other parts of the program. Some Democrats thought such big spenders could afford to be more generous with drug coverage. They proposed setting the drug bill budget target at $528 billion, funded by sharp reductions in the size of the president's tax cuts. Fiscally conservative Blue Dog Democrats were willing to live with the $400 billion drug bill cap but wanted much smaller tax-cut targets to hold deficits down. Both parties wanted yet more spending for physicians, home health agencies, and other health care vendors to ease some of the cuts still to be implemented as a result of the huge series of annual reductions set into law in the 1997 BBA. Indeed, Republicans particularly wanted those increases as a way of garnering physicians' support for their drug bill and potentially pressuring some AMA-supported members of Congress to move toward the Republican bill, as they had in the last Congress.

Both sets of Democratic proposals were spurned by the Republican House majority, and the House ultimately passed the budget resolution 215-212 on March 21, after a day of what the *Congressional Quarterly Almanac* (2003, 5-10) called "arm twisting" and phone calls from the vice president to individual lawmakers. The Senate also passed the resolution, but only after what House members charged was a broken promise. House conservatives wanted a large tax cut—ideally, as large as the president had proposed—while Senate moderates were determined not to let the tax cut exceed $350 billion. House leaders told their members to hold their noses and vote for a smaller cut, with the expectation that the conference committee would set the cuts higher than the Senate was proposing. And the conference committee did—sort of. The conferees set the tax-cut targets at $550 billion, but only conditionally: if the Senate did not raise a point of order, the higher number would go through. So the conference bill in a sense had two tax-cut targets: $550 billion (or higher) and $350 billion if the Senate objected to higher numbers. But as soon as the conference report passed the House with that conditional language, the Senate's Finance Committee chair Charles Grassley announced that he and the other Republican Senate leaders had agreed that the tax cut would be kept at $350 billion. House conservatives were furious. They would exact their revenge later.

Although the budget resolution is not signed by the president, because it is not a law, and although it is seldom actually honored in the final spending decisions made as Congress passes its reconciliation act at the end of a session, the numbers in the resolution were of vital importance to both the would-be tax cutters and the would-be Medicare drug bill spenders, for one particular reason: the amounts in the budget resolution are included in the reconciliation bill. And reconciliation bills cannot be filibustered. Thus, lowering the target for the Bush tax cuts below his request was an important decision made as a budget target long before the statutory language was written. With that decision, the institution's rules would, as rational choice theorists have suggested, constrain and in part determine the legislative outcome. Sticking to budget resolution targets would shield the majority from filibusters. This was the House plan.

However, Senate Republicans would not agree to passing such an important bill as part of reconciliation. The $400 billion reserve provision was thus agreed to, but the legislation spelling out the provisions of the new drug program would be kept separate from the budget resolution (*Congressional Quarterly Almanac* 2003). Thus the drug bill, when it eventually came to a vote in the Senate, could be filibustered unless its supporters could cut off debate with a 60-vote majority. If it passed, it would be the first major health initiative in years that was not enacted as a provision in a reconciliation bill.

The budget resolution and its accompanying projections of huge budget deficits and rapidly growing debt were also critical to the drug bill for another reason: anyone looking at the projected budget shortfalls could see that for the drug bill, it was now or never. The $400 billion earmarked for the program over 10 years would guarantee a very solid starting point on which Democrats might someday be able to build.

In this sense, the budget resolution defined the terms of the coming

Medicare drug bill debate. Despite vast ideological differences, the two parties would have to find ways to compromise on a bill costing an estimated $400 billion, or they could probably expect Medicare prescription drug coverage to go the way of the patients' bill of rights—meeting its death on the floor of one house or the other or in conference committee, never to be heard of again.

Despite constraints imposed by the budget limit, both parties brought to the legislation certain goals they wanted to achieve. Neither party wanted to meet the voters in the next election with no drug coverage to offer. Both knew that if they waited until the second year of the 108th Congress, passage would become harder, probably impossible, because 2004 was an election year. But Republicans also had a broader agenda. Many, including the president, wanted the new drug program to serve as a vehicle to reform Medicare, to make it means-tested and competitive, to limit the future obligations of the federal government, and to give the private sector a broader role in the program's administration. Republicans had wanted these same program changes since Medicare was debated and passed in 1965.

With control of both houses and the White House, with the drug bill on the agenda, and with Medicare falling short of funds for the long term, Republicans were perhaps in a position to get what they wanted. Democrats had successfully fought these very same changes in 1965, winning by just one vote in the House Ways and Means Committee before passing what became the non-means-tested Medicare program. Now the means-testing issue was back on the reform agenda. Most Democrats wanted no part of the Republicans' means-testing plans. "Medicare is not a welfare program. If these benefits are based on income, you're compromising the philosophy of Medicare," said Benjamin L. Cardin (D-MD) (*Congressional Quarterly Almanac* 2003, 11-4).

Democrats were more receptive to employing private plans to administer the new drug program, much as they had acquiesced to involving private insurance plans as bill payers in the original Medicare plan to neutralize industry opposition to Medicare. But they wanted these new plans to provide uniform benefits.

The White House also wanted to push beneficiaries into managed care as a vehicle for restructuring the entire Medicare program into a "premium support" plan. Managed care firms would be paid a premium to cover a minimal set of benefits. Individuals who wanted better coverage would have to pay more. But rural members of Congress—in particular Senate Finance Committee chair Charles Grassley of Iowa—feared that rural constituents would be short-changed by the lack of private managed care plans in rural areas. These legislators insisted that benefits be available either through fee-for-service options or through fallback plans if an area had insufficient managed care plans. By March 1, the White House had backed down (Adams 2003b).

Two other sticking points were drug prices and what to do about the fact that many retirees already had drug coverage from their employers, and no one wanted to see it lost. Both wanted to use some funds to give employers tax incentives to keep up existing coverage. To bring down prices, Democrats, and many Republicans, were eager to endorse drug reimportation from Canada or elsewhere. (*Reimportation* refers to the fact that many drugs sold in Canada are made in the United States, exported to Canada, and sold at regulated prices lower than those for the same drugs sold in the United States. Americans then "reimport" the drugs—against FDA rules—back into the United States to save money.)

SENATE ACTION 2003

Finance Committee Action

A major boost to the prescription drug bill came in the Senate Finance Committee when long-time health policy entrepreneur Edward Kennedy (D-MA) announced that he would support the bill. "This is not the bill we would have written, but to finally get something moving is a major step forward," Kennedy said (*Congressional Quarterly Almanac* 2003, 11-5). He was confident that with this modest start, Democrats in future Congresses would be able to build a more comprehensive program. Kennedy had mellowed from the days in the 1970s when he had opposed his own party's president, who wanted to pass a minimalist national health insurance program that would have granted catastrophic coverage to all Americans.

Conservative Republican Jon Kyl of Arizona, probably encouraged by the success of the Arizona Health Care Cost Containment System, operating since the 1980s via competitively selected Medicaid plans in each county, offered an amendment requiring competition in Medicare plan selection with no link to fee-for-service payments. Committee chair Grassley persuaded him to withdraw this amendment, with the promise that he would cooperate with Kyl on the bill before it passed the Senate. Don Nickles (R-OK) tried to reduce the cost of the bill. This attempt failed. Olympia J. Snowe (R-ME) proposed an amendment to adjust drug premiums to regional use rates, an outcome that would favor her rural constituents. It passed.

Minority leader Tom Daschle offered an amendment limiting Medicare premium increases to no more than 5 percent annually. It lost 7-14. John D. Rockefeller (D-WV), who strongly opposed the gap in coverage in the Republican bill, offered an amendment aimed at making the drug plan a government-run program. It, too, lost 7-14.

On June 12, 2003, the Senate Finance Committee voted 16-5 to approve the bill and send it to the Senate floor.

Senate Floor Debate on the Senate Bill

Democrats offered 23 amendments during the floor debate, trying to expand the bill and make its benefits more generous, especially by eliminating the donut hole. None was adopted. Among those rejected was a proposal by Illinois Democrat Richard Durbin that would have given the Medicare program the authority to use its nationwide clout to negotiate lower drug prices from the drug companies. Senator Rockefeller sought to minimize the gap for retirees by counting toward their out-of-pocket payments the contributions of their employer health plans. That amendment, too, was rejected, as was one by Bob Graham that would have suspended Medicare drug premiums once a beneficiary's spending had reached the donut hole amount.

Where the two parties did compromise was over a joint proposal by Grassley and Max Baucus (D-MT) for spending $12 billion of the $400 billion spending cap that had not already been allocated. They agreed on a five-year demonstration project in which traditional Medicare would compete with private plans, on a separate decision to grant major subsidies to managed care plans to help them enroll a larger share of the Medicare population, and on extra preventive and chronic care services for traditional Medicare beneficiaries (*Congressional Quarterly Almanac* 2003).

An important Democratic-sponsored amendment to permit reimportation of drugs from Canada was adopted, but it was amended by a Republican provision requiring HHS to certify that the imported drugs would not pose a health hazard. This kind of provision had killed implementation of earlier laws permitting reimportation, because they were not accompanied by the new agency staff positions, authority, and funding required to implement them.

A bipartisan amendment proposing that wealthy seniors pay higher premiums nearly stopped the bill in its tracks. To Senator Kennedy and others, introducing means testing into Medicare would be far worse than not changing it at all. He threatened to personally prevent the bill's passage if the amendment were not defeated. When a roll-call vote to table the amendment failed by a substantial margin of 38-59 (*Congressional Quarterly Almanac* 2003), Democrats called for a voice vote and succeeded in defeating the provision by shouting "no" so loudly that they drowned out Republicans. Since presiding officers sometimes exercise discretion in interpreting who wins on voice votes, and since presiding officers invariably are members of the majority party, it can be assumed that Republican Senate leaders must have decided that this issue was not worth a major roll-call vote and battle.

The full bill passed the Senate floor on June 27, 2003, by a vote of 76-21.

EYES TURN TO THE HOUSE

While the Senate debated its bill, the House wrote its own version, moving it through markup sessions in two committees in mid-June. Ways and Means Republicans prized a provision that offered higher subsidies to managed care plans in hopes of attracting them to serve rural areas. Their bill included no fallback provision to ensure that a substitute source of drug coverage was available if managed care plans didn't emerge or if, as in the past, they left the market when they were disappointed with their profits. Republicans also pushed a provision to require broad competition between Medicare and private plans beginning in 2010. Much of the debate centered on these issues of the role of the federal government in managing the new benefit, with Republican members strongly favoring a reduced public role and an expanded role for private insurance plans. Democratic Ways and Means members called the bill a device to force seniors into private plans, stripping Medicare of its government-plan status.

The Democrats, led by former Ways and Means Health Subcommittee chair Pete Stark (D-CA), now ranking minority member on the full committee, offered a substitute that would completely replace the GOP-written committee bill. His plan would set premiums at $25 per month, charge seniors a $1,000 annual deductible, and limit their out-of-pocket drug spending for co-payments to $2,000 per year, after which Medicare would take over. His substitute was estimated to cost twice as much as the Republican version. It lost in a committee vote by 14-26 (*Congressional Quarterly Almanac* 2003). Other Democratic proposals met a similar fate. All 39 members present were happy to support another amendment, however. This one, offered by a Midwestern Republican, tacked onto the drug bill a hike in pay for Medicare physicians working in underserved areas.

Energy and Commerce Committee Action

Under the chairmanship of Louisiana Republican Billy Tauzin, the House Energy and Commerce Committee spent three days on its markup of the Ways and Means bill, ending on June 19, 2003, with a 29-20 approving vote (*Congressional Quarterly Almanac* 2003). Tauzin was quick to gavel quiet Democratic charges that the bill was a gift to the drug companies. Only weeks later, with the bill passed, Tauzin resigned from his position as committee chair, and he later became CEO of PhRMA, the drug manufacturers' lobby group. Many votes in the committee were party-line, especially Democrats' attempts to strike requirements for competition between Medicare and private plans and their attempts to replace the GOP vision of several or many regional private plans offering different drug benefits with one nationwide Medicare plan offering the same benefits to all beneficiaries. Also defeated were Democratic proposals to eliminate means testing altogether and to eliminate asset considerations from means testing. The Republican plan required that those qualifying for premium subsidies must have few assets as well as low income. As in the Ways and Means Committee, a Democratic proposal to count toward a beneficiary's out-of-pocket costs the contributions of an employer health insurance plan was offered and defeated.

House Floor Vote on the House Bill

The Republican leadership began counting noses, meeting with potential "no-voters" in the party and offering sweeteners as the last week of June 2003 unfolded. On Thursday, June 26, HHS secretary Tommy D. Thompson and Vice President Dick Cheney took up stations in the Capitol and were making the case for the GOP prescription drug bill. One recalcitrant legislator was offered a meeting with the president but turned it down. Another said no, while acknowledging that he could have demanded any number of pork projects for his Minnesota district (J. Allen and Graham-Silverman 2003). Majority leader Tom DeLay (R-TX) cornered his party's opposition members in groups of one, two, and three. Leaders as well as rank-and-file supporters buttonholed opponents. This was, after all, the party that in recent Congresses had delivered an all-time high party allegiance (see chapter 1).

Democrats again tried to replace the $400 billion Republican drug bill with their own $800 billion version, capping out-of-pocket spending at $2,000, no donut hole, and 80 percent coverage between a $100 annual deductible and the $2,000 maximum personal spending limit. When that proposal failed, Democrats from rural areas agreed to support the Republican bill because it contained substantial spending—$28 billion—for providers in their areas. But even with this Democratic support, the bill teetered on the verge of defeat. House leaders, Republican supporters, and the vice president all cornered reluctant Republicans and hammered at them on switching their votes. A single copy of the nearly 700-page bill, unread by most legislators, was being passed around among those being buttonholed, with language changes penciled into the margins as they were agreed to in exchange for support. "I got a little bit of the language in the bill that I wanted," one first-year legislator said, still nervous about the overall bill, but feeling good enough about it to switch his vote to yes (J. Allen and Graham-Silverman 2003, 1614). Another opponent agreed to switch his vote to "present" to offset the missing yes vote of Appropriations Committee chair C. W. Bill Young (R-FL), who was out of town.

As the House clock ticked past 2:30 a.m., nearly an hour after the final vote on the bill had begun, House leaders still did not have the votes they needed to gain a one-vote margin and pass the bill (J. Allen and Graham-Silverman 2003). Half an hour later, two Midwestern holdouts switched their votes: one on the promise of a vote on a bill to permit reimports from Canada, the other perhaps in support of a last-minute expansion of health savings account provisions, to permit charging the costs of uncovered drugs against these tax-free savings accounts. The bill passed in the wee hours of Friday, June 27, 2003, with a vote of 216-215 and one "present," after setting a record for the time a vote was held open.

CONFERENCE COMMITTEE 2003

The two bills sent to the conference committee had a number of similarities but differed in important ways that would make compromise difficult. Both bills provided poor beneficiaries with subsidies, and near-poor beneficiaries would pay premiums on a sliding scale tied to income, though the two houses differed slightly in how they defined "near poor." Both bills required nonpoor beneficiaries to pay a deductible of $250 to $300 before coverage started and monthly premiums of between $35 and $40, and both left a gap in coverage before stop-loss catastrophic coverage started. Both required about $3,600 or $3,700 of out-of-pocket spending before the stop-loss cap was reached, but the House version would cover below-average to average spending ($2,000 per year) rather generously (80 percent of spending), while the Senate would cover a much broader range of spending (up to $4,500) but only half of those costs. After the stop-loss level, the Senate version still required beneficiary co-payments of 5 percent of spending; the House version covered all costs above the stop-loss level.

Reflecting the Grassley-Baucus concern with managed care penetration into rural areas, the Senate version of the bill required a government-run plan to be offered if there were fewer than two managed care firms competing in an area. The House offered no government-run option. The House bill required head-to-head price competition, starting in 2010, between Medicare fee-for-service plans and managed care plans, while the Senate had approved only competition among private plans, setting Medicare fee-for-service prices as their ceiling payments. The House had tucked in a provision expanding health savings accounts, while the Senate had not needed this provision to win votes (CQ Weekly 2003a).

Democrats were appointed to the conference committee but were summarily cut out of the negotiations, except for two supporters of the bill. These were ranking minority Senate Finance Committee member Max Baucus, who had helped draft the Senate bill, and John Breaux, who with Bill Thomas had co-chaired the earlier National Bipartisan Commission on the Future of Medicare, which had proposed pharmacy coverage similar to that in the current bills. Nonetheless, hammering out a conference report took many months and came to the brink of disaster at several points.

Working through the many issues that differed between House and Senate versions of the bill would require co-chairs Grassley and Thomas to be prepared to give in or stick to their guns on points that would gain or lose important support in one or the other house. Both houses would have to feel that they had walked away with important victories. Thomas and Grassley gave it a try, but they failed. They could work through the easy stuff, but when it came to the hard issues where one or the other co-chair knew he would lose supporters in his house, they not only couldn't come to agreement—they couldn't even talk to each other. Thomas in particular was unyielding, perhaps because he had by now lived with versions of this bill for more than three years since he had co-chaired the national commission charged with restructuring Medicare with prescription drug coverage as the sweetener.

Weeks dragged into months without resolution. Acrimony among negotiators rose—especially between the co-chairs. By November 27, meetings had come to a complete halt. Thomas, according to later news reports, "stormed out of the Capitol," cancelled further negotiations, and announced that he had booked himself on a 6 p.m. flight home to California. Three and a half hours later he was back at the negotiating table. Reached on his cell phone by both Speaker Dennis Hastert and House majority leader Tom DeLay, Thomas was bluntly told that failure to pass the Medicare bill was simply too high a price to pay (A. Goldstein 2003). Besides the implication that he could be replaced, perhaps he was also reminded that he had persuaded Hastert and other House leaders to make him the House Ways and Means chair because he was a man who could pass legislation, despite his reputation for a prickly personality. Thomas was also simply preempted on some points of the negotiations. House Speaker Hastert and Senate majority leader Frist personally took over some aspects of the negotiations, working together to negotiate sensitive points with selected conferees and influential interest-group representatives. When they finished, the conference report that emerged shared provisions of each of the two versions.

Conference Report on the House Floor

To gain the support of some recalcitrant members of its party, the GOP leadership had to agree, in an evening meeting in the basement of the Capitol, to a change in Medicare payment policy that had taken money out of oncologists' pockets by restricting payment for cancer drugs. Oncologists' supporters wanted the money put back, and the leadership agreed. That picked up a few votes, reflecting the savvy performance of the House whip in knowing what it would take to tote up the needed votes. But still the House leaders' nose counts came up short. One leadership appeal pointed out that the basic idea of drug coverage was still a good one and was supported by the $400 billion set aside. The money would disappear if not used this year and might not be found again next year, when the House and a third of the Senate would be facing reelection and might be unwilling to push federal deficit totals even higher. But conservatives of both parties were already furious about the estimated cost of the bill, even at $400 billion, and few if any believed that the true cost would actually be kept that low. (Later events would prove them correct as cost estimates in the coming months moved closer and closer to a trillion dollars over 10 years.)

House Democrats, with few exceptions, were strongly united against the bill, making it mandatory that the president, vice president, Speaker, majority leader, whip, and committee and subcommittee chairs use every ounce of their power and persuasive zeal to demand loyalty from their partisan fellows. But the Democratic exceptions were important. California Democrat Calvin M. Dooley had reportedly told a GOP colleague that if the Republicans could muster 208 votes, he and other Democrats would give them an additional 15 votes, enough to ensure a substantial victory. Dooley, described as a moderate, was slated to retire the next year (Broder 2003).

Debate on the House floor was declared over, and voting began at 3 a.m. on November 22, many hours after the House had been called to order. But rather than the brief, 15-minute electronic interlude that usually constitutes a vote, the process was destined to drag on for a historic length of time. At 4 a.m. the leadership was still 2 votes short: 216 for the conference report, 218 against. Pressure mounted on leaders and Republican no-voters alike, with promises and threats delivered and rebuffed until nearly 6 a.m. At several points the majority leader started toward the rostrum to change his vote to no, so that the lost vote could be moved for reconsideration (reconsideration must be moved by someone who voted in the majority). But each time he did, someone would pull him aside and suggest one more way to try to move a wavering colleague. The HHS secretary Tommy D. Thompson broke precedent and roamed the House floor, making the case for the bill and trying to win over more votes. Deals offered included money for a specific hospital in Tennessee promised to Rep. Harold Ford, Jr. (D-TN), to win his vote. (When he then voted against the bill, the White House said the money would be withheld.) Doctors in Alaska got money for a specific cancer treatment, the product for which is made in Georgia, home of two Republican representatives (Pear and Janofsky 2003).

At 5 a.m., the White House legislative liaison decided it was time to call in the president again, who was just back from London and likely hadn't had time for his biological clock to reset, so he would be up even earlier than his usual rising time (Broder 2003). Though the president had already made a dozen calls the night before on his way home from the airport, he now made five or six morning calls to members on their cell phones and tried to persuade them. The crucial switches came as the clock neared 6 a.m., when a group of several no-voting Republicans met with the leadership and the White House liaison just off the House floor to discuss rumors that if the Republicans lost the vote, the Democrats would initiate a "discharge petition" (an order signed by 218 members to bring a bill directly to the floor without committee approval) to revive and pass their own earlier-defeated version of the bill (Broder 2003).

It is not clear whether the rumor had any substance, or whether the deed could be done, especially in a short time, but the rumor seemed to do the trick. Two more Republicans switched from no to yes. "We didn't know what they [the Democrats] might do, but this was a logical step for them. We couldn't get the votes we needed by promising bridges or roads. The conservatives opposed this bill on policy grounds, so we had to give them a policy reason to be for it," a GOP leadership aide told the *Washington Post* (Broder 2003) in an interview the day after the vote.

With the outcome determined, one more Democrat changed his vote to yes, giving the Republicans one more vote than needed to assure passage—2 hours and 51 minutes after voting began. Democrats howled that they had been cheated, but Speaker Hastert rejected the criticism: "They criticize me for keeping the vote open so long," he said, "but I've been working that issue for 20 years, and seniors have been waiting through three Congresses for a prescription drug benefit. So I don't think waiting three hours to get it done is too much" (Broder 2003).

Just how strong the pressure got would not be known until after the vote, when war stories of the long, nail-biting night began to seep out. The pressure had been fierce, GOP conservatives agreed, as they held out firmly against their president, their party, and their leadership, refusing to budge from their opposition to the drug bill because of its lack of strong competitive mechanisms and its high price tag (R. J. Smith 2003). One member recounted that he had been told he would face primary opposition in his next campaign if he voted against the leadership's bill. Another was told that voting against the bill would cost him his subcommittee chair. Health care industry lobbyists called many holdouts and pressured them to change their votes. But 69-year-old Nick Smith (R-MI), who hoped his son would take over his seat when he retired after the current session, topped all these stories when he reported that he had been offered "substantial financial sums" (later he said, and then denied, that the sum was $100,000) for his son's congressional campaign. If he declined, determined efforts to work against his son would come, instead of money. Nonetheless, he would not change his vote. "I told them, not very politely, to get away from me," Smith said. "Threatening your kids is beyond the pale. It caught me by surprise. It made me mad" (R. S. Smith 2003). When he later wrote about his experience in a Michigan newspaper, Democrats demanded a criminal investigation of influence pedaling and bribery. Smith recanted, attributing it all to miscommunication.

Conference Report on the Senate Floor

Now the action shifted to the Senate, where Democrats tried to stop the conference report passage. Given that the original bill had passed by 70 votes, it was an uphill struggle for the dissenters. But Senator Kennedy, who had supported the Senate bill and was crucial to its passage, was now furious about the conference report, especially the prohibition against the government's negotiating prices, the heavy reliance on insurance companies to implement the program, and the bonuses to managed care firms. "The Senate is on trial . . . Let us not reverse the historic decision our country made in 1965. Let us not turn our back on our senior citizens so that insurance companies and pharmaceutical companies can earn even higher profits," Kennedy told the Senate (Zuckman 2003).

Kennedy then called for a filibuster but was cut off by a 70-29 vote, well over the 60 votes needed to invoke cloture, stop debate, and force a vote. Kennedy's problem was that he could not hold Democrats together on his points of objection. Sen. Dianne Feinstein (D-CA) was a case in point. She countered her fellow party members' concerns on three important points. First, she supported higher premiums for beneficiaries to make them share more of the program's costs, since she was concerned that entitlement costs were already pushing out other program options. Second, she noted that employers were already dropping retiree drug coverage at the rate of 10 to 12 percent per year, suggesting that expanded public coverage would produce a better outcome even if some employers used it as an excuse to drop coverage. Finally, she argued that higher payments to HMOs to encourage higher participation rates among elderly people would be a good thing, so the rest of the country would catch up with California's high rate of HMO penetration, potentially stabilizing premiums through better cost control. Her fellow California senator Barbara Boxer, also a Democrat, did not agree, saying that the bill "begins the privatization of Medicare and in many ways its dismantling" (Lockhead 2003).

Minority leader Tom Daschle raised a point of order. The price of the drug bill, with health savings accounts and the demonstration projects on competition added by the House to win needed votes, exceeded the limits set in the budget resolution. But points of order, like filibusters, can be turned aside by a supermajority. The Senate voted 61-39 to waive all points of order (*Congressional Quarterly Almanac* 2003). With these two procedural hurdles out of the way, and the Senate, by implication, on record as supporting passage, the conference report was sure to pass the next day, November 25, 2003. And it did.

WINNERS AND LOSERS

President Bush

As he signed the MMA into law on December 8, 2003, President Bush fulfilled a major promise from his campaign. He lauded the bill as "the greatest advance in health care coverage for America's seniors since the founding of Medicare" (*Congressional Quarterly Almanac* 2003, 11-8).

Some of his preferences and demands had been ignored or rebuffed by Republican congressional leaders at several points, steps they thought necessary to win passage of the bill. The president intended the bill to be a vehicle for transforming and reforming Medicare to make consumers more aware of prices by replacing Medicare's defined benefits with a defined contributions plan. Medicare services would be provided through managed care plans. They would offer a standard government-subsidized benefits package. If middle- and upper-class beneficiaries wanted better coverage they would have to pay higher premiums to get it. Plans would compete for enrollees by making additional services available at varying prices. House conference committee co-chair Thomas supported this approach; Senate co-chair Grassley did not. Grassley was from a rural state, where few managed care plans are available to compete. Nonetheless, pushing beneficiaries into managed care might yet happen, because managed care is heavily subsidized by the new law. Thus managed care firms may be able to offer better benefits than traditional fee-for-service plans.

Another departure from the president's initial position was the decision to offer drug coverage through the national Medicare program. His early program plan had offered drugs to poor people through the state-federal Medicaid program.

But these were details. President Bush would be credited with enacting a piece of legislation that Democrats had promised for years without being able to deliver. The president's willingness to let the congressional leadership do its job and to respond to calls for help only when asked would be remembered as a major contributor to the success of the legislation.

Republican Leadership

House and Senate leaders had proven themselves able to deliver major legislation. "Hastert and Frist drove the process . . . just through sheer force," one congressional source told the *Washington Post*'s Amy Goldstein (2003). Since January, the two men had rebuffed—and in a few instances, reneged on agreements with—the White House, congressional Democrats, and even GOP lawmakers, she reported. But they had done so in the interests of accomplishing the larger goal of getting the bill passed. The victory would help strengthen congressional party leadership and give both Speaker Hastert and majority leader Frist a running start on the coming election-year legislative session by making them look like leaders who could work in tandem to get things done.

Of Senator Frist, fellow Tennessee Republican senator Lamar Alexander said, "I have tried to think of anyone else on the Republican side who could have helped the Senate accomplish as much, and I don't think there is anyone" (Brosnan 2003). Of Speaker Hastert, a veteran reporter wrote, "Mr. Hastert, an imposing former wrestling coach, was literally leaning on recalcitrant lawmakers to win their support" (Hulse 2003).

Yet critics frequently pointed out that the leaders accomplished this by running roughshod over Democrats and by violating decorum. The Brookings Institution's Thomas Mann, who has closely watched and written about Congress for his whole career, said, "If you were to judge this Congress by how it operated, the process by which it operated, and the quality of the legislative product, I would give it a D minus. This session of Congress may be remembered more for the death of regular order than for anything else" (*Milwaukee Journal Sentinel* 2003).

Republican Conservatives

Even though they ultimately voted overwhelmingly against the bill, Republican House conservatives got a few deals struck into the bill during leaders' efforts to woo some of their votes. One would bar the prescription drug benefit from becoming a new entitlement program by requiring that premiums be raised if government subsidies to Medicare's Parts B and D combined were about to exceed 40 percent of total Parts B and D spending. This would also help usher in higher premiums, would bar expansion of the program to fill the donut hole, and might even encourage additional means testing when

Congress found, very soon, that the limit would be triggered. Conservatives also got a demonstration project on competition, though a paltry one—much less than the reform to a fully competitive Medicare program that they had wanted. While the planned demonstration project was a start, some health policy experts doubted it would ever get off the ground, noting that several attempts to make Medicare competitive in the past had failed to find any managed care providers to participate (Freudenheim 2003).

Structuring the program so that only the poor and near poor have full or nearly full coverage, leaving a donut hole in the middle, and then picking up coverage again at the catastrophic-cost level of more than $5,000 meant that consumers, not the government, would still be making a market for drugs. This was essential to market-oriented conservatives and a boon to PhRMA manufacturers' pricing policies, since only in the United States are prices allowed to be set largely by the drug companies.

Yet conservatives were unhappy, having been promised a competitive Medicare program rather than just a demonstration. One conservative described himself as "apoplectic" over the level of spending in the drug bill and other major programs approved by the Bush administration. Some suggested they would carry their resentment on to other battles. Nonetheless, a leading conservative think tank assessed the level of anger as too low to cost the president conservatives' support in the next election: "People are upset about it, but they weigh it against what they consider to be Bush's leadership in Iraq and elsewhere . . . They say, 'Well, we don't like this, but it's not enough to cause us to bolt.'" (D. Milbank 2003).

Democrats

Liberals and most Democrats were unhappy with the bill, having lost a major platform plank to the Republicans and having been defeated in their efforts to make the bill more generous. But as a venerated House Speaker once said, political feasibility is getting 218 votes, and for that the majority did not need votes from House Democratic liberals. In the Senate, where so many senators represent states that are predominately rural, rural interests were so well served that getting 60 votes was not difficult, partisanship notwithstanding.

Some Democrats came over to the Republican side because specific interest groups important to their campaigns asked them to do so—including Sen. Dianne Feinstein, who supported the bill after California physicians asked her to. Other Democratic senators represented states that voted for the Republican president in the last election. They were not about to cross him on such a high-stakes issue and have him come to their state during the next election campaign and denounce them as liberal obstructionists. Party loyalty is important, but, in the end, party is but a tool for reelection. When loyalty will hurt rather than help back home, party must take a back seat to other factors.

Also hurt by party cohesion among Republicans and a lack of it among Democrats was health policy champion Sen. Ted Kennedy. His efforts on the original Senate bill turned out to be a major embarrassment for himself and his party. His initial support of the Senate version had allowed other Democrats to support it and send it to conference, where it underwent substantial change, much of it in the direction of the more conservative House bill. "Republicans controlled the House, they controlled the Senate and they controlled the presidency," he said. "And they used that power in an abusive way . . . There was just a recognition that they could ram this thing through, rather than work out the historical give-and-take of the legislative process . . . I'm not charging bad faith so much as I'm charging an abuse of power" (Von Drehle 2003). Kennedy said he would work for outright repeal of the law. But with the loss of additional Democrats in the next election, stronger Republican control of both Houses, and reelection of President Bush, that prospect seemed unlikely.

Of course, the next election took place before most major provisions of the bill had kicked in, as they would in January 2006. Most seniors did not understand the bill, complex as it was. Yet even some of the most ardent Bush critics, once they had figured out what they would get from the new law, had to give the devil his due. "It's better than what I've got now," one senior said.

Interest Groups

Long-time Washington, D.C., reporter Daniel Schorr (2003) editorialized on the bill a few days after its passage:

> Big lobbies also had spectacular success in the drafting of the Medicare bill, which has burgeoned from the original idea of helping the elderly pay for prescription drugs into a sweeping overhaul of the program. Built into the 681-page bill is $125 billion over 10 years in subsidies for the health industry and related businesses. The largest item is $86 billion to subsidize the benefits that employers already provide to their workers. There are benefits for doctors,

for hospitals, for managed health organizations. The winners of these goodies were the American Medical Association and the lobbies for the pharmaceutical industry, for business, and for HMOs and hospitals. Where, in this high-powered mix of healthcare providers, was the lobby for the consumers? That should have been the 35-million member AARP. But the AARP had other fish to fry. No longer confined to being an advocate for the elderly, the AARP is itself in the insurance business. It endorsed the now-passed administration bill, to the dismay of many of its members.

"There's a tremendous amount of money floating in this bill," said Judith Feder, Public Policy School dean at Georgetown University and a former Clinton administration health official. "While we think it's about prescription drugs, the promoters of this bill put money into every interest group: physicians, hospitals, rural providers, cancer doctors, on the drug side, the pharmaceutical and insurance industries" (Toner 2003). While *Wall Street Journal* reporters reached similar conclusions of windfalls to insurers, providers, and drug makers in the short run, their experts saw potential problems in the longer term. "Congress will start worrying about the retiring baby boomers and the rising costs of the drug benefit, and will do something about containing costs," an investment firm analyst predicted (McGinley et al. 2003).

AARP

Once the bill had finally emerged from conference committee, it faced tough tests on both house floors as interest groups, parties, and party factions assessed what they had gained and lost. Among the most important interest groups was the AARP. Surprising most experts, the deal was quickly endorsed by the AARP, a move that would be absolutely critical to getting final approval of the conference report in the two houses of Congress. Many observers would ask why this happened. Why would this most influential of interest groups support a bill that many retirees would come to see as extremely flawed, and quite likely one that AARP representatives had not even read in its final form (because it was not yet fully completed)?

Some suggested that the AARP simply did not want to see the money set aside for the drug bill spurned, fearful that it would be much harder to find a similar amount in the future. Others speculated that AARP CEO Bill Novelli would personally benefit by playing the role of power broker on this important bill, giving his organization additional clout in Washington, especially if he were perceived by Republicans as a potential ally on subsequent issues. Some accused the organization of selling out to insurance or other business interests.

Some AARP members were angry with the association's decision to support the conference report and dropped their memberships—10,000 to 15,000 immediately (*Madison Capital Times* 2003). "It's a firestorm out there. I am absolutely convinced that on this issue AARP doesn't speak for their membership," said Edward Coyle, executive director of the Alliance for Retired Americans, which represents more than 3 million retirees (Associated Press 2003). "We have some repair work to do with the Medicare legislation and members' views of it," William Novelli, AARP CEO, told a reporter (Cook 2003, 3).

Democrats accused the AARP of having a conflict of interest because it sells insurance. But interviews with reporters Stolberg and Freudenheim (2003) suggested a broader motivation. "Boomers," Novelli told the reporters, "are the future of the AARP." James Parkel, AARP president, added that "we had to change." He meant that the organization had to change the target population to which its policy choices would appeal. It had to get younger. The group had already changed its focus over the past decade from retired seniors to the aging baby boomers, most of whom were employed. Changing its name from American Association of Retired Persons to simply AARP, it sought to recruit potential members starting at age 45 and to enroll them at its newly reduced membership age of 50 and over, wanting to be no longer dominated by retirees. Indeed, 2003 marked the first time in its history that a majority of the AARP's membership was still employed rather than retired.

"In polls and focus groups, the organization learned that boomers would support an experiment with private competition in the government-run Medicare program—a contentious provision that many elderly people, AARP's traditional constituency, bitterly oppose" (Stolberg and Freudenheim 2003). The AARP's board and officers decided to throw their support behind a bill that appealed to the organization's younger membership, even at the cost of losing many older members.

Both Senate majority leader Frist and House Speaker Hastert claimed credit for wooing the AARP, and the final version of the bill may reflect some of that effort. Two provisions in areas that the organization had put as its top priorities were changed in the final weeks of negotiations after Hastert and Frist took over. The House-passed plan for competition between Medicare and private plans (crucial to House conservatives) was scaled back to only a demonstration project—with a long time delay before it would begin. And employers were given strong financial incentives to continue offering drug coverage to retirees.

With these changes, the AARP said it would support the deal. Both Hastert and especially Frist had been wooing the group's leadership for months, even years, including intense meetings with leaders of both houses and culminating in a private meeting of AARP president James Parkel with President Bush on October 29, 2003. "The AARP endorsement 'didn't happen overnight,'" said Thomas A. Scully, administrator of the agency that runs Medicare and Medicaid. "We spent a lot of time working with them over the last three years" (Broder and Goldstein 2003).

PhRMA

Drug companies were perhaps the biggest winners. They carried the day on all three major issues: defeating government price setting for drugs, stymieing reimportation, and weakening states' bargaining positions in price negotiations.

To prevent government price setting, the drug companies demanded that the CMS be prohibited from negotiating with companies over price. Instead, the new program would be administered by much smaller entities, subnational PBMs, which would compete for consumers and negotiate prices with drug companies. (The PBMs, likely to team up with insurance companies, would be happy too, facing many new business opportunities.) This was a major victory for PhRMA and eloquent testimony to the ability of lobby groups to use creative strategies to snatch victory from the jaws of defeat. At one point, PhRMA's heavy-handed tactics had become so belligerent and intolerable that even the group's Republican allies wanted nothing to do with it. Tactics had included use of a Christian church group, the Traditional Values Coalition, to send out letters actually written by a PhRMA lobbyist (VandeHei and Eilperin 2003). The letters claimed to have been motivated by "sanctity-of-life" concerns about proposed drug reimportation, which, so the letters claimed, would make the abortion pill RU-486 "as easy to obtain as aspirin." To combat the negative image engendered by these moves, PhRMA used the PBMs as a front group to achieve its own ends (Heaney 2005). This was similar to the way in which PhRMA had used the United Seniors Association, which, though claiming to speak for consumers, was running ads supporting the proposed bill and PhRMA with money provided through a more than $4 million grant from PhRMA (M. Gerber 2002). PhRMA's refurbishing of its image had started when it replaced the limos that drug company executives used to shuttle to meetings in Washington, D.C., with more modest town cars, after press attention to their mode of travel. Other strategies included ad campaigns, hiring a public relations staff, changing the name of the trade group by adding *research* (it was formerly the Pharmaceutical Manufacturers' Association), and running ads promoting the benefits of drug company research (Cusack 2003).

The new law also very effectively got the monkey of states' discount demands off PhRMA's back, through the so-called clawback provision. That little heralded section of the new law served the interests of PhRMA in particular at the expense of the states. The MMA took over drug-program management, purchasing, and delivery responsibility for all Medicare beneficiaries, including those served by state Medicaid programs. But the clawback provision demanded that states continue to pay most of the costs of drugs used by these beneficiaries, even though the federal government took over most other aspects of the program. In other words, by supporting passage of the MMA, the drug industry very quietly and very effectively stopped states' aggressive demands for price discounts—demands that had been upheld in a number of court decisions when PhRMA sued the states as its first strategy for stopping the discount demands (W. Weissert and Miller 2005).

Unable to win in the courts, PhRMA had changed venue and gotten a much more favorable outcome from Congress, which, acting under authority of the U.S. Constitution, can preempt state law. Fiscal conservatives also were pleased with the provision, since it cut down federal government costs. Only states would suffer, and perhaps some patients too, who would now be forced to accept a new set of drug rules and choices, not to mention the transaction costs of choosing a new drug vendor from among the PBMs competing for Medicare beneficiaries' business.

PhRMA had also feared that consumers and PBMs would be permitted to import drugs from abroad. Consumers were demanding it. Even the Republican rank-and-file membership in Congress supported it. A reimportation provision passed both Houses in 2000 but could not meet the standards of a provision requiring the FDA to assure the safety and efficacy of reimported drugs (Schuler 2004b). Reimportation again passed the Republican-controlled House in 2001 against the leadership's objections, but it was dropped in conference with the Senate (J. Davis 2001). Reimportation then passed again in an agricultural appropriations bill (*CQ Weekly* 2003b). But once again, what Congress gave it also took back in the same provision, requiring FDA approval of any drugs imported but giving the FDA no new authority, staffing, or funds to make safe importation possible.

Doctors

Physicians got a payment hike and are (along with hospitals) eligible for performance bonuses under a quality improvement provision included in the new law. The bill included a request for the Institute of Medicine to formulate quality standards and develop a method for paying bonuses to physicians who meet the standards.

Hospitals

Hospitals were very big winners, walking away from their lobbying efforts with a 1.5 percent reimbursement hike instead of the 4.5 percent cut they would have suffered without the new law. They also got an additional 4 percent in higher payments for every Medicare patient in exchange for voluntarily turning over quality assurance data to the CMS. But an even bigger hospital victory came in a blow dealt to general hospitals' most aggressive competitors: specialty hospitals. The roughly 100 specialty hospitals across the nation took a major hit, sought by the general hospitals. Sometimes called boutique providers, and often owned in part or in whole by physician investors, these hospitals specialize in profitable conditions such as heart disease. The MMA prevents physicians from newly investing in these facilities for 18 months while experts study the impact on patients and the Medicare program.

This ban was inserted as a single paragraph in the huge piece of legislation at the behest of American Hospital Association lobbying on behalf of the nation's community hospitals. The group's leaders focused their lobbying efforts on John Breaux, one of the two Democratic senators allowed by the GOP to participate in the conference committee's redrafting of the House and Senate bills. The AHA argued that investments in specialty hospitals represented a loophole in a Medicare law that, based on conflicts of interest, prohibits physicians from investing in clinics to which they might refer patients. Obstetricians, for example, could invest in fertility clinics and then refer their patients to them for fertility treatments. Other physicians invested in laboratories that they then used for patients' lab tests. The conflict-of-interest law, written largely by House Ways and Means Health Subcommittee ranking Democrat Pete Stark, permits physicians' investments only in "whole hospitals." That became the nub of the argument. The AHA argued that specialty hospitals are not whole hospitals.

"It's a David and Goliath story . . . And little David got creamed," a spokesperson for a chain of heart-specialty hospitals told the *Washington Post* (A. Goldstein 2003). AHA hospitals "hide behind their community mission," the spokesperson said, and that "stifles competition." Her group—which was ably represented by its own lobbyists, including former HHS secretary Tommy Thompson and Birch Bayh, former Democratic senator from Indiana—argued that specialty hospitals perform a wide range of hospital services, often including services to uninsured patients, and should qualify as whole hospitals.

But the AHA spent $100,000 on advertising and threatened to decline to endorse the Medicare drug bill if it did not get the anti-specialty-hospital provision. Nonetheless, the 18-month investment ban was only a partial victory for the AHA, which had wanted a permanent ban. Senator Breaux's efforts on the association's behalf ran into opposition from House Energy and Commerce Committee chair Billy Tauzin, also a conferee. The two Louisianans settled on the time-limited ban as a compromise between no ban and a permanent one.

States

The states were big losers. They had wanted Medicare to take over responsibility for the drug costs of Medicaid-eligible Medicare beneficiaries, letting state budgets off the hook for these "dual eligibles." But in the MMA, Congress required the states to pay most of the costs for the foreseeable future by charging them most of what they would have spent for these beneficiaries had the MMA not passed. States were very unhappy with this outcome, which on the one hand gave them little relief from prescription drug costs and on the other took away their self-determination by moving the program under federal control. Many states feared that their net costs would actually rise as more people joined Medicaid than might otherwise have done. A few states vowed to take the issue to the courts, saying Congress had no business ordering them to pay for Medicare (Pear 2005d).

CONCLUSION

Control of both houses and the presidency set the stage for a major legislative victory by the Republicans, snatching a traditional agenda item from the Democrats. But victory was by no means guaranteed. Strong congressional leadership was a key factor. Neutralizing interest-group opposition was equally important, pulled off largely by the same congressional leadership that wrangled just enough votes from its own majority party to win the day. In each case, giveaways played critical roles. Presidential cheerleading, minimal meddling in leadership decisions, and firm control over the bureaucracy were important contributing factors. The legislation itself reflects a conservative ideology; budget constraints, but only in the context of lavish deficit spending; and a very deft use and sometimes abuse of congressional rules. A key tool of leadership was the ability to rein in the most powerful committee chairs at crucial moments—this achieved by House and Senate leaders when they took over the final steps in the conference negotiations to break an impasse between the houses. Republican decisions in 1994 to permit the caucus to choose committee chairs, rather than allowing seniority rules to reign unchecked, may have been an essential precursor to bringing chairs to heel at critical times. Nonetheless, many key provisions of the law reflect chairs' preferences, especially those of Senate Finance Committee chair Charles Grassley of Iowa, who was determined to protect rural interests.

Still, party control was not perfect. Key votes were almost lost when Republican conservatives refused to support their leaders. Most House conservatives' votes simply could not be switched, necessitating deals to win over others. In most cases this meant giving in to yet another demand—of a committee chair, an interest group, or, in the wee hours of the House conference vote, individual members. Some Democrats also switched sides, giving Republicans the narrow margin they needed to offset their own defections.

It helped enormously that the problem had peaked, that it was well defined and quantified, that a presidential commission, many think tanks, and two Congresses had helped write earlier versions of the bill, and that a majority of Americans supported Medicare prescription drug coverage. But in the end, leaders ready, willing, and able to do whatever had to be done to make the bill pass were as important as any other ingredient—and probably more important. At every turn it was leadership's hand that removed roadblocks, whether these were interest-group demands or congressional rules limiting participation in conference negotiations or time allowed for voting.

Deals were clearly cut, quietly in some cases, either in the initial drafting or at the last minute, with PhRMA, the AARP, physicians, hospitals, managed care firms, employers, and others. In the case of prescription drugs, congressional leaders—and a president who let them do their job—delivered a substantially unified party and, despite a tiny majority in each House, delivered the bill for presidential signature. Democrats were left to lick their wounds and wait for their day to come, when once again they might be able to use their majority status to wield raw power over a Republican minority, blocking their initiatives, rejecting their amendments, and shunning their participation in conference committees. Picking up cues from the Republicans, they might decide to pass around a single copy of a major piece of legislation, making notes in the margins to reflect deals cut and provisions to be added or deleted.

But when the Democrats' day does come, they may have to do some soul searching to decide what their core Medicare principles now include, given the legacies left by the MMA. Means testing is now an important feature of Medicare policy that was not there before the MMA. Important Democrats supported it. Major steps toward private sector competition in Medicare created another institutional change not likely to be rolled back. Enrollment of Medicare beneficiaries in managed care is likely to accelerate and, with it, a diminution of the government role in setting fees—the quintessence of Medicare policy for two decades or more. This approach to setting prices was scrapped by the MMA. So was the uniformity of Medicare benefits across the land. Private firms will now make choices about which drugs to offer, while negotiating with drug companies for the best prices they can get.

The big unanswered question for the future of health care policy is what employers will do about retiree health plans now that drug coverage is available in Medicare. When it was not available, retirees could not be convinced that Medicare was a viable alternative to retiree coverage by employers. Will the subsidy they got in the MMA be sufficient to encourage employers to keep up their own plans? Or will they gradually drop retiree health coverage as a benefit of employment, driving more and more seniors into Medicare, aggravating its already strapped financial condition? When the majority party does switch to Democratic, as it will given sufficient time, will there be any choice but to push for more middle-class gaps in coverage, more means testing, and more premium support or defined contributions approaches to make Medicare affordable? If not, where will the money come from to meet the needs of the growing army of uninsured younger workers? Did the MMA change more than Medicare drug coverage? Did it also change the future of Medicare?

Conclusion

In the decade since the first edition of this book, the United States has seen a sea change in its health care politics and policy—particularly the institutions that form, shape, and put in place our public policies: Congress, political parties, the presidency, interest groups, the bureaucracy, and the states.

Congressional leadership is much stronger, more skilled, and very much in charge of writing the laws and designing the programs proposed by the president, even though the president has worked hard to strengthen the presidency. The office of the presidency was strengthened by the presidency of George W. Bush as he successfully put into place the policies he desired. In terms of making laws, he chose to focus on his agenda-setting role while leaving much of the detailed business of legislation writing to the legislative branch. This served both institutions well in terms of their effectiveness.

Of course, both institutions were greatly helped by control of both by the same party. And the two major political parties are much more homogeneous, disciplined, and partisan than they were 10 years ago. The interest groups are less divisive and more closely involved in congressional (and sometimes administration) decisions throughout the policy process. The influence of the bureaucracy has been undermined by the proliferation of information (not necessarily balanced) and by efforts to politicize bureaucrats' findings and positions. Finally, the states have seen their efforts to innovate used against them as the federal government preempts some policies and imposes expensive mandates (and, in one case, repayment to Washington, D.C.).

In contrast, the problems plaguing the health care system and public health remain substantially the same as a decade ago, and many are even more acute: high and rising costs, growing millions of uninsured (though the actual estimates are in some dispute), badly strained safety-net providers, frequent medical errors and other patient-safety problems, racial and ethnic disparities, and regional variations in access and outcomes—to name only the most obvious.

Meanwhile, of course, the baby boomers continue to move inexorably toward retirement age, Medicare eligibility, and the accompanying high costs of treating chronic disease. Scholars are a bit more optimistic than most pundits about the effect of increased longevity and the burgeoning numbers of seniors, noting that the coming crop enters older age with more wealth and better health than its predecessors. Indeed, it is the subsequent groups of future seniors that may be the most worrisome, because so many of them are obese or overweight now. They may be sicker in old age following a lifetime of weight-related problems, and if the market for health care works as most expect it to, they are likely to be offered expensive treatments for their chronic conditions.

Even in the short run, however, projected Medicare deficits, Medicaid outlays, and general fund obligations of both national and state governments loom ever larger. Both government and the private sector now think about solutions much differently than a decade ago. Fewer and fewer employers are willing to assume any responsibility for their employees' health care costs. When they do, they prefer subsidies designed as defined contributions—an agreement to pay a fixed subsidy and no more, regardless of any additional services or costs needed by the beneficiary and leaving the choice of health plan scope and coverage, as well as supplementary costs, to the beneficiary. Eventually, these kinds of plans are likely to replace the traditional employer-sponsored plans that paid for everything, or close to it.

In this same spirit, a provision in the Medicare Prescription Drug, Improvement and Modernization Act of 2003 sets the stage for shifting more of the burden for Medicare costs to beneficiaries. The new law leaves a major gap in coverage for the middle class, fully covers only poor beneficiaries, and charges near-poor individuals premiums based on income, with everyone else paying full premiums. Incentives in the law seem likely to lead inexorably to increased enrollment in managed care of this last holdout of the fee-for-service population, once beneficiaries realize that better coverage at lower out-of-pocket costs is now available via managed care (due to substantial managed care subsidies) than via fee-for-service plans.

Once enrolled in managed care, beneficiaries may be ripe for being required to pay premiums and deductibles if their income is above poor or near-poor levels. This precedent has already been set in the MMA, which ties public subsidy amount to seniors' ability to pay their own costs. Even some Democratic senators supported this provision, providing premium subsidies for the new prescription drug coverage only to those making less than or little more than the federal poverty level and having only the smallest assets. In the past, rightly or wrongly, Medicare paid equally for all beneficiaries, regardless of income or assets, the well-heeled and even millionaires included. Now, discussions of means testing for all of Medicare are becoming relatively common. Some would say this policy change is inevitable if Medicare is to be kept solvent.

It seems more true than ever that the business community wants an end to its historical obligation to provide health care coverage for its workforce, but CEOs continue to shun the idea of comprehensive national health insurance. Meanwhile, foundations continue to sponsor the lunches at which national health insurance advocates and detractors meet to find common ground for a coalition effort. But the gap between them seems to widen rather than narrow. Worse, the solutions offered are the same limited and ineffectual state insurance pools and tax discounts for buying health insurance that are likely to do very little for the large population of uninsured who lack sufficient funds or the awareness of risk to buy coverage. Wal-Mart employees, who work for the nation's largest corporation, now account for an important share of Medicaid enrollees in some states.

The Republican Party continues to press the case for health savings accounts—tax-free savings plans with a huge consumer-paid deductible for health care services. These are designed to instill consumer buying power into the health care market, as consumers use their own money from the accounts to buy their health care, up to an insured catastrophic level. Democrats are quick to point out that health savings accounts must eventually lead to adverse selection, since takers are likely to be those who need little care (they can save money, tax-free). To the extent that this leaves an increasing percentage of high-risk individuals in the general insurance pool or uninsured, the premiums of those remaining in the general pool will rise, encouraging still more of the least sick to exit the pool and move to self-insured accounts. If left unchecked, the much feared death spiral and eventual collapse of the general insurance pool is likely to follow.

To avoid similar developments in the auto insurance industry, state legislatures enacted individual mandates requiring every driver to have his or her own policy. Is that the future for health care? Will individual mandates to carry insurance, catastrophic or otherwise, become the nation's health care coverage policy to solve the adverse selection and free-rider problems of the decaying employer-sponsored approach? If so, how might it be enforced? Drivers who get into an accident and are found to lack insurance lose their registration, license, or both. Some states and virtually all providers of auto loans won't issue license plates or make a loan without proof of insurance. Will mortgage companies, rental agents, or others with a stake in their customers' income stability come to require proof of health insurance? They may have a special incentive to do this now that filing for personal bankruptcy is much harder, due to changes in federal bankruptcy law. Health care bills have long been a leading cause of bankruptcy. If people must pay those hospital bills, will they stop paying their rent, mortgage, or auto loan? As hospitals come under increasing pressure to hold down costs, will they quietly seek repeal or bureaucratic reinterpretation of EMTALA (the Emergency Medical Treatment and Active Labor Act) of the mid-1990s, which requires emergency departments to render stabilizing care before they can ask about a patient's ability to pay the bill?

While both these ideas—individual mandates for health insurance and EMTALA repeal or reinterpretation—may seem outrageous and unlikely, so did means testing in Medicare not so long ago, or charging the states the cost of a federal program (as the MMA does on behalf of poor and near-poor individuals who qualify for drug coverage under both Medicare and Medicaid). What's different now seems to be a change in both public attitudes and the ability of the two major political parties to design and enact a legislative program consistent with their own ideology. The public seems to have a substantial willingness to see adoption of market-oriented approaches to health care. True, the public has apparently drawn the line at Social Security reform, so there are limits; but in health care the limits seem quite broad.

Another idea that has not gained much traction so far, one supported by business, is the proposal for Association Health Plans supported by the National Federation of Independent Business. It would do for smaller businesses what ERISA (the Employee Retirement Income Security Act) does for large businesses: allow their health and benefit plans to pool across state lines, thereby vitiating state regulation. The proposal passed the House of Representatives in both the 108th and 109th Congresses, but although introduced in the Senate by the chair of the Small Business and Entrepreneurship Committee, Olympia J. Snowe (R-ME), it has received little support there so far. But its key supporting interest group, the NFIB, is a powerful and determined advocate. This group wants the new law because it would immunize small business from state insurance regulation, as ERISA does for large business. Removal of this regulation would free small businesses of many state insurance-coverage mandates and oversight of various consumer protections.

The Republican Party seems to be endowed with ideas, such as this one, that grow logically from a system of beliefs about the role of the market versus government. In a word, they believe in competition rather than regulation to bring down prices and raise quality. Democrats don't seem to have much faith in competition, but they are apparently at a loss to propose a better alternative, and deficit spending closes off most publicly financed options (though deficits don't seem to be a problem for some other priorities—defense, homeland security, transportation, energy, hurricane relief, to name a few big-ticket items financed through deficits).

The possibility of a national health insurance of the traditional comprehensive, universal variety seems faint indeed, and likely to be kept off the agenda for many years to come by huge budget deficits—and an absence of public support. Today's solutions are market-based, ideological, and often innovative, reflecting the political and policy institutions from which they come. Health care reform is always somewhere on the policy agenda, frequently debated broadly but changed narrowly. *Health* is nearly always a major subheading in the Congressional Quarterly publication *CQ Weekly,* and *New York Times* domestic correspondent Robert Pear goes few days without an important story on health policy somewhere in the front section of the *Times.* But lately there is little pressure for a comprehensive expansion to universal health care coverage. The list of reasons for this is short, but impressive in its intractability:

— Americans inherently fear health services provided, authorized, or subsidized by government, sure that they will result in poor quality, long queues, and restricted access, despite many examples to the contrary—including Medicare, which enjoys remarkably low administrative costs and high levels of satisfaction.

— The two political parties differ fundamentally in how they and their supporters view the role of government. Republicans view government's dictating the scope of coverage, or setting health professionals' fees, or performing the insurance risk-pooling function as an inefficient tampering in the market. Democrats believe access to health care is so fundamental that relying on the market is simply inadequate. Republicans want plans to be voluntary, while Democrats consider mandatory participation is the only way to assure that risk is equally shared.

— Comprehensive change is especially hard to produce, because it concentrates costs on many separate interests, large and small, while thinly spreading the benefits to taxpayers and the insured in general. Payment sources for a comprehensive health care system have always been elusive. Small (and some large) employers, especially those in the growing service industry, do not want to pay premiums for their workers, even though economists argue that it is the workers who pay the cost through foregone wages. By outsourcing customer call services and many production functions to firms overseas, employers can avoid health care, other fringe benefits, and even some wage costs altogether. The only remaining payment source, higher taxes, is even less appealing. Few Americans—especially among the 85 to 88 percent who have health insurance—are willing to pay substantially higher taxes to ensure access to health care for the 12 to 15 percent who do not.

— Government seems to be moving toward a more market-oriented approach to health care policy, coupled with a desire to limit government's financial liability for health care costs. These steps reflect a growing and determined unwillingness to create open-ended financial obligations for government, a sea change in policy from the days of the Great Society. Concomitantly, the MMA expressly limits the use of government to set or even negotiate drug prices, relying instead on private sector competition to hold down prices—another sea change, even from the time of the Reagan administration, when hospital prospective budgeting and physician payment schedules were put in place.

— Many interest groups profit under the existing system, including health care providers, which are generally well paid; drug and specific-disease researchers, who are generously supported; insurance companies, which either sell in the private sector or process claims for the public sector; manufacturers of all sorts, which know they can create a market by selling to providers or by winning the battle to insert a few words into a regulation or, failing that, through a court case or congressional mandate.

— A steep learning curve confronts those who would tackle the many facets of national health insurance reform, and periodic bursts of saliency and public support for real change tend to be temporary and waning, hardly justifying the investment in learning. The crest of the wave passes before solutions can be formulated, and ideological differences over the role of government in a reformed system become sound-bite bursts of partisan warfare as election times approach.

— Campaign contributions to key committee and subcommittee chairs and party leaders make it unlikely that those legislators with a stake in the way things are now done will have to change their ways.

— States increasingly find themselves stymied by the budget-busting burden of Medicaid costs and by federal laws prohibiting them from exacting participation from employers in insurance reform plans, or even using innovative negotiating strategies to win better deals. When a major reform passes, it is, as often as not, soon repealed when costs are reconsidered.

Most important, most middle-class Americans continue to be relatively content with their health care, whether they should be or not, given the many European systems in which care is free to the patient and typically ranked higher in quality. To a large extent this contentment reflects the fact that, for most Americans, health care is low cost or close to free, because someone else pays the bill. Business is trying to change this in the private sector, and Republicans have tried to change it in the public sector. Business has met with some success. Republicans may yet do so.

Meanwhile, the Republican Party has proved that it can do at least as effective a job (some would say a much more effective job) of running the national legislature as did the Democrats when they controlled the White House and held a majority in one or both houses of Congress. One reason is party discipline. Republicans have been able to exact very high levels of party loyalty from their congressional parties on many crucial votes.

The House and Senate Republican leaderships have shown themselves to be determined, skilled, adaptive, and, when needed, ruthless in gaining support for major pieces of legislation and ensuring passage, often by very thin but sufficient margins. The White House has repeatedly shown that the president and his staff have learned to do what congressional party leaders ask them to do, and to stay out of the way the rest of the time, when legislative battles come down to a few votes. Those familiar with the Balanced Budget Act battles under President Clinton may note the contrast to the prevailing feeling that congressional Democrats were largely left out of the negotiations between the White House and congressional Republicans.

Perhaps Republican leaders have been most ruthless in the way they have used congressional powers, especially their power to manage the conference process. Democrats have found themselves largely cut out of conference negotiations. Republican leaders have expanded the time allotted for counting votes—stretched at times, for lobbying purposes, to nearly three hours from the usual quarter-hour needed to merely count noses. And they have threatened severe retribution for fellow Republicans who balk at casting a desired party vote, hitting them in two important goals: reelection and status in the Congress. They have told recalcitrant members that they will seek out and support opponents in upcoming elections and will see that desired committee or subcommittee leadership positions are taken away. Republicans have also been successful in working with their party counterparts in state legislatures to make effective use of redistricting, so that the number of Republicans is maximized while incumbent Democrats must run against each other, leaving the way clear for adding to the size of the Republican congressional majority. Had Democrats been as goal-oriented and strategic in their management of Congress and their party, they might not have lost their majorities in House and Senate elections, or at least not lost so badly.

Republican leaders have also developed new and daring relationships with interest groups. While Democrats have long been cozy with some interest groups, they have often fought openly with others. Republicans seem more willing to negotiate with anybody, more willing to give and take, to gain not just support but active lobbying, television advertising, and campaign support from groups across the political spectrum, though they are closest to groups that share their ideological view of limited government involvement in business. The "daring" component relates to the systematic effort to place staunch Republicans—often former staffers of House members and leaders—in lobbyist positions and in leadership roles in associations in Washington. These groups are then naturally aligned with Republican thinking. In case they are not, Republicans have sometimes refused to meet with them—taking away the access that is key to successful lobbying. For groups accepted by the Republican leadership, the reward is unprecedented access throughout the policy process.

Often, party leaders now start negotiations even before a bill is drafted, identifying key sticking points and making deals to include provisions in the bill or agreeing on amendments that will be introduced if things seem to be heading in a wrong direction. For example, when the House adopted an amendment authorizing drug reimportation as part of the MMA, another amendment was introduced and passed that guaranteed the effects of the reimportation amendment would be neutralized by safety contingencies. The price of these compromises often seems to raise the total cost of whatever piece of legislation is being considered ("rifle shots" bestowing benefits on a particular member) or to limit the law's effectiveness in critical ways (no national negotiations for drug prices; no increase in automobile gas mileage standards; immunity for gun makers). But most often, the higher prices and concessions on key provisions sought by groups ranging from PhRMA to the AARP, to the American Hospital Association, to the American Medical Association, to automobile and gun manufacturers, lead to support from the groups and their congressional allies, with little response from the public.

Also changed over the past decade are the role and relationship of the major political parties in setting the agenda for health policy. Democrats, who once owned the health policy agenda, now seem largely at a loss for next steps. It is little wonder that they have found themselves in a quandary over what exactly to do, given that Republicans have seized what was the Democrats' major middle-class health care issue—Medicare prescription drug coverage—and effectively mortgaged future social initiatives with deficit spending. The Republican policy agenda, focusing on market-based approaches and consumer empowerment, is clear and well-known by party members, think tanks, the press, and the public. There does not seem to be a clear Democratic alternative vision.

President George W. Bush showed himself at various points to be an almost exact opposite to his predecessor in his approach to health policy: targeting only a few areas of interest, following the tenets of a market-based ideology, setting the broad outlines of his goals but leaving the details to Congress, and a willingness to compromise on key issues to get past roadblocks. The George W. Bush White House proved much more dedicated to, and effective at, framing policy issues to help its agenda than many of its predecessors. The legacies of victories and defeats of earlier administrations seemed to be taken seriously in crafting policy and legislative strategies.

Health-related interest groups also seem to have matured and changed their strategy from the largely one-dimensional "no-change" positions of the past to more nuanced approaches. They are likely to seek and find compromise positions that allow them to support the president's program while getting in return their top-priority limits on policy proposals. Compromise is back in congressional, presidential, and interest-group politics.

One explanation is the lingering effects of the 1997 BBA. That act cut health care providers so severely that they have been back to Congress as supplicants every year since, begging to have some cuts restored and others delayed or eliminated. This has strengthened the hands of congressional leaders, who are able to condition their givebacks on support for the party agenda (as well as promises of generous campaign contributions). The price for the nation has been a switch back from declining rates of increase in health care spending to rising rates of increased spending. Government clearly has the ability to cut costs when it wants to. But interest groups have the persistence needed to make sure that many of the cuts get restored.

Bureaucracy has taken a black eye over several years, with false alarms and cumbersome procedures from the new Department of Homeland Security, flu vaccine shortages, and passivity in response to major catastrophic events. But other, more subtle, changes have also occurred in the bureaucratic role. There is some evidence that the health bureaucracy has been weakened in the past decade. It is no longer the primary source (or even one of the primary sources) of expertise for the White House and Congress. Each branch has its own staff and relies heavily on think tanks, academics, and interest groups that may have some vested interest in policy outcomes. Even cabinet secretaries complain that they are being circumvented and are out of the policy loop. Advice from experts at the FDA has been ignored, and there is some concern that scientific information in general is under attack, if not viewed skeptically. A long history of bad estimates of future costs, unintended consequences of health policies adopted with good intentions, and limited oversight of implementation may have contributed to some of these changes. But so has the change in party composition that has increased the ideological purity in Congress. Congressional enacting coalitions used to be temporary, fleeting, and with little capacity to follow through to see how the bureaucracy implemented things. Now there is a pretty good bet that those who voted for a bill share the same views as those who serve on the committees that pay attention to how the bureaucrats are interpreting it.

The state role in health care has taken an important turn as well. The states' traditional role as program implementers and innovators has been greatly curtailed in the MMA provision related to poor and near-poor beneficiaries and the increasing reliance on private sector firms such as PBMs and managed care organizations to implement programs. States' market power to demand discount prices for drugs has been substantially diminished now that they are no longer parties to negotiations over which drugs will be made available to those eligible for both Medicare and Medicaid—even though the states will pay most of the bill for these so-called dual eligibles.

History suggests that Republicans, as they remain longer in power, will lose some of their homogeneity and with it their discipline and willingness to let their leaders run the show. The seeds of that unraveling have appeared from time to time, especially in battles over deficit spending. The Iraq war has also cost the party support among the public. But for the foreseeable future, there seems little likelihood that the major change that has taken place in the health policy agenda will move back to the Roosevelt-to-Johnson era, with its huge growth in the federal role in social programs. All three editions of this book have repeatedly demonstrated that much change takes place in health policy even in the most seemingly quiescent of times. But for those who remember the days when national health policy meant broad new initiatives with broader ones still on the horizon, times and the programs they bring will be quite different.

We continue to contend that these new directions reflect prevailing public sentiment. The neglected though burgeoning army of the uninsured, the broad gap in coverage in the Medicare prescription drug bill, the costs of war and tax cuts—all were known to the electorate when it voted into power—and even expanded the majority of—the party that has determinedly called for a more limited role for public involvement in health care. When offered national health insurance, the public has repeatedly rejected it. Of course, it could all be attributed to the influence of interest groups, and surely it was interest groups, not the public, that, year after year, wanted the patients' bill of rights killed and drug companies immunized from government price negotiations. But who is in those interest groups if not the American people and their businesses?

If one follows the arc of public health policy from Lyndon Johnson to George W. Bush, it seems hard to deny that what is really behind the change is public attitudes. When the public favored an active and involved government working to press the case for social equity and government as an instrument of solving problems, it got an active government willing to take on almost any problem. Now government seems to be viewed as President Reagan viewed it, not the solution but rather the problem. Perhaps in a decade or two these attitudes will shift back in the other direction, as they did from Roosevelt-Truman to Eisenhower, then back again with Kennedy-Johnson, and back again with Bush through to Bush. In the meantime, health politics and policy reflect these shifts, but nonetheless remain fascinating, important, and incredibly expensive as health care becomes an ever-larger share of the GDP, no matter who is in charge, and is likewise ever evolving, unmindful of party control.

A few things to watch for in the next decade include more attention to performance-based payment in health care, conditioning the amount paid for care on performance indicators of quality for hospitals and physicians; expanded voluntary efforts to cover uninsured groups, including contributions to insurance premiums by counties, employers, providers offering discount prices, and individuals sharing a larger burden of their own care costs; expansion of health savings accounts, becoming available from more employers and chosen by more employees; further diminution of the state role in health care regulation; more market-oriented approaches to, and reduced funding for, Medicaid services; malpractice insurance reform, including caps on liability payments, limits on premium increases, and broadened immunity from liability conditioned on adherence to practice protocols; technological improvements in health and medical records; broadened health education roles for schools to battle the obesity epidemic, and a concomitant response by food processors and restaurants to reduce caloric and fat intake; expanded means testing of Medicare premium subsidies; more price competition among providers; more Americans traveling abroad for major health care procedures; no major change in long-term care quality, costs, or delivery settings other than continued expansion of assisted living facilities; national health care expenditures moving closer and closer to a quarter of GDP; and health care providers, drug companies, and medical device companies continuing to be disproportionately represented among the top campaign contributors to congressional and presidential races.

Abbreviations

AAMC	Association of American Medical Colleges
AAO	American Academy of Ophthalmology
AARP	formerly known as the American Association of Retired Persons
ACIR	Advisory Commission on Intergovernmental Relations
ACT-UP	AIDS Coalition to Unleash Power
ADA	American Dental Association
AFDC	Aid to Families with Dependent Children
AHA	American Hospital Association
AHCCCS	Arizona Health Care Cost Containment System
AHRQ	Agency for Healthcare Research and Quality (formerly the Agency for Health Care Policy and Research, AHCPR)
AIDS	acquired immune deficiency syndrome
AMA	American Medical Association
AMPAC	American Medical Association political action committee
ANA	American Nurses Association
AOA	American Optometric Association
ASCO	American Society of Clinical Oncology
BBA	Balanced Budget Act
BCRA	Bipartisan Campaign Reform Act
BEA	Budget Enforcement Act
BoB	Bureau of Budget (became OMB in 1970)

CBO	Congressional Budget Office
CDC	Centers for Disease Control and Prevention
CHA	Catholic Health Association
CMS	Centers for Medicare and Medicaid Services
CRS	Congressional Research Service
DRGs	diagnosis-related groups
DSH	disproportionate share hospital
EPA	Environmental Protection Agency
EMTALA	Emergency Medical Treatment and Active Labor Act
ERISA	Employee Retirement Income Security Act
FDA	Food and Drug Administration
FEC	Federal Election Commission
FEMA	Federal Emergency Management Agency
FTC	Federal Trade Commission
GAO	Government Accountability Office (formerly the General Accounting Office)
GDP	gross domestic product
GSA	General Services Administration
HCFA	Health Care Financing Administration (became CMS in 2001)
HEW	(U.S. Department of) Health, Education, and Welfare (became HHS)
HHS	(U.S. Department of) Health and Human Services
HIAA	Health Insurance Association of America
HIFA	Health Insurance Flexibility and Accountability
HIPAA	Health Insurance Portability and Accountability Act
HIV	human immunodeficiency virus
HMO	health maintenance organization
HRSA	Health Resources and Services Administration
HSA	health savings account (formerly known as medical savings account)
HUD	(Department of) Housing and Urban Development
IRS	Internal Revenue Service
MADD	Mothers Against Drunk Driving
MedPAC	Medicare Payment Advisory Commission

MMA	Medicare Modernization Act (in full, Medicare Prescription Drug, Improvement and Modernization Act of 2003)
MMCAP	Minnesota Multi-State Contracting Alliance for Pharmacy
NAFTA	North American Free Trade Agreement
NASBO	National Association of State Budget Officers
NCSL	National Conference of State Legislatures
NEPPS	National Environmental Performance Partnership System
NFIB	National Federation of Independent Business
NGA	National Governors Association
NIH	National Institutes of Health
NRA	National Rifle Association
OMB	Office of Management and Budget
OSHA	Occupational Safety and Health Administration
PAC	political action committee
PBMs	pharmacy benefit managers
PhRMA	Pharmaceutical Research and Manufacturers of America
PHS	Public Health Service
PPRC	Physician Payment Review Commission
PPS	(Medicare) Prospective Payment System
ProPAC	Prospective Payment Assessment Commission
PRWORA	Personal Responsibility and Work Opportunity Reconciliation Act
PSROs	professional standards review organizations
RBRVS	Resource-Based Relative Value Scale
SAMHSA	Substance Abuse and Mental Health Services Administration
S-CHIP	State Children's Health Insurance Program
SSI	Supplemental Security Income
TANF	Temporary Assistance for Needy Families
TEL	tax and expenditure limit
UPL	upper payment limit

References

Aberbach, Joel D. 2000. A Reinvented Government, or the Same Old Government? In *The Clinton Legacy*, ed. Colin Campbell and Bert A. Rockman. New York: Chatham House.

Abrahms, Boud. 2006. Lawmakers Seek to Rein in Pork. *Tallahassee Democrat*, Feb. 5, 2A.

Abramson, Jill. 1998. The Business of Persuasion Thrives in Nation's Capital: Issues in Depth: Lobbying—The Influence Industry. *New York Times*, Sept. 29. www.nytimes.com

AcademyHealth. 2003. State of the States: Bridging the Health Coverage Gap. Jan. www.statecoverage.net

———. 2005. State of the States: Finding Alternative Routes. Jan. www.statecoverage .net

Adams, Rebecca. 1999. Clinton's Medicare Drug Subsidy Plan Is Criticized for Scope and Cost. *CQ Weekly*, July 3, 1612.

———. 2003a. For First Time, Fighting Odds for Malpractice Awards Cap. *CQ Weekly*, Mar. 1, 484–91.

———. 2003b. Many Skirmishes Lie ahead for Medicare Overhaul as Major Constituencies Remain Billions Apart. *CQ Weekly*, Mar. 1, 481.

———. 2005a. Cries Grow to Increase FDA's Drug Oversight. *CQ Weekly*, Feb. 21, 438–39.

———. 2005b. Heavy Lifting Ahead: Federal and State Outlook on Health. *Governing* and *CQ Weekly*, June, 22–23.

———. 2005c. A Low Dose of FDA Oversight. *CQ Weekly*, Apr. 11, 886–92.

Adams, Rebecca, and Joseph J. Schatz. 2004. GOP Weighs Politically Iffy Plan: Cut Medicare Provider Payments. *CQ Weekly*, Nov. 13, 2694–95.

Advisory Commission on Intergovernmental Relations (ACIR). 1985. *The Question of State Government Capability.* Washington, DC: Government Printing Office.

Agency for Healthcare Research and Quality (AHRQ). 2006. AHRQ Mission: Mission and Budget. www.ahrq.gov/about/budgtix.htm

AHA Launches Massive Grassroots Effort. 1994. *Medicine and Health* 48 (Mar. 7): 2.

Ainsworth, Scott. 2002. *Analyzing Interest Groups: Group Influence on People and Policies.* New York: W. W. Norton.

Aldrich, John H., and David W. Rohde. 1995. Conditional Party Government Revisited: Majority Party Leadership and the Committee System in the 104th Congress. In *Extension of Remarks: The New Republican Congress: Explanations, Assessments, and Prospects,* ed. Lawrence C. Dodd, 1–2. Newsletter of the Legislative Studies Section. Dec. Washington, DC: American Political Science Association.

———. 2000. The Republican Revolution and the House Appropriations Committee. *Journal of Politics* 62:1–33.

———. 2005. Congressional Committees in a Partisan Era. In *Congress Reconsidered,* 8th ed., ed. Lawrence C. Dodd and Bruce I. Oppenheimer. Washington DC: CQ Press.

Allen, Johnathan, and Adam Graham-Silverman. 2003. Hour by Hour, Vote by Vote, GOP Breaks Tense Tie on Medicare. *CQ Weekly,* June 28, 1614.

Allen, Mahalley D., Carrier Pettus, and Donald P. Haider-Markel. 2004. Making the National Local: Specifying the Conditions for National Government Influence on State Policymaking. *State Politics and Policy Quarterly* 4 (3): 318–44.

Alpert, Bruce. 2004. Bill Tauzin: The Cajun Ambassador. *New Orleans Times-Picayune,* Dec. 12, 1.

Anderson, J. E. 1994. *Public Policymaking: An Introduction,* 2d ed. Boston: Houghton Mifflin.

Anderson, Odin W. 1990. *Health Services as a Growth Enterprise in the United States since 1875,* 2d ed. Ann Arbor: Health Administration Press.

Andres, Gary. 2004. Lobbying's Changed, So Why Haven't Our Perceptions of It? *Roll Call,* May 17. www.rollcall.com

Annas, George J. 2002. Bioterrorism, Public Health, and Human Rights. *Health Affairs* 21 (6): 94–97.

Ansolabehere, Stephen, James M. Snyder, Jr., and Charles Stewart III. 2001. The Effects of Party and Preferences on Congressional Roll-Call Voting. *Legislative Studies Quarterly* 26 (4): 533–72.

Anton, Thomas. 1989. *American Federalism and Public Policy.* New York: Random House.

Appleby, Paul H. 1945. *Big Democracy.* New York: Knopf.

Arnold, R. Douglas. 1990. *The Logic of Congressional Action.* New Haven, CT: Yale University Press.

Artiga, Samantha, and Cindy Mann. 2005. New Directions for Medicaid Section 1115 Waivers: Policy Implications of Recent Waiver Activity. Kaiser Commission on Medicaid and the Uninsured. Mar. www.kff.org/KCMU

Associated Press. 1992. Inquiry Discounts Texas H.I.V. Cases. New York Times, Aug. 2, C6.

———. 1999. Tough Rules Are Approved for New Paint. May 15. www.ap.org

———. 2003. AARP Faces Rebellion over Medicare Bill Support. FoxNews.com, Nov. 26.

———. 2005a. AARP Endorsement Angers Members—Democrats Predict a Revolt within the 45-Year-Old Group. Telegraph Herald (Dubuque, IA). http://infoweb.newsbank

———. 2005b States Seek to Regulate "Black Boxes" in Autos. *New York Times,* Mar. 27, 16.

Bach, Stanley, and Steven Smith. 1988. *Managing Uncertainty in the House of Representatives: Adaptation and Innovation in Special Rules.* Washington, DC: Brookings Institution.

Balla, Steven J. 1998. Administrative Procedures and Political Control of the Bureaucracy. *American Political Science Review* 92:663–73.

Barber, James David. 1985. *The Presidential Character: Predicting Performance in the White House.* Englewood Cliffs, NJ: Prentice-Hall.

Baron, David P. 2000. *Business and Its Environment,* 3d ed. Upper Saddle River, NJ: Prentice-Hall.

Baumgartner, Frank R., and Bryan D. Jones. 1993. *Agendas and Instability in American Politics.* Chicago: University of Chicago Press.

Baumgartner, Frank R., and Beth L. Leech. 2001. Interest Niches and Policy Bandwagons: Patterns of Interest Group Involvement in National Politics. *Journal of Politics* 63:1191–1213.

Beamer, Glenn. 2004. State Health Care Reform Politics and the Unfortunate End of the 1990s. *Journal of Health Politics, Policy, and Law* 29:293–304.

Becker, Elizabeth. 1999. V.A. Chief, under Fire, Is Said to Plan an Early Departure. *New York Times,* July 9. www.nytimes.com

Benda, Peter, and Charles Levine. 1986. OMB and the Central Management Problem: Is Another Reorganization the Answer? *Public Administration Review* 46:379–91.

Bendavid, Naftali, T. R. Goldman, and Sheila Kaplan. 1993. Handicapping Health Care's Major Players. *Legal Times,* Oct. 11, S28–S45.

Benenson, Bob. 1987. Savvy "Stars" Making Local TV a Potent Tool. *Congressional Quarterly Weekly Report,* July 18, 1551–55.

Berke, Richard. 1995. Republicans Rule Lobbyists' World with Strong Arm. *New York Times,* Mar. 20, A1.

———. 1998. Sierra Club Ads in Political Races Offer a Case Study of "Issue Advocacy." *New York Times,* Oct. 24. www.nytimes.com

Berrens, Robert P., Alok K. Bohara, Amy Baker, and Ken Baker. 1999. Revealed Preferences of a State Bureau: Case of New Mexico's Underground Storage Tank Program. *Journal of Policy Analysis and Management* 18:303–26.

Berry, Jeffrey M. 1984. *The Interest Group Society.* Boston: Little, Brown.

Best, J. 1988. Missing Children, Misleading Statistics. *Public Interest* 92:84–92.

Beyle, Thad. 1989. From Governor to Governors. In *The State of the States,* ed. Carl Van Horn. Washington, DC: Congressional Quarterly Press.

Binder, Sarah A. 1999. The Dynamics of Legislative Gridlock, 1947–96. *American Political Science Review* 93:519–33.

———. 2003. *Stalemate: Causes and Consequences of Legislative Gridlock.* Washington, DC: Brookings Institution.

Binder, Sarah A., Eric D. Lawrence, and Forrest Maltzman. 1999. Uncovering the Hidden Effect of Party. *Journal of Politics* 61:815–31.

Birnbaum, Jeffrey H. 2004. Capitol Hill Listens to Coalitions. *Washington Post,* May 3, E1.

Blumenthal, Sidney. 1994. The Education of a President. *New Yorker,* Jan. 24, 31–43.

Bond, Jon R., and Richard Fleisher. 1990. *The President in the Legislative Arena.* Chicago: University of Chicago Press.

Boodman, Sandra G. 1994. Health Care's Power Player. *Washington Post National Weekly Edition,* Feb. 14–20, 6–7.

Borins, Sandford. 1999. *Innovating with Integrity: How Local Heroes Are Transforming American Government.* Washington, DC: Georgetown University Press.

Bosso, Christopher. 1994. The Contextual Bases of Problem Recognition. In *The Politics of Problem Recognition,* ed. David Rochefort and Roger Cobb. Lawrence: University Press of Kansas.

Bosso, Christopher J., and Michael Thomas Collins. 2002. Just Another Tool? How Environmental Groups Use the Internet. In *Interest Group Politics,* 6th ed., ed. Allan J. Cigler and Burdett A. Loomis. Washington, DC: CQ Press.

Bottom, William P., Cheryl L. Eavey, Gary J. Miller, and Jennifer Nicoll Victor.

2000. The Institutional Effect on Majority Rule Instability: Bicameralism in Spatial Policy Decisions. *American Journal of Political Science* 44:523–40.

Bowler, M. Kenneth. 1987. Changing Politics of Federal Health Insurance Programs. *PS* 20:202–11.

Bozeman, Barry, and Leisha DeHart-Davis. 1999. Red Tape and Clean Air: Title V Air Pollution Permitting Implementation as a Test Bed for Theory Development. *Journal of Public Administration Research and Theory* 9:141–77.

Brandon, William, Rosemary Chaudry, and Alice Sardell. 2001. Launching SCHIP: The States and Children's Health Insurance. In *The New Politics of State Health Policy*, ed. Robert B. Hackey and David A. Rochefort. Lawrence: University Press of Kansas.

Bresnahan, John, and Erin Billings. 2003. Democrats Fume at AARP: GOP Hails Key Endorsement of Medicare Reform Package. *Roll Call*, Nov. 18. www .rollcall.com

Brinkley, Joel. 1993. Cultivating the Grass Roots to Reap Legislative Benefits. *New York Times*, Nov. 11, A1, A14.

Brisbin, Richard A., Jr. 1998. The Reconstitution of American Federalism? The Rehnquist Court and Federal-State Relations, 1991–1997. *Publius: The Journal of Federalism* 28 (1): 189–215.

Broder, David S. 1993. Who Does the Senate Represent? *Washington Post National Weekly Edition*, Aug. 23–29, 4.

———. 1994a. Can We Govern? *Washington Post National Weekly Edition*, Jan. 31–Feb. 6, 25.

———. 1994b. Congress Cranks up Its Health Reform Sausage-Maker. *Washington Post National Weekly Edition*, Apr. 25–May 1, 10.

———. 1994c. Congressional Staffers Wield Power in Health Care Reform. *Ann Arbor News*, July 13, A9.

———. 2003. Time Was GOP's Ally on the Vote. *Washington Post*, Nov. 23, A01, final edition.

Broder, David S., and Stephen Barr. 1993. Going over the Top on Oversight? *Washington Post National Weekly Edition*, Aug. 2–8, 31.

Broder, David S., and Amy Goldstein. 2003. AARP Decision Followed a Long GOP Courtship. *Washington Post*, Nov. 20, A01, final edition.

Brodie, Mollyann, and Robert J. Blendon. 1995. The Public's Contribution to Congressional Gridlock on Health Care Reform. *Journal of Health Politics, Policy, and Law* 20:403–10.

Brosnan, James. 2003. Reluctant Frist Basks in Victory. *Commercial Appeal* (Memphis), Nov. 28, A1.

Brott, Armin A. 1994. Battered-Truth Syndrome. *Washington Post*, July 31, C1.

Brown, Clyde, and Herbert Waltzer. 2002. Lobbying the Press: "Talk to the People Who Talk to America." In *Interest Group Politics,* 6th ed., ed. Allan J. Cigler and Burdett A. Loomis. Washington, DC: CQ Press.

Browne, William. 1991. Issue Niches and the Limits of Interest Group Influence. In *Interest Group Politics,* 3d ed., ed. Allan J. Cigler and Burdett A. Loomis. Washington, DC: Congressional Quarterly Press.

———. 1993. Group Leaders, Grassroots Confidants, and Congressional Responses. Paper presented at the Annual Meeting of the Midwest Political Science Association, Chicago, Apr. 6–8.

Brownlow, Louis. 1949. *The President and the Presidency.* Chicago: University of Chicago Press.

Burgin, Eileen. 2003. Congress, Health Care, and Congressional Caucuses: An Examination of the Diabetes Caucus. *Journal of Health Politics, Policy, and Law* 28:789–820.

Burns, James MacGregor. 1984. *The Power to Lead.* New York: Simon and Schuster.

Bush, George W. 2004. Speech Accepting Republican Nomination for President at the Republican National Convention. Sept. 2. *CQ Weekly,* Sept. 4, 2072.

Butler, Patricia A. 2000. *ERISA Preemption Primer.* Washington, DC: Alpha Center.

———. 2004. *ERISA Update: The Supreme Court Texas Decision and Other Recent Developments.* Washington, DC: National Academy for State Health Policy.

Califano, Joseph A. 1994. Imperial Congress. *New York Times Magazine,* Jan. 23, 40–41.

Calvert, Randall L., Mark J. Moran, and Barry R. Weingast. 1987. Congressional Influence over Policymaking: The Case of the FTC. In *Congress: Structure and Policy,* ed. Mathew D. McCubbins and Terry Sullivan. New York: Cambridge University Press.

Campaign for Tobacco-Free Kids. 2005. A Broken Promise to Our Children: The 1998 State Tobacco Settlement Six Years Later. http://tobaccofreekids .org/reports/settlements/2005/fullreport.pdf

Campbell, John C. 1992. *How Policies Change: The Japanese Government and the Aging Society.* Princeton: Princeton University Press.

Campion, Frank D. 1984. *The AMA and U.S. Health Policy.* Chicago: Chicago Review Press.

Canes-Wrone, Brandice, and Scott de Marchi. 2002. Presidential Approval and Legislative Success. *Journal of Politics* 64:491–509.

Carey, John M., Richard Niemi, and Lynda Powell. 2000. *Term Limits in the State Legislatures.* Ann Arbor: University of Michigan Press.

Carey, Mary Agnes. 2000a. Both Parties Step up Efforts on Medicare Prescription Benefit, with Universality a Key Issue. *CQ Weekly*, Mar. 25, 665.

———. 2000b. Drug Proposals Compared. *CQ Weekly*, May 13, 1107.

———. 2000c. GOP Drug Plan Prevails. *CQ Weekly*, July 1, 1584.

———. 2000d. Prescription Drug Proposal Unveiled by House GOP: Democrats Say It Overlooks Middle Class. *CQ Weekly*, Apr. 15, 900.

———. 2001a. Bush Proposes Drug Discount Card as Key Element of His Medicare Plan. *CQ Weekly*, July 14, 1690.

———. 2001b. Drug Plan's Low-Key Launch Signals Bush May Be Open to Deal. *CQ Weekly*, Feb. 3, 281.

———. 2001c. A New Take on Health Care. *CQ Weekly*, Jan. 13, 102.

———. 2002a. Complex Drug Bill May Prove More Difficult for GOP to Sell. *CQ Weekly*, June 22, 1667.

———. 2002b. GOP Bets on Private Insurers with Medicare Drug Bill. *CQ Weekly*, June 29, 1737.

———. 2003. Small Issues Add up to Big Headaches for Medicare Prescription Drug Conference. *CQ Weekly*, Oct. 11, 2508–10.

Carey, Mary Agnes, and Rebecca Adams. 1999. Medicare Panel a Year Later: Deadlocked at Deadline. *CQ Weekly*, Feb. 27, 481.

Carey, Mary Agnes, and John Reichard. 2005. The Call to eConnect: Outlook on Health Care. *Governing* and *CQ Weekly*, June, 10–16.

Carney, Eliza Newlin. 1998. The Ailing AMA. *National Journal*, Oct. 3. www.nationaljournal.com

Carter, Jimmy. 1981. President Jimmy Carter's Farewell Address. *Congressional Quarterly Weekly Report* 39 (Jan. 17): 196.

———. 1982. *Keeping the Faith: Memoirs of a President.* New York: Bantam Books.

Casamayou, Maureen Hogan. 2001. *The Politics of Breast Cancer.* Washington DC: Georgetown University Press.

Ceaser, Douglass. 1988. The Reagan Presidency and American Public Opinion. In *The Reagan Legacy: Promise and Performance,* ed. Charles O. Jones. Chatham, NJ: Chatham House.

Center for Responsive Politics. 2000. PAC Contributions to Federal Candidates, 1999–2000. www.opensecrets.org/pacs/indus/2000/HO1.htm

———. 2005. 2004 Election Overview. www.opensecrets.org/overview/incumbs.asp?cycle-2004

Centers for Medicare and Medicaid Services (CMS). 2004. 2004 Medicaid Managed Care Enrollment Report June 30. www.cms.hhs.gov/medicaid/mcaidsad.asp

————. 2005. CMS Oral History Interview with Donna Shalala. www.cms.hhs
.gov/about/historyshalala.asp

Chiou, Fang-Yi, and Lawrence S. Rothenberg. 2003. When Pivotal Politics Meets
Partisan Politics. *American Journal of Political Science* 47:503–22.

Cigler, Allan J., and Burdett A. Loomis. 1991. Organized Interests and the Search
for Certainty. In *Interest Group Politics*, 3d ed., ed. Allan J. Cigler and Burdett A. Loomis. Washington, DC: Congressional Quarterly Press.

Citizens Against Government Waste (CAGW). 2004. CAGW Slams $388 Billion
Omnibus Bill. Nov. 22. www.councilfor.cagw.org

————. 2005a. CAGW Appalled by Swelling Cost of Drug Benefit. Feb. 10. www
.councilfor.cagw.org

————. 2005b. CAGW Slams Medicare Coverage for Impotence Drugs. Jan. 28.
www.cagw.org/site/News2?page=NewsArticle&id=86022/18/2005

Clapp, Charles L. 1963. *The Congressman: His Work as He Sees It*. Garden City,
NY: Anchor Books.

Clark, Peter B., and James Q. Wilson. 1961. Incentive Systems: A Theory of
Organizations. *Administrative Science Quarterly* 6:129–66.

Clarke, Gary J. 1981. The Role of the States in the Delivery of Health Services.
American Journal of Public Health 71:59–69.

Clymer, Adam, Robert Pear, and Robin Toner. 1994. For Health Care, Time Was
a Killer. *New York Times*, Aug. 29, A1, A8–A9.

Cobb, Roger W., and Charles D. Elder. 1972. *Participation in American Politics:
The Dynamics of Agenda-Building*. Boston: Allyn and Bacon.

Cochran, John. 2004. George W. Bush: Another Shot at His Legacy. *CQ Weekly*,
Aug. 28, 1944–55.

Cohen, Jeffrey. 1994. Presidential Rhetoric and the Public Agenda. *American
Journal of Political Science* 39:87–107.

Cohen, Michael D., James G. March, and Johan O. Olsen. 1972. A Garbage
Can Model of Organizational Choice. *Administrative Science Quarterly*
17:1–25.

Cohn, Peter. 2005. House Considers Budget Cuts Package. *National Journal*,
Nov. 19, 3638.

Colamosca, Anne. 1979. The Trade Association Hustle. *New Republic*, Nov. 3,
16–19.

Collier, Ken. 1995. The President, the Public and the Congress. Paper presented
at the annual meeting of the Midwest Political Science Association, Chicago, Apr. 6–8.

Confessore, Nicholas. 2003. Welcome to the Machine: How the GOP Disciplined
K Street and Made Bush Supreme. *Washington Monthly* 35 (78): 30–38.

Congressional Budget Office (CBO). 1998. How Increased Competition from Generic Drugs Has Affected Prices and Returns in the Pharmaceutical Industry. July. Washington, DC: CBO. www.cbo.gov/ftpdocs/6xx/doc655/pharm.pdf

———. 2002. Issues in Designing a Prescription Drug Benefit for Medicare. Oct. Washington, DC: CBO. www.cbo.gov/showdoc.cfm?index=3960&sequence=0

———. 2005a. An Introduction to the Congressional Budget Office. www.cbo.gov

———. 2005b. Payments for Prescription Drugs under Medicaid. Statement of Douglas Holtz-Eakin, Director, before the Special Committee on Aging, United States Senate. July 20. Washington, DC: CBO. www.cbo.gov/showdoc.cfm?index=6564&sequence=0

Congressional Quarterly. 1997. *Congressional Quarterly Almanac.* Washington, DC: CQ Press.

———. 2001. *Congressional Quarterly Almanac.* Washington, DC: CQ Press.

———. 2003. *Congressional Quarterly Almanac.* Washington, DC: CQ Press.

Conlan, Timothy J., and Francosi Vergniolle De Chantal. 2001. The Rehnquist Court and Contemporary American Federalism. *Political Science Quarterly* 116:253–75.

Consumers Union. 2001. Consumers Union Reaction to President Bush's Immediate Helping Hand. Sept. 19. www.consumersunion.org

Cook, David. 2003. The Point Man on AARP's Controversial Medicare Move: The Senior Group Has Lost Thousands of Members, but Maintains the Drug Plan Was a Step Forward. *Christian Science Monitor,* Dec. 11, 3.

Cotterell, Bill. 2004. Tallahassee Is a Prime Habitat for Lobbyists. *Tallahassee Democrat,* Feb. 22, E1.

———. 2005. State Workers Need Health Incentives. *Tallahassee Democrat,* June 13, B1.

Cox, Gary W., and Mathew D. McCubbins. 1993. *Legislative Leviathan: Party Government in the House.* Berkeley: University of California Press.

———. 1997. Toward a Theory of Legislative Rules Changes: Assessing Schickler and Rich's Evidence. *American Journal of Political Science* 41:1376–86.

———. 2002. Agenda Power in the U.S. House of Representatives, 1877–1986. In *Party, Process, and Political Change in Congress: New Perspectives on the History of Congress,* ed. David W. Brady and Mathew D. McCubbins. Palo Alto, CA: Stanford University Press.

CQ Weekly. 1984. Summary of Major 1984 Congressional Action: Health. Oct. 20, 2713.

———. 2001. Bush Pledges to Seek Unity: Appeals for Compassion, Renewed Sense of Civic Duty. Jan. 27, 239.

———. 2003a. Medicare Bills Differ in Details. June 28, 1617.

———. 2003b. 2003 Legislative Summary: Agricultural Appropriations. Dec. 13, 3096.

Craig, Steven G. 1996. Should States Be Responsible for New Directions in Health Provision? Lessons from Other Policy Areas. In *Health Policy, Federalism, and the American States,* ed. Robert F. Rich and William D. White. Washington, DC: Urban Institute Press.

Crain Communications. 1997. Outliers: Asides and Insides: Congress Made One Cut Too Many for Hospital, Physician Pay Boards. *Modern Healthcare,* Mar. 17, 40.

Crawford, Craig. 2005. Craig Crawford's 1600: A Fortified White House. *CQ Weekly,* May 23, 1406.

Cronin, Thomas, and Michael A. Genovese. 1998. *The Paradoxes of the American Presidency.* New York: Oxford University Press.

Cusack, Bob. 2003. Drug Industry Does Battle: Policymakers Say Drug Makers Must Improve Standing with an Image. *The Hill,* Sept. 17, 3.

Davidson, Roger H. 1984. The Presidency and the Congress. In *The Presidency and the Political System,* ed. Michael Nelson. Washington, DC: Congressional Quarterly Press.

———. 1995. Building a Republican Regime on Capitol Hill. In *Extension of Remarks: The New Republican Congress: Explanations, Assessments, and Prospects,* ed. Lawrence C. Dodd, 1–2. Newsletter of the Legislative Studies Section. Dec. Washington, DC: American Political Science Association.

Davidson, Roger H., and Walter J. Oleszek. 1994. *Congress and Its Members.* Washington, DC: Congressional Quarterly Press.

Davis, Julie Hirschfeld. 2001. House Passes Agriculture Spending Bill with Drug Re-importation Language, Increases for Research and Farm Loans. *CQ Weekly,* July 14, 1698.

Davis, Patricia. 1990. U.S. Releases First Study on Missing Children: 4,600 Taken by Strangers in '88, Report Says. *Washington Post,* May 4, A1.

DeClercq, Eugene, and Diana Simmes. 1997. The Politics of "Drive-through Deliveries": Putting Early Postpartum Discharge on the Legislative Agenda. *Milbank Quarterly* 75:175–202.

DeGregorio, Christine A. 1999. *Network of Champions.* Ann Arbor: University of Michigan Press.

———. 2000. Leaders and Advocates in Pursuit of Policy: Some Consequences of Changing Majorities in the U.S. House of Representatives. Paper presented at the annual meeting of the Midwest Political Science Association, Chicago, Apr. 26–30.

Derthick, Martha. 1975. *Uncontrollable Spending for Social Services Grants.* Washington, DC: Brookings Institution.

———. 1990. *Agency under Stress.* Washington, DC: Brookings Institution.

Dery, David. 1984. *Problem Definition in Policy Analysis.* Lawrence: University Press of Kansas.

de Tocqueville, Alexis. [1835] 1956. *Democracy in America.* Ed. Richard D. Heffner. New York: Mentor Books.

Diamond, Martin. 1985. What the Framers Meant by Federalism. In *American Intergovernmental Relations: Foundations, Perspectives, and Issues,* ed. Laurence O'Toole, Jr. Washington, DC: Congressional Quarterly Press.

Dodd, Lawrence C., and Bruce I. Oppenheimer. 2005. A Decade of Republican Control: The House of Representatives, 1995–2005. In *Congress Reconsidered,* 8th ed., ed. Lawrence C. Dodd and Bruce I. Oppenheimer. Washington, DC: CQ Press.

Doherty, Carroll J. 1999. Senate Acquits Clinton. *CQ Weekly,* Feb. 13, 361.

Donnelly, John M. 2005. Bipartisan House Resolution Brings Unease over Iraq War into Public View. *CQ Weekly,* June 17, 0657.

Downs, Anthony. 1967. *Inside Bureaucracy.* Boston: Little, Brown.

———. 1972. Up and Down with Ecology: The "Issue-Attention Cycle." *Public Interest* 28:38–50.

Drew, Christopher, and Richard Oppel, Jr. 2004. How Power Lobby Won Battle of Pollution Control at E.P.A. *New York Times,* Mar. 6, A1.

Drew, Elizabeth. 2005. Selling Washington. *New York Review of Books* 52 (June 23), 11. www.nybooks.com/articles/18075

Dubay, L. C., G. G. Kenney, and J. Holahan. 1989. Should Medicare Compensate Hospitals for Administratively Necessary Days? *Milbank Quarterly* 67:137–67.

Duncan, Phil. 1993. *Politics in America, 1994: The 103d Congress.* Washington, DC: Congressional Quarterly Press.

Dwyre, Diana. 2002. Campaigning outside the Law: Interest Group Issue Advocacy. In *Interest Group Politics,* 6th ed., ed. Allan J. Cigler and Burdett A. Loomis. Washington, DC: CQ Press.

Dye, T. R. 1984. *Understanding Public Policy,* 5th ed. Englewood Cliffs, NJ: Prentice-Hall.

Edelman, Murray. 1964. *The Symbolic Uses of Politics.* Urbana: University of Illinois Press.

Edsall, Thomas B. 1996. Issue Coalitions Take on Political Party Functions: Alliances on Left, Right Gain Power. *Washington Post,* Aug. 8, A1.

Edwards, George C. 1980. *Presidential Influence in Congress.* San Francisco: W. H. Freeman.

———. 1989. *At the Margins: The Presidential Leadership of Congress.* New Haven, CT: Yale University Press.

———. 2000. Campaigning Is Not Governing: Bill Clinton's Rhetorical Presidency. In *The Clinton Legacy,* ed. Colin Campbell and Bert A. Rockman. New York: Chatham House.

Edwards, George, and B. Dan Wood. 1999. Who Influences Whom? The President, the Congress, and the Media. *American Political Science Review* 93:327–45.

Eilperin, Juliet. 1999. Beer Lobby Keeps Anti-Drug Drive Alcohol-Free: In Battle over Ads, Big Brewers Tapped Political Leverage. *Washington Post,* July 23, A27.

———. 2000. GOP Group Discloses Fundraising Sources. *Washington Post,* Oct. 21, A9.

———. 2005. Professor at Harvard Is Being Investigated: Fluoride-Cancer Link May Have Been Hidden. *Washington Post,* July 13, A3.

Eisler, Kim Isaac. 1999. Almost Every Business Has Its Man—or Woman—in Washington: Here Are the 50 Association Heads with Real Clout. *Washingtonian Magazine,* Sept., 97.

Elazar, Daniel. 1984. *American Federalism: A View from the States,* 3d ed. New York: Harper and Row.

Ellwood, John, and James Thurber. 1977. The New Congressional Budget Process. In *Congress Reconsidered,* ed. Lawrence Dodd and Bruce Oppenheimer. New York: Praeger.

Epstein, David, and Sharyn O'Halloran. 1994. Administrative Procedures, Information, and Agency Discretion. *American Journal of Political Science* 38:697–722.

Epstein, Samuel. 1979. *Politics of Cancer.* Garden City, NY: Anchor Press.

Express Scripts. 2004. Exhibit 1. National Health Expenditures for Selected Healthcare Accounts: 1990 and 1994 to 2003. *Drug Trend Report,* 5. Maryland Heights, MO: Express Scripts. www.express-scripts.com

Eyestone, R. 1978. *From Social Issues to Public Policy.* New York: John Wiley.

Falk, Erika. 2003. *Legislative Issue Advertising in the 107th Congress.* Washington, DC: Annenberg Public Policy Center of the University of Pennsylvania. www.annenbergpublicpolicycenter.org

Feder, Barnaby. 1993. Medical Group Battles to Be Heard over Others on Health-Care Changes. *New York Times,* June 11, A12.

Feder, Judith M. 1977. *Medicare: The Politics of Federal Hospital Insurance.* Lexington, MA: D. C. Heath.

Feder, Judith, John Holahan, Randall Bovbjerg, and Jack Hadley. 1982. Health. In *The Reagan Experiment,* ed. John L. Palmer and Isabel V. Sawhill. Washington, DC: Urban Institute Press.

Federal Election Commission. 2005. *FEC Issues Semi-Annual Federal PAC Count.* www.fec.gov

Feldstein, Paul J. 1977. *Health Associations and the Demand for Legislation.* Cambridge, MA: Ballinger.

Fenno, Richard. 1973. *Congressmen in Committees.* Boston: Little, Brown.

———. 1978. *Home Style: House Members in Their Districts.* Boston: Little, Brown.

Fineberg, Harvey V. 1988. Education to Prevent AIDS: Prospects and Obstacles. *Science* 239:592–96.

Fiorina, Morris. 1981. Congressional Control of the Bureaucracy: A Mismatch of Incentives and Capabilities. In *Congress Reconsidered,* 2d ed., ed. Lawrence C. Dodd and Bruce Oppenheimer. Washington, DC: Congressional Quarterly Press.

Fiscella, Kevin. 2003. Assessing Health Care Quality for Minority and Other Disparity Populations. Washington D.C.: Agency for Healthcare Research and Quality. www.ahrq.gov/qual/qdisprep.pdf

Ford, Julie L., Beth H. Olson, and Amy J. Baumer. 2004. Michigan Residents "Weigh In" on Health Issues. IPPSR-SOSS Bull. 04-01. http://ippsr.msu .edu/Publications/b0401.pdf

Foreman, Christopher. 1995. Grassroots Victim Organizations: Mobilizing for Personal and Public Health. In *Interest Group Politics,* 4th ed., ed. Allan J. Cigler and Burdett A. Loomis. Washington, DC: Congressional Quarterly Press.

Forgette, Richard, and Lindsey Scruggs. 2005. Committee Assignments and House Republicans: Have Party Effects Increased? Paper presented at the 2005 Southern Political Science Association Meeting, New Orleans, Jan. 6–9.

Fox, Daniel, and Daniel Schaffer. 1989. Health Policy and ERISA: Interest Groups and Semipreemption. *Journal of Health Politics, Policy, and Law* 14:239–60.

Foxhall, Kathryn. 2005. Managed Care in It for the Long Term. *State Legislatures,* June, 32–34.

Frank, Richard, and Thomas McGuire. 1996. Health Care Financing Reform and State Mental Health Systems. In *Health Policy, Federalism, and the American States,* ed. Robert F. Rich and William D. White. Washington, DC: Urban Institute Press.

Freudenheim, Milt. 2003. Experts Question Competition for Medicare. *Milwaukee Journal Sentinel,* Nov. 28, 1D.

Fritsch, Jane. 1995. The Grass Roots, Just a Free Phone Call Away. *New York Times,* June 23, A1, A11.

Furlong, Scott R. 2005. Exploring Interest Group Participation in Executive Policymaking. In *The Interest Group Connection: Electioneering, Lobbying and Policymaking in Washington,* 2d ed., ed. Paul S. Herrnson, Ronald G. Shaiko, and Clyde Wilcox. Washington, DC: CQ Press.

Gais, Thomas. 1998. *Improper Influence.* Ann Arbor: University of Michigan Press.

Gais, Thomas, and James Fossett. 2005. Federalism and the Executive Branch. In *The Executive Branch,* ed. Joel D. Aberbach and Mark A. Peterson. Institutions of American Democracy Series, ed. Jaroslav Pelikan. New York: Oxford University Press, 2005.

Gardner, Jonathan. 1999. Barely Breaking Even: Industry-Sponsored Report Projects Hospitals Will Post Miniscule Margins in Medicare in '99. *Modern Healthcare,* Mar. 15, 2.

Gelles, R. J. 1984. Parental Child Snatching. *Journal of Marriage and the Family* 46:735–39.

Gerber, Elisabeth. 1999. *The Populist Paradox.* Princeton, NJ: Princeton University Press.

Gerber, Michael S. 2002. Hostility Erupts over Drug Bill; Advocacy Groups Square off As Senate Debates Benefits. *The Hill,* July 24, 35. web.lexis-nexis.com

Gerth, Jeff. 2000. Agency Plans to Study Drug Makers' Records to See Whether Deals Delay Generics. *New York Times,* Oct. 12. www.nytimes.com

Gewirtz, Paul, and Chad Golder. 2005. So Who Are the Activists? *New York Times,* July 6, A23.

Gilmour, John B. 1990. *Reconcilable Differences: Congress, the Budget Process, and the Deficit.* Berkeley: University of California Press.

———. 2002. Institutional and Individual Influences on the President's Veto. *Journal of Politics* 64:198–218.

Glazer, Nathan. 1975. Towards an Imperial Judiciary? *Public Choice* 41 (fall): 104–23.

Glick, Henry R., and Amy Hutchinson. 2001. Physician-Assisted Suicide: Agenda Setting and the Elements of Morality Policy. In *The Public Clash of Private Values: The Politics of Morality Policy,* ed. Christopher Z. Mooney. New York: Chatham House.

Goldstein, Amy. 2003. For GOP Leaders, Battles and Bruises Produce Medicare Bill. *Washington Post,* Nov. 30, A08, final edition.

Goldstein, Amy, and Helen Dewar. 2003. Congress Poised to Pass Medicare Bills: Prescription Drug Benefit Is Centerpiece of Biggest Revamp in 28 Years. *Washington Post,* June 27, A6.

Goldstein, Kenneth M. 1999. *Interest Groups, Lobbying, and Participation in America.* New York: Cambridge University Press.

Goode, Erica. 2001. Nine Million Gaining Upgraded Benefit for Mental Care. *New York Times,* Jan. 1. www.nytimes.com

Goodman, Ellen. 1988. AIDS "Experts" Spread Risk of High Anxiety. *Newsday,* Mar. 11, 92.

Goodstein, Laurie. 1999. Coalition's Woes May Hinder Goals of Christian Right. *New York Times,* Aug. 2. www.nytimes.com

Gordon, Joshua. 2005. The (Dis)Integration of the House Appropriations Committee: Revisiting the Power of the Purse in a Partisan Era. In *Congress Reconsidered,* 8th ed., ed. Lawrence C. Dodd and Bruce I. Oppenheimer. Washington, DC: CQ Press.

Gormley, William T., Jr. 1982. Alternative Models of the Regulatory Process: Public Utility Regulation in the States. *Western Politics Quarterly* 25:297–317.

Government Accountability Office / General Accounting Office (GAO). 1992. *Access to Health Insurance.* GAO/HRD-92-90. Washington, DC: Government Printing Office.

———. 2000. *Medicaid and SCHIP: Comparisons of Outreach, Enrollment Practices, and Benefits.* GAO/HEHS-00-86. Washington, DC: Government Printing Office.

———. 2003. Medical Malpractice: Implications of Rising Premiums on Access to Health Care. Aug. 8. GAO-03-836. Washington, DC: Government Printing Office.

———. 2004. HHS Bioterrorism Preparedness Programs: States Reported Progress but Fell Short of Program Goals for 2002. GAO-04-360R. Washington, DC: Government Printing Office.

———. 2005. GAO at a Glance. www.gao.gov/about/gglance.html

Government Printing Office. 2005. State of the Union. www.gapaccess.gov/sou

Grant, Daniel, and Lloyd Omdahl. 1993. *State and Local Government in America,* 6th ed. Madison, WI: WCG Brown and Benchmark.

Greenstein, Fred. 2004. *The Presidential Difference: Leadership Style from FDR to George W. Bush.* Princeton, NJ: Princeton University Press.

Greif, Geoffrey L. 1993. *When Parents Kidnap: Families behind the Headlines.* New York: Free Press.

Grier, Kevin B., and Michael Munger. 1993. Comparing Interest Group Contributions to House and Senate Incumbents, 1980–86. *Journal of Politics* 55:615–43.

Gutermuth, Karen. 1999. The American Medical Political Action Committee: Which Senators Get the Money and Why? *Journal of Health Politics, Policy, and Law* 24:357–82.

Haass, Richard N. 1994. Bill Clinton's Adhocracy. *New York Times Magazine,* May 29, 40–41.

Hackey, Robert B. 1998. *Rethinking Health Care Policy: The New Politics of State Regulation.* Washington, DC: Georgetown University Press.

———. 2001. State Health Policy in Transition. In *The New Politics of State Health Policy*, ed. Robert B. Hackey and David A. Rochefort. Lawrence: University Press of Kansas.

Hadley, Jack, and John Holahan. 2003/2004. Is Health Care Spending Higher under Medicaid or Private Insurance? *Inquiry* 40:323–42.

Hall, Richard L. 1996. *Participation in Congress*. Ann Arbor: University of Michigan Press.

Hall, Richard L., and Kris C. Miler. 1999. Paying the Costs of Costly Signaling: Legislators as Group Agents in Agency Rulemaking. Paper presented at the annual meeting of the Midwest Political Science Association, Chicago, Apr. 15–18.

Hall, Richard, and Frank Wayman. 1990. Buying Time: Moneyed Interests and the Mobilization of Bias in Congressional Committees. *American Political Science Review* 84:797–820.

Hammond, Thomas, and Jack Knott. 1996. Presidential Power, Congressional Dominance, Legal Constraints, and Bureaucratic Autonomy in a Model of Multi-institutional Policymaking. *Journal of Law, Economics, and Organization* 12:121–68.

Hammond, Thomas H., and Gary J. Miller. 1987. The Core of the Constitution. *American Political Science Review* 81:1155–74.

Harris, Gardiner. 2005. F.D.A. Moves toward More Openness with the Public. *New York Times*, Feb. 20, 19.

Harris, John F. 1999. OMB Chief Hits GOP Tax, Spending Plans: Lew Projects 50 Pct. Agency Budget Cuts. *Washington Post*, Aug. 14, A7.

Harris, Richard. 1966. *A Sacred Trust*. New York: New American Library.

Hayes, Michael T. 1992. *Implementation and Public Policy*. White Plains, NY: Longman.

Health and Human Services, Department of (HHS). 2000. HHS Announced Final Regulation Establishing First-Ever National Standards to Protect Patients' Personal Medical Records. Press Release. Dec. 20. www.hhs .gov/news/press/2000pres/20001220.html

———. 2005a. HHS Announces $1.3 Billion in Funding to States for Bioterrorism Preparedness. News Release. May 13. www.hhs.gov/news/press/ 2005pres/20050513.html

———. 2005b. Organizational Chart. www.hhs.gov/about/orgchart.html

Heaney, Michael T. 2003. What Was in It for Them. *Washington Post*, Nov. 30, B4.

———. 2004a. Outside the Issue Niche: The Multidimensionality of Interest Group Identity. *American Politics Research* 32 (6): 611–51.

———. 2004b. Reputation and Leadership Inside Interest Group Coalitions. Paper presented at the annual meeting of the American Political Science Association, Chicago, Sept. 2–5.

———. 2005. Coalition of the Willing? Party Leaders, Lobbying Coalitions and the Medicare Overhaul of 2003. Paper presented at the annual meeting of the American Political Science Association, Washington, DC, Sept. 2.

Heclo, Hugh. 1977. *A Government of Strangers.* Washington, DC: Brookings Institution.

———. 1978. Issue Networks and the Executive Establishment. In *The New American Political System,* ed. Anthony King. Washington, DC: American Enterprise Institute.

Heffler, Stephen, Sheila Smith, Sean Keehan, Christine Borger, M. Kent Clemens, and Christopher Truffler. 2005. U.S. Health Spending Projections for 2004–2014. *Health Affairs* 23, w5-74 (web-exclusive). www.healthaffairs.org

Hegner, Richard E. 1998. The State Children's Health Insurance Program: How Much Latitude Do the States Really Have? *National Health Policy Forum Issue Brief,* Oct. 1.

Heilprin, John. 2004. EPA to Pursue Clean-Air Lawsuits. *Tallahassee Democrat,* Jan. 10, 5A.

Heinz, John P., Edward O. Laumann, Robert H. Salisbury, and Robert L. Nelson. 1990. Inner Circles or Hollow Cores? Elite Networks in National Policy Systems. *Journal of Politics* 52:356–90.

Heinz, John P., Edward O. Laumann, Robert L. Nelson, and Robert H. Salisbury. 1993. *The Hollow Core: Private Interests in National Policy Making.* Cambridge. MA: Harvard University Press.

Herbert, Bob. 2004. Malpractice Myths. *New York Times,* June 21, A19.

Herrick, Rebekah, and Michael K. Moore. 1993. Political Ambition's Effect on Legislative Behavior: Schlesinger's Typology Reconsidered and Revised. *Journal of Politics* 55:765–76.

Herrnson, Paul S. 2005. The Bipartisan Campaign Reform Act and Congressional Elections. In *Congress Reconsidered,* 8th ed., ed. Lawrence C. Dodd and Bruce I. Oppenheimer. Washington, DC: CQ Press.

Hill, Jeffrey, and Carol S. Weissert. 1995. Implementation and the Irony of Delegation: The Politics of Low-Level Radioactive Waste Disposal. *Journal of Politics* 57:344–69.

Hinckley, Barbara. 1990. *The Symbolic Presidency.* New York: Routledge.

Hojnacki, Marie. 1997. Interest Groups' Decisions to Join Alliances or Work Alone. *American Journal of Political Science* 41:61–87.

Hojnacki, Marie, and David C. Kimball. 1998. Organized Interests and the

Decision of Whom to Lobby in Congress. *American Political Science Review* 92:775–90.

———. 1999. The Who and How of Organizations' Lobbying Strategies in Committee. *Journal of Politics* 61:999–1024.

Holahan, John, and Len Nichols. 1996. State Health Policy in the 1990s. In *Health Policy, Federalism, and the American States,* ed. Robert F. Rich and William D. White. Washington, DC: Urban Institute Press.

Holtz-Eakin, Douglas. 2005. The Cost and Financing of Long-Term Care Services. Testimony before the Subcommittee on Health, Committee on Energy and Commerce, U.S. House of Representatives. Apr. 27. www.cbo.gov

Hord, Bill. 2001. Food Industry Hungry for Biotech Companies Look for Ways to Quickly and Accurately Identify Gene Altered Crops. *Omaha World-Herald,* Feb. 11, 1M.

Horn, Murray. 1995. *The Political Economy of Public Administration.* New York: Cambridge University Press.

Hrebenar, Ronald, Matthew Burbank, and Robert Benedict. 1999. *Political Parties, Interest Groups, and Political Campaigns.* Boulder, CO: Westview Press.

Hulse, Carl. 2003. Fight to Pass Medicare Measure Raised House Speaker's Profile. *New York Times,* Dec. 6, A1, late edition, East Coast.

———. 2005. Two "Bridges to Nowhere" Tumble Down in Congress. *New York Times,* Nov. 17, 19.

Iglehart, John K. 1977. The Hospital Lobby Is Suffering from Self-inflicted Wounds. *National Journal,* Oct. 1, 1526–31.

Ingram, Helen. 1977. Policy Implementation through Bargaining. *Public Policy* 25:449–501.

Initiative and Referendum Institute. 2005. What Is the Initiative and Referendum Process? www.iandrinstitute.org

Jacobs, Lawrence R. 1993a. *The Health of Nations: Public Opinion and the Making of American and British Health Policy.* Ithaca, NY: Cornell University Press.

———. 1993b. Health Reform Impasse: The Politics of American Ambivalence toward Government. *Journal of Health Politics, Policy, and Law* 18:629–55.

Jacobs, Lawrence R., and Robert Y. Shapiro. 1995. Don't Blame the Public for Failed Health Care Reform. *Journal of Health Politics, Policy, and Law* 20:411–23.

———. 2000. *Politicians Don't Pander: Political Manipulation and the Loss of Democratic Responsiveness.* Chicago: University of Chicago Press.

Jacobson, Gary C. 1987. *The Politics of Congressional Elections,* 2d ed. Boston: Little, Brown.

Janiskee, Brian. 1995. Bicameralism and Health Legislation in Michigan. Paper presented at the annual meeting of the Midwest Political Science Association, Chicago, Apr. 6–8.

Johnson, Cathy Marie. 1992. *The Dynamics of Conflict between Bureaucrats and Legislators.* Armonk, NY: M. E. Sharpe.

Johnson, Charles A. 1976. Political Culture in American States: Elazar's Formulation Examined. *American Journal of Political Science* 20:491–509.

Johnson, Linda. 2005. Abstinence Advocates Want Condom Correction. *Tallahassee Democrat,* June 30, 6A.

Johnson, Lyndon Baines. 1971. *The Vantage Point.* New York: Holt, Rinehart, and Winston.

Jones, Charles O. 1984. *An Introduction to the Study of Public Policy.* Monterey, CA: Brooks/Cole.

———. 1994. *The Presidency in a Separated System.* Washington, DC: Brookings Institution.

Jones, Mark P., and Wonjae Hwang. 2005. Party Government in Presidential Democracies: Extending Cartel Theory beyond the U.S. Congress. *American Journal of Political Science* 49:267–82.

Jost, Kenneth. 2003. Medical Malpractice: Are Lawsuits out of Control? *CQ Researcher* 13 (6, Feb. 14): 129–52.

Joyce, Amy. 2005. Bill Targets Wal-Mart's Health Care. *Tallahassee Democrat,* June 23:4A.

Judis, John B. 1999. Deregulation Run Riot. *American Prospect,* Sept.–Oct., 16–19.

Jump, Linda. 2005. Cities Turn to Lobbyists for Fed Voice. Florida Today.Com, Aug 26. www.floridatoday.com

Justice, Glen. 2005. Ads Will Seek to Turn DeLay's Powerful Network into His Downfall. *New York Times,* Mar. 20, A11.

Kaiser Commission on Medicaid. 1999. *Medicaid: A Primer.* San Francisco: Kaiser Commission on Medicaid.

Kaiser Family Foundation. 2005a. Americans Value the Health Benefits of Prescription Drugs, but Say Drug Makers Put Profits First, New Survey Shows. Feb. 25. www.kff.org/kaiserpolls/pomr022505nr.cfm

———. 2005b. Medicaid Enrollment and Spending Trends. www.kff.org/medicaid/upload/Medicaid-enrollment-and-spending-trends-fact-sheet .pdf

———. 2005c. The President's FY 2006 Budget Proposal: Overview and Briefing Charts. www.kff.org/uninsured/7294.cfm

———. 2005d. State Health Facts. www.statehealthfacts.org

———. 2005e. Trends and Indicators in the Changing Health Care Marketplace. Exhibit 1.7: Relative Contributions of Different Types of Health Services to Total Growth in National Health Expenditures, 1993–2003. Publication 7031. Feb. 17. www.kff.org/insurance/7031

Kaufman, Herbert. 1977. *Red Tape.* Washington, DC: Brookings Institution.

Kaufman, Marc. 2004. Study Cites Crestor Concerns. *Tallahassee Democrat,* May 24, 1A.

———. 2005. FDA Was Told of Viagra-Blindness Link Months Ago: Senator Criticizes DeLay in Alerting Consumers after Safety Officer Warned Agency about Drug. *Washington Post,* July 1, A2.

Kearns, Doris. 1976. *Lyndon Johnson and the American Dream.* New York: Harper and Row.

Keefe, William J. 1984. *Congress and the American People,* 2d ed. Englewood Cliffs, NJ: Prentice-Hall.

Keiser, K. Robert, and Woodrow Jones, Jr. 1986. Do the American Medical Association's Campaign Contributions Influence Health Care Legislation? *Medical Care* 24:761–66.

Kelly, Michael. 1993. David Gergen, Master of the Game. *New York Times Magazine,* Oct. 31, 62–71, 80, 94, 97.

Kelman, Steven. 1980. Occupational Safety and Health Administration. In *The Politics of Regulation,* ed. James Q. Wilson. New York: Basic Books.

Kennedy, Edward M. 2005. Perspective: The Role of the Federal Government in Eliminating Health Disparities: Strong Federal Action Is Crucial to Marshaling the Resources and Political Will to End Minority Health Disparities. *Health Affairs* 24 (2): 452–58.

Kenyon, Daphne A. 1996. Health Care Reform and Competition among the States. In *Health Policy, Federalism, and the American States,* ed. Robert F. Rich and William D. White. Washington, DC: Urban Institute Press.

Kernell, Samuel. 1984. The Presidency and the People. In *The Presidency and the Political System,* ed. Michael Nelson. Washington, DC: Congressional Quarterly Press.

———. 1991. Facing an Opposition Congress: The President's Strategic Circumstance. In *The Politics of Divided Government,* ed. Gary Cox and Samuel Kernell. Boulder, CO: Westview Press.

Kernell, Samuel, Peter W. Spelich, and Aaron Wildavsky. 1975. Public Support for Presidents. In *Perspectives on the Presidency,* ed. Aaron Wildavsky. Boston: Little, Brown.

Kersh, Rogan, and James Morone. 2002. The Politics of Obesity: Seven Steps to Government Action. *Health Affairs* 21 (6): 142–53.

Kerwin, Cornelius. M. 2003. *Rulemaking: How Government Agencies Write Law and Make Policy,* 3d ed. Washington, DC: CQ Press.

Kiewiet, Roderick, and Mathew McCubbins. 1991. *The Spending Power: Congress, the President, and the Appropriations Process.* Chicago: University of Chicago Press.

King, James D. 2000. Changes in Professionalism in U.S. State Legislatures. *Legislative Studies Quarterly* 25:327–43.

Kingdon, John. 1977. *Congressmen's Voting Decisions.* New York: Harper and Row.

———. 1995. *Agendas, Alternatives, and Public Policies,* 2d ed. New York: Harper Collins.

Knott, Jack, and Gary Miller. 1987. *Reforming Bureaucracy: The Politics of Institutional Choice.* Englewood Cliffs, NJ: Prentice-Hall.

Kollman, Ken. 1998. *Outside Lobbying: Public Opinion and Interest Group Strategies.* Princeton, NJ: Princeton University Press.

Kondracke, Morton M. 2001. AARP's Agenda at Odds with Bush Priorities. *Roll Call,* Feb. 19. www.rollcall.com

———. 2002. Congress Set to Aid Medicare Providers, Not Seniors—Why? *Roll Call,* June 20. www.rollcall.com

Kosterlitz, Julie. 1992. Survival Tactics. *National Journal,* Oct. 24, 2428–32.

———. 1994. The Big Sell. *National Journal,* May 14, 1118–23.

Kraft, Michael E., and Denise Scheberle. 1998. Environmental Federalism at Decade's End: New Approaches and Strategies. *Publius: The Journal of Federalism* 28 (1): 131–46.

Krane, Dale. 2003. The State of American Federalism 2002–03: Division Replaces Unity. *Publius: The Journal of Federalism.* 33 (1): 1–44.

Krane, Dale, and Heidi Koenig. 2005. The State of American Federalism, 2004: Is Federalism Still a Core Value? *Publius: The Journal of Federalism* 35 (1): 1–40.

Krause, Brendan. 2005. State Purchasing Pools for Prescription Drugs: What's Happening and How Do They Work? National Governors Association Center for Best Practices. www.nga.org/center/divisions/1,1188,C_ISSUE_BRIEF^D_7244,00.html

Krehbiel, Keith. 1992. *Information and Legislative Organization.* Ann Arbor: University of Michigan Press.

———. 1998. *Pivotal Politics: A Theory of U.S. Lawmaking.* Chicago: University of Chicago Press.

Kurtz, Howard. 1994a. Over Easy on the Opposition. *Washington Post National Weekly Edition,* Sept. 12–18, 24.

———. 1994b. Rolling with the Punches from the Press Corps. *Washington Post National Weekly Edition,* Jan. 24–30, 10.

Kurtz, Karl. 1989. State Legislatures in the 1990s. *Handbook on State Government Relations.* Washington, DC: Public Affairs Council.

———. 1990. The Public Standing of the Legislature. Paper presented at the Eagleton Institute of Politics Symposium on the Legislature in the Twenty-First Century, Williamsburg, VA, Apr. 27–29.

Lacy, Marc. 2000. Blocked by Congress, Clinton Wields a Pen. *New York Times,* July 5, A11.

Ladenheim, Kala. 1997. Health Insurance in Transition: The Health Insurance Portability and Accountability Act of 1996. *Publius: The Journal of Federalism* 27 (2): 33–51.

Lambert, David A., and Thomas McGuire. 1990. Political and Economic Determinants of Insurance Regulation in Mental Health. *Journal of Health Politics, Policy, and Law* 15:169–89.

Lamm, Richard D. 1990. The Ten Commandments of Health Care. In *The Nation's Health,* 3d ed., ed. P. R. Lee and C. L. Estes. Boston: Jones and Bartlett.

Lasker, Eric G. 2005. Position on Federal Preemption Consistent with Law and Public Health. *Legal Backgrounder* 20:9. www.web.lexis-nexis.com.proxy.lib.fsu.edu

Layton, Charles, and Mary Walton. 1998. Missing the Story at the Statehouse. *American Journalism Review,* July–Aug., 42–63.

Lee, Christopher. 2003. Medicare Bill Partly a Special Interest Care Package. *Washington Post,* Nov. 23, A11.

———. 2006. Bush Seeks to Increase Health Savings Accounts. *Washington Post,* Feb. 6, A13.

Leingang, Matt. 2005. States Revisit Universal Health Care. *Tallahassee Democrat,* July 10, 4A.

Lemov, Penelope. 1994. An Acute Case of Health Care Reform. *Governing* 7:44–50.

———. 2005. Setting Limits on Medicaid. *Governing,* Mar., 50.

Lewis, Neil A. 1994. Lobby for Small-Business Owners Puts Big Dent in Health Care Bill. *New York Times,* July 6, A1, A9.

Light, Paul. 1984. The Presidential Policy Stream. In *The Presidency and the Political System,* ed. Michael Nelson. Washington, DC: Congressional Quarterly Press.

———. 1991. *The President's Agenda: Domestic Policy Choice from Kennedy to Reagan,* rev. ed. Baltimore: Johns Hopkins University Press.

———. 1999. *The True Size of Government.* Washington, DC: Brookings Institution.

Lindblom, Charles. 1980. *The Policy-Making Process.* Englewood Cliffs, NJ: Prentice-Hall.

Lipman, Larry. 2004. Lawmakers Seek to Block Florida from Medicare Test. *Palm Beach Post,* Feb. 26, 5A.

Locker, Richard. 2005. A True Tennessee Titan. *State Legislatures* 31 (7): 56–59.

Lockhead, Carolyn. 2003. Prescription Benefit Clears Logjam: Feinstein, 21 Other Democrats Vote to Break Filibuster. *San Francisco Chronicle,* Nov. 25, A1, final edition.

Lohmann, Susanne. 1998. An Information Rationale for the Power of Special Interests. *American Political Science Review* 92:809–27.

Long, Norton E. 1949. Power and Administration. *Public Administration Review* 9:257–64.

Long, Stephen H. 1994. Prescription Drugs and the Elderly: Issues And Options. *Health Affairs,* spring (2): 157–74.

Loomis, Burdett A. 1988. *The New American Politician.* New York: Basic Books.

———. 1995. Organized Interests, Paid Advocacy, and the Scope of Conflict. Paper presented at the annual meeting of the Midwest Political Science Association, Chicago, Apr. 6–8.

Loven, Jennifer. 2005. Bush Says He Would Veto Changes to New Medicare Drug Plan. *Tallahassee Democrat,* Feb. 12, A4.

Lovern, Ed. 2002. Ready, Aim, Litigate: AHA Takes Feds to Court to Stop HHS from Eliminating Medicaid Loophole. *Modern Healthcare,* Mar. 11, 8–11.

Lowi, T. J. 1964. American Business, Public Policy, Case-Studies and Political Theory. *World Politics* 16:677–715.

———. 1969. *The End of Liberalism: Ideology, Policy, and the Crisis of Public Authority.* New York: Norton.

MacKuen, Michael B., and Calvin Mouw. 1992. The Strategic Configuration, Personal Influence, and Presidential Power in Congress. *Western Political Quarterly* 45:579–608.

Madison Capital Times. 2003. Retiree Group Facing Rebellion. Nov. 28, 3c.

Mann, Thomas E. 2005. Redistricting Reform. *National Voter* 54 (3): 4–6.

Marchione, Marilynn. 2005. Being Overweight Still Not Good. *Tallahassee Democrat,* June 3, 3A.

Marcus, Ruth. 1998. Big Tobacco Quietly Tries to Grow Grass Roots: Industry's Sophisticated Lobbying Tactics Strike Some Critics as Deceptive. *Washington Post,* May 16, A1.

Marini, John. 1992. *The Politics of Budget Control: Congress, the Presidency, and the Growth of the Administrative State.* Washington, DC: Crane, Russak.

Markowitz, Gerald, and David Rosner. 2004. Emergency Preparedness, Bioterrorism, and the States: The First Two Years after September 11. www.milbank.org/reports/SEPT110406/SEPT110406.html

Marmor, Theodore. 1970. *The Politics of Medicare*. Chicago: Aldine.

Martin, Andrew D. 2001. Congressional Decision Making and the Separation of Powers. *American Political Science Review* 95:361–78.

Martinez, Gebe, and Mary Agnew Carey. 2004. Erasing the Gender Gap Tops Republican Playbook. *CQ Weekly*, Mar. 6, 564–70.

Matherlee, Karen. 2000. HCFA's Outpatient PPS: Finally Ready to Roll? *National Health Policy Forum Issue Brief*, June 16.

Matlack, Carol, James A. Barnes, and Richard E. Cohen. 1990. Quid with Quo? *National Journal* 22:1473–74, 1479.

Mayer, Kenneth R. 2001. *With the Stroke of a Pen: Executive Orders and Presidential Power*. Princeton, NJ: Princeton University Press.

Mayhew, David. 1974. *Congress: The Electoral Connection*. New Haven, CT: Yale University Press.

———. 1987. The Electoral Connection and the Congress. In *Congress: Structure and Policy*, ed. Mathew McCubbins and Terry Sullivan. New York: Cambridge University Press.

———. 1991. *Divided We Govern: Party Control, Lawmaking, and Investigations, 1946–1990*. New Haven, CT: Yale University Press.

McCall, Nelda, and Thomas Rice. 1983. Factors Influencing Physician Assignment Decisions under Medicare. *Inquiry* 20:45–56.

McCoy, Kevin. 2000. Flurry of Regulations Set to Kick in as Clinton Exits: New Rules Affect Many Industries. *USA Today*, Nov. 27, 4B.

McCubbins, Mathew, and Thomas Schwartz. 1984. Congressional Oversight Overlooked: Police Patrols vs. Fire Alarms. *American Journal of Political Science* 28:165–79.

McCutcheon, Chuck. 2001. Unveiling a Bit Too Much. *CQ Weekly*, Mar. 3, 449.

McFarlane, Deborah R., and Kenneth J. Meier. 2001. *The Politics of Fertility Control: Family Planning and Abortion Policies in the American States*. New York: Chatham House.

McGinley, Laurie, Barbara Martinez, Leila Abboud, Vanessa Fuhrmans, Sarah Lueck, Peter Landers, and Matt Murray. 2003. A Guide to Who Wins and Loses in Medicare Bill. *Wall Street Journal*, Nov. 18, B1.

McGrory, Mary. 1999. The Corner on Caring. *Washington Post*, Aug. 26, A3.

McNeil, Donald G., Jr. and Alexei Barrionuevo. 2005. Washington's Handling of Mad Cow Tests Angers Ranchers and Consumers. *New York Times*, June 26, 16.

Medical News Today. 2005. Total Sales of Generic Drugs Surpass the Sales of Brand Name Drugs in US. July 24. medicalnewstoday.com

Meier, Kenneth. 1985. *Regulation: Politics, Bureaucracy, and Economics.* New York: St. Martin's.

Meinke, Scott R. 2005. Long-Term Change and Stability in House Voting Decisions: The Case of the Minimum Wage. *Legislative Studies Quarterly* 30:103–26.

Merrill, Richard A. 1999. Modernizing the FDA: An Incremental Revolution. *Health Affairs,* Mar.–Apr., 96–111.

Michigan Consumer Health Care Coalition. 2005. *Facts about Drug Advertising: Its Effectiveness and Impact* 5 (1): 2.

Milbank, Dana. 2003. Conservatives Criticize Bush on Spending: Medicare Bill Angers Some Allies. *Washington Post,* Dec. 6, A01, final edition.

Milbank Memorial Fund, the National Association of State Budget Officers, and the Reforming States Group. 2005. 2002–2003 State Health Expenditure Report. www.milbank.org/reports/05NASBO/index.html

Miller, Gary J. 1993. Formal Theory and the Presidency. In *Researching the Presidency,* ed. George C. Edwards III, John H. Kessel, and Bert A. Rockman. Pittsburgh: University of Pittsburgh Press.

Milwaukee Journal Sentinel. 2003. Legislators Break Bearing Grudges. Nov. 28, 2A.

Moe, Terry. 1985. The Politicized Presidency. In *The New Direction in American Politics,* ed. John E. Chubb and Paul E. Peterson. Washington, DC: Brookings Institution.

Mooney, Christopher Z. 2001. The Public Clash of Private Values. In *The Public Clash of Private Values: The Politics of Morality Policy,* ed. Christopher Z. Mooney. New York: Chatham House.

Morandi, Larry. 2005. Staying ahead of the Feds: EPA Proposes Cap-and-Trade to Cut Back on Mercury Emissions but Many States Think They Have a Quicker, Better Solution. *State Legislatures,* June, 14–17.

Morgan, Dan. 1994. The Medicaid Time Bomb. *Washington Post National Weekly Edition,* Feb. 7–13, 6–8.

Morone, James A. 1990. *The Democratic Wish: Popular Participation and the Limits of American Government.* New York: Basic Books.

———. 1993. The Health Care Bureaucracy: Small Changes, Big Consequences. *Journal of Health Politics, Policy, and Law* 18:723–39.

———. 1995. Nativism, Hollow Corporations, and Managed Competition: Why the Clinton Health Care Reform Failed. *Journal of Health Politics, Policy, and Law* 20:391–98.

Morone, James A., and Andrew B. Dunham. 1985. Slouching toward National Health Insurance: The New Health Care Politics. *Yale Journal on Regulation* 2:263–91.

Moy, Ernest, Elizabeth Dayton, and Carolyn M. Clancy. 2005. Compiling the Evidence: The National Healthcare Disparities Reports: These Important Reports Contribute to the Infrastructure Needed to Track Progress toward Eliminating Disparities. *Health Affairs* 24 (2): 376–87.

Mueller, Keith J. 1992. State Government Policies and Rural Hospitals: Facilitating Change. *Policy Studies Journal* 20:168–81.

Nathan, Richard P. 1983. *The Administrative Presidency.* New York: John Wiley.

———. 1993. *Turning Promises into Performance.* New York: Twentieth Century Fund.

Nather, David. 2004. Congress as Watchdog: Asleep on the Job? *CQ Weekly,* May 22, 1190–95.

National Association of State Budget Officers (NASBO). 2002. *Budget Processes in the States.* Washington, DC: NASBO. www.nasbo.org/Publications/PDFs/budpro2002.pdf

———. 2004. State Expenditures 2003. www.nasbo.org/Publications/PDFs/2003ExpendReport.pdf

National Bipartisan Commission on the Future of Medicare. 1999. Facts about the National Bipartisan Commission on the Future of Medicare. http://medicare.commission.gov

National Commission on the State and Local Public Service. 1993. *Frustrated Federalism: Rx for State and Local Health Care Reform.* Albany, NY: Nelson A. Rockefeller Institute of Government.

National Conference of State Legislatures (NCSL). 2005a. Recall of State Officials. www.ncsal.org/programs/legman/elect/recallprovision.htm

———. 2005b. State Medical Malpractice Reform: 2005 Numbers at a Glance. www.ncsl.org/standcomm/sclaw.medmalataglance.htm

———. 2005c. The Term Limited States. www.ncsl.org/programs/legman/about/states.htm

National Governors Association (NGA). 2002. Addressing the Medical Malpractice Insurance Crisis. *Issue Brief,* Dec. 5.

———. 2005. Medicaid Reform: A Preliminary Report. June 15. www.nga.org

National Institutes of Health (NIH). 2005. Institutes, Centers and Offices. www.nih.gov/icd

National Journal. 2005. Helping the Poor, Polishing the Image. Apr. 9. www.nationaljournal.com.proxy.lib.umich.edu

National Public Radio. 2000. *Morning Edition.* Nov. 3. www.npr.org

NBC News/Wall Street Journal Survey. 2005. http://online.wsj.com/public/resources/media/pol120050518.pdf

Nelson, Suzanne. 2000. Brooks Voted out but Not Silenced. *Roll Call,* Dec. 14. http://rollcall.com

Neustadt, Richard E. 1960. *Presidential Power.* New York: John Wiley.

———. 1990. *Presidential Power and the Modern Presidents.* New York: Free Press.

New, Michael J. 2005. Analyzing the Impact of State Level Anti-Abortion Legislation in the Post-Casey Era. Paper presented at the annual meeting of the Midwest Political Science Association, Chicago, Apr. 7–10.

Nexon, David. 1987. The Politics of Congressional Health Policy in the Second Half of the 1980s. *Medical Care Review* 44:65–88.

Noah, Timothy. 1993. AMA Lavishly Courts Congressional Staffers Who Will Affect Outcome of Clinton's Health Plan. *Wall Street Journal,* June 30, A16.

Norrander, Barbara, and Clyde Wilcox. 2001. Public Opinion and Policymaking in the States: The Case of Post-Roe Abortion Policy. In *The Public Clash of Private Values: The Politics of Morality Policy,* ed. Christopher Z. Mooney. New York: Chatham House.

Office of the Clerk, U.S. House of Representatives. 2005. Congressional History. http://clerk.house.gov/histHigh/Congressional>History/index.html

Office of Management and Budget (OMB). 2000. *A Citizen's Guide to the Federal Budget, Budget of the United States Government, Fiscal Year 2001.* Chart 2-3: The Federal Government Dollar—Where It Comes From. Washington, DC: OMB. www.access.gov/usbudget

———. 2005. The Budget for Fiscal Year 2006, Historical Tables. www.whitehouse.gov/omb/budget/fy2006/pdf/hist.pdf

O'Leary, Rosemary. 1989. The Impact of Federal Court Decisions on the Policies and Administration of the U.S. Environmental Protection Agency. *Administrative Law Review* 41:549–76.

Oleszek, Walter J. 1989. *Congressional Procedures and the Policy Process,* 3d ed. Washington, DC: Congressional Quarterly Press.

———. 2004. *Congressional Procedures and the Policy Process,* 6th ed. Washington, DC: CQ Press.

Oliver, Thomas, and Pam Paul-Shaheen. 1997. Translating Ideas into Actions: Entrepreneurial Leadership in State Health Care Reforms. *Journal of Health Politics, Policy, and Law* 22:721–83.

Olson, Mancur, Jr. 1968. *The Logic of Collective Action.* New York: Schocken.

OMB Director Lew Calls GOP Budget a "Bankrupt Approach," Threatens Vetoes. 2000. *Tax Management Financial Planning Journal,* May 16, 137–38.

Oppenheimer, Bruce I. 2005. Deep Red and Blue Congressional Districts: The Causes and Consequences of Declining Party Competitiveness. In *Congress Reconsidered*, 8th ed., ed. Lawrence C. Dodd and Bruce I. Oppenheimer. Washington, DC: CQ Press.

Ornstein, Norman. 2004. Lobbyists Often Get More Shakedowns Than They Give. *Roll Call*, Feb. 25. www.rollcall.com

Ornstein, Norman J., Thomas E. Mann, and Michael J. Malbin. 2002. *Vital Statistics on Congress 2001–2002*. Washington, DC: AEI Press.

Ostrom, Elinor. 1999. Institutional Rational Choice: An Assessment of the Institutional Analysis and Development Framework. In *Theories of the Policy Process*, ed. Paul A. Sabatier. Boulder, CO: Westview Press.

Pal, Leslie A., and R. Kent Weaver. 2003. Conclusions. In *The Government Taketh Away: The Politics of Pain in the United States and Canada*, ed. Leslie A. Pal and R. Kent Weaver. Washington, DC: Georgetown University Press.

Parker, Glenn. 1989. *Characteristics of Congress*. Englewood Cliffs, NJ: Prentice-Hall.

Patterson, Samuel. 1983. Legislators and Legislatures in the American States. In *Politics in the American States*, 4th ed., ed. Virginia Gray, Herbert Jacob, and Kenneth Vines. Boston: Little, Brown.

Patterson, Thomas E. 2003. *The American Democracy*. Columbus, OH: McGraw-Hill Higher Education.

Paul-Sheehan, Pamela. 1998. The States and Health Care Reform: The Road Traveled and Lessons Learned from Seven That Took the Lead. *Journal of Health Politics, Policy, and Law* 23:319–61.

Pear, Robert. 1993. Drug Industry Gathers a Mix of Voices to Bolster Its Case. *New York Times*, July 7, A1, A6.

———. 1994. Report Criticizes the Objectivity of the Federal Watchdog Agency. *New York Times*, Oct. 17, A1.

———. 1996. U.S. Shelves Plan to Limit Rewards to H.M.O. Doctors. *New York Times*, July 8, A1.

———. 1997. Battle Lines Form in Medicare Fight. *New York Times*, May 27, A1.

———. 1998. Congress Alarmed at Failure of Medicare to Bring Change. *New York Times*, Sept. 27, 1, 24.

———. 1999. Ruling on Medicare Splits White House. *New York Times*, Jan. 21, A22.

———. 2000a. Clinton to Order Medicare to Pay New Costs. *New York Times*, June 7. www.nytimes.com

———. 2000b. Drug Company Executives Drop Opposition to Medicare Coverage of Prescription Drugs. *New York Times*, Jan. 14. www.nytimes.com

———. 2000c. One Step at a Time, Clinton Seeks More Help for Poor and Elderly. *New York Times,* Feb. 7. www.nytimes.com

———. 2000d. White House Raises Expected Cost of Medicare Drug Plan. *New York Times,* Feb. 10. www.nytimes.com

———. 2003a. Bill on Medicare Drug Benefit Is Stalled by House-Senate Republican Antagonism. *New York Times,* Aug. 27, 15.

———. 2003b. Drug Companies Increase Spending to Lobby Congress and Governments, *New York Times,* June 1.

———. 2003c. Florida Elderly Feel Let Down by Medicare Drug Benefit. *New York Times,* Nov. 30, 1.34, late edition, East Coast.

———. 2004a. Bush's Aides Put Higher Price Tag on Medicare Law. *New York Times,* Jan. 30, A1.

———. 2004b. In a Shift, Bush Moves to Block Medical Suits. *New York Times,* July 25, A1.

———. 2005a. Cost-Cutting Medicare Law Is a Money Loser for States. *New York Times,* Mar. 25, A12.

———. 2005b. Judge Blocks Rule Allowing Companies to Cut Benefits When Retirees Reach Medicare Age. *New York Times,* Mar. 31, A14.

———. 2005c. Panel Seeks Better Disciplining of Doctors. *New York Times,* Jan. 5, A21.

———. 2005d. States Rejecting Demand to Pay for Medicare Cost. *New York Times,* July 4, A9.

———. 2006. Slowing the Growth of Medicare. *New York Times,* Feb. 7, A1.

Pear, Robert, and James Dao. 2004. States Trying New Tactics to Reduce Spending on Drugs. *New York Times,* Nov. 21, 27.

Pear, Robert, and Carl Hulse. 2003. A Final Push in Congress: The Overview: Senate Removes Two Roadblocks to Drug Benefit. *New York Times,* Nov. 24, A1, A17.

Pear, Robert, and Michael Janofsky. 2003. Broad Bills Stuffed with Lawmakers' Pet Items. *New York Times,* Nov. 28, 7.

Perine, Keith. 2004. "Heightened Tensions" Fray Judicial-Legislative Relations. *CQ Weekly,* Sept. 13, 2148–53.

Pershing, Ben, Erin P. Billings, and Emily Pierce. 2003. Drug Votes Open Rifts. *Roll Call,* June 30. www.rollcall.com

Peters, B. Guy. 1981. The Problem of Bureaucratic Government. *Journal of Politics* 43:56–82.

Peters, Charles. 1994. Tilting at Windmills. *Washington Monthly* 26 (Jan.–Feb.): 5.

Peterson, Mark. 1990. *Legislating Together: The White House and Capitol Hill from Eisenhower to Reagan.* Cambridge, MA: Harvard University Press.

——. 2000. Clinton and Organized Interests: Splitting Friends, Unifying Enemies. In *The Clinton Legacy*, ed. Colin Campbell and Bert A. Rockman. New York: Chatham House.

Peterson, Paul. 1995. *The Price of Federalism*. Washington, DC: Brookings Institution.

Petracca, Mark. 1992. The Future of an Interest Group Society. In *The Politics of Interests: Interest Groups Transformed*, ed. Mark Petracca. Boulder, CO: Westview Press.

Pfiffner, James P. 1987. Political Appointees and Career Executives: The Democracy-Bureaucracy Nexus in the Third Century. *Public Administration Review* 47:57–65.

PhRMA. 2004a. Cost-Sharing Trends for Medicines in Managed Care Plans: Copayments Increasing at a Much Faster Rate than Prescription Prices. www.phrma.org

——. 2004b. In the Courts: Overview. www.phrma.org/issues/courts

Pierson, Paul, 2000. The Limits of Design: Explaining Institutional Origins and Change. *Governance: An International Journal of Policy and Administration* 13:475–99.

Pollan, Michael. 2002. *The Botany of Desire: A Plant's-Eye View of the World*. New York: Random House.

PollingReport. 2005. ABC News/Washington Post Poll. www.pollingreport.com/BushJob.htm

Poole, Isaiah J. 2004. Party Unity Vote Study: Votes Echo Electoral Themes. *CQ Weekly*, Dec. 11, 2906–8.

Posner, Paul. 1997. Unfunded Mandates Reform Act: 1996 and Beyond. *Publius: The Journal of Federalism* 27 (2): 53–71.

Preston, Mark. 2000. Senate Still Tied in Knots. *Roll Call*, May 22. www.rollcall.com

Price, David E. 1971. Professionals and "Entrepreneurs": Staff Orientations and Policy Making on Three Senate Committees. *Journal of Politics* 33:316–36.

——. 1978. Policy Making in Congressional Committees: The Impact of "Environmental" Factors. *American Political Science Review* 72:548–74.

Price, Raymond. 1977. *With Nixon*. New York: Viking Press.

Priest, Dana, and David S. Broder. 1994. The Pen as a Mighty Sword. *Washington Post National Weekly Edition*, Jan. 31–Feb. 6, 11.

Publius [Alexander Hamilton, James Madison, and John Jay]. [1787–88] 1961. *The Federalist Papers*. New York: New American Library.

Pugh, Tony. 2005. Ex-Cabinet Official Slams White House. *Tallahassee Democrat*, Mar. 25, 4A.

Purdum, Todd S. 2000. A New Player Enters the Campaign Spending Fray. *New York Times,* Apr. 2. www.nytimes.com

Quirk, Paul. 1981. *Industry Influence in Federal Regulatory Agencies.* Princeton, NJ: Princeton University Press.

Quirk, Paul J., and William Cunion. 2000. Clinton's Domestic Policy: The Lessons of a "New Democrat." In *The Clinton Legacy,* ed. Colin Campbell and Bert A. Rockman. New York: Chatham House.

Rabe, Barry G. 2004. *Statehouse and Greenhouse: The Emerging Politics of American Climate Change Policy.* Washington, DC: Brookings Institution.

Ratan, Suneel. 1993. How to Really Cut the Budget Deficit. *Fortune,* Oct. 4, 101–4.

Rawls, John. 1971. *A Theory of Justice.* Cambridge, MA: Harvard University Press.

Regenstein, Marsha, and Jennifer Huang. 2005. Stresses to the Safety Net: The Public Hospital Perspective. Kaiser Commission on Medicaid and the Uninsured. www.kff.org/medicaid

Reilly, Patrick. 2002. Special Treatment: The CHA Says It's Leading the Fight for All Not-for-Profit Hospitals to Receive Fair Compensation for Being Nation's Healthcare Safety Net. *Modern Healthcare,* Nov. 18, 8.

Relman, Arnold. 1980. The New Medical-Industrial Complex. *New England Journal of Medicine* 303:963–70.

Rice, Thomas. 1998. *The Economics of Health Reconsidered.* Chicago: Health Administration Press.

Rich, Robert F., and William D. White. 1996. Health Care Policy and the American States: Issues of Federalism. In *Health Policy, Federalism, and the American States,* ed. Robert F. Rich and William D. White. Washington, DC: Urban Institute Press.

Riddlesperger, James W., Jr. 2005. Redistricting Politics in Texas 2003. Paper presented at the meeting of the Southern Political Science Association, New Orleans, Jan. 8–10.

Ripley, Randall B., and Grace A. Franklin. 1986. *Policy Implementation and Bureaucracy,* 2d ed. Chicago: Dorsey Press.

Rivers, Douglas, and Nancy L. Rose. 1985. Passing the President's Program: Public Opinion and Presidential Influence in Congress. *American Journal of Political Science* 29:183–96.

Robinson, Chester A. 1991. *The Bureaucracy and the Legislative Process: A Case Study of the Health Care Financing Administration.* Lanham, MD: University Press of America.

Rochefort, David A., and Roger W. Cobb. 1994. *The Politics of Problem Definition.* Lawrence: University Press of Kansas.

Rockman, Bert. 1984. Legislative-Executive Relations and Legislative Oversight. *Legislative Studies Quarterly* 9:387–440.

Rogers, David. 1999. Speaking Up: Hastert Finds Leading in House Isn't the Same as Being in Charge—GOP Rifts, Tough Rivals, and His Own Low Profile Have Bred Frustration—The Budget Brings Limelight. *Wall Street Journal,* Nov. 8, A1.

Rohde, David. 1990. Divided Government, Agenda Change, and Variations in Presidential Support in the House. Paper presented at a conference in honor of William H. Riker, Rochester, NY, Oct. 12–13.

———. 1991. *Parties and Leaders in the Postreform House.* Chicago: University of Chicago Press.

Rohde, David, and Dennis Simon. 1985. Presidential Vetoes and Congressional Response: A Study of Institutional Conflict. *American Journal of Political Science* 29:397–427.

Roll Call. 2003. BCRA Half-Full. Dec. 15. www.rollcall.com

Romano, Michael. 2003. 100 Most Powerful. *Modern Healthcare,* Aug. 25, 6.

Romer, Thomas, and James Snyder. 1994. An Empirical Investigation of the Dynamics of PAC Contributions. *American Journal of Political Science* 38:745–69.

Rosenberg, Gerald N. 1991. *The Hollow Hope: Can Courts Bring about Social Change?* Chicago: University of Chicago Press.

Rosenblatt, Rand E. 1993. The Courts, Health Care Reform, and the Reconstruction of American Social Legislation. *Journal of Health Politics, Policy, and Law* 18:439–76.

Rosenblatt, Roger. 1994. How Do Tobacco Executives Live with Themselves? *New York Times Magazine,* Mar. 20, 34–41, 55, 73–74, 76.

Rosenbloom, David H. 1981. The Judicial Response to the Bureaucratic State. *American Review of Public Administration* 50:29–51.

Rosenheck, R., P. Gallup, and C. A. Leda. 1991. Vietnam Era and Vietnam Combat Veterans among the Homeless. *American Journal of Public Health* 81:643–46.

Rosenthal, Alan. 1993. *The Third House: Lobbyists and Lobbying in the States.* Washington, DC: Congressional Quarterly Press.

———. 2004. *Heavy Lifting: The Job of the American Legislature.* Washington, DC: CQ Press.

Rosenthal, Elisabeth, 1997. US to Pay New York Hospitals Not to Train Doctors, Easing Glut. *New York Times,* Feb. 18, A1.

Ross, Sonya. 1994. AARP Members Irate when Leaders Back Bills. *Ann Arbor News,* Aug. 12, A2.

Roth, Bennett. 2005. Experts Sound Medicare Alarm. *Houston Chronicle,* Feb. 6, 1.

Rourke, Francis. 1984. *Bureaucracy, Politics, and Public Policy,* 3d ed. Boston: Little, Brown.

———. 1991. American Bureaucracy in a Changing Political Setting. *Journal of Public Administration Research and Theory* 2:111–29.

Rubin, Alissa. 1993. Special Interests Stampede to Be Heard on Overhaul. *Congressional Quarterly,* May 1, 1081–84.

———. 1999. Business Joins Fight against Health Reform: Legislation: Lawmakers Can Expect a Full-Court Press by Lobbyists Who Fear Passage of a Patients' Bill of Rights in Congress. *Los Angeles Times,* Aug. 8, A1.

Rudder, Catherine E. 2005. The Politics of Taxing and Spending in Congress. In *Congress Reconsidered,* 8th ed., ed. Lawrence C. Dodd and Bruce L. Oppenheimer. Washington, DC: CQ Press.

Ruethling, Gretchen. 2005. 5 Drug-Importing States Add 2 Countries as Source. *New York Times,* July 19, A15.

Ryan, Jennifer, and Nora Super. 2003. Dually Eligible for Medicare and Medicaid: Two for One or Double Jeopardy? *National Health Policy Forum Issue Brief,* Sept. 30.

Sabatier, Paul, and Hank Jenkins-Smith. 1988. Special Issue: Policy Changes and Policy-Oriented Learning: Exploring an Advocacy Coalition Framework. *Policy Sciences* 21:123–278.

———. 1993. *Policy Change and Learning: An Advocacy Approach.* Boulder, CO: Westview Press.

Sabato, Larry. 1985. *PAC Power.* New York: W. W. Norton.

———. 1991. *Feeding Frenzy: How Attack Journalism Has Transformed American Politics.* New York: Free Press.

Salamon, Lester M., and Alan J. Abramson. 1984. Governance: The Politics of Retrenchment. In *The Reagan Record,* ed. John L. Palmer and Isabel V. Sawhill. Washington, DC: Urban Institute Press.

Salant, Jonathan D. 1998. No Expense Spared to Defeat Patients' Bill of Rights. *Buffalo News,* Nov. 29, 12A.

Salisbury, Robert H. 1969. An Exchange Theory of Interest Groups. *Midwest Journal of Political Science* 13:1–32.

———. 1992. *Interests and Institutions: Substance and Structure in American Politics.* Pittsburgh: University of Pittsburgh Press.

Salisbury, Robert H., John P. Heinz, Edward O. Laumann, and Robert L. Nelson. 1987. Who Works with Whom? Interest Group Alliances and Opposition. *American Political Science Review* 81:1217–34.

Salisbury, Robert, and Kenneth Shepsle. 1981. U.S. Congressman as Enterprise. *Legislative Studies Quarterly* 6:559–76.

Sanford, Terry. 1967. *Storm over the States.* New York: McGraw-Hill.

Savage, David. 2001. Judgment Call: The Supreme Court Steps In. *State Legislatures,* Feb. 21–23.

Schattschneider, E. E. 1960. *The Semi-sovereign People.* New York: Holt, Rinehart, and Winston.

Schatz, Joseph J. 2004. Presidential Support Vote Study: With a Deft and Light Touch, Bush Finds Ways to Win. *CQ Weekly,* Dec. 11, 2900–2904.

Schatz, Tom, and Leslie Paige. 1997. Politics Trumps Science at the FDA. *Wall Street Journal,* July 21.

Scheberle, Denise. 2005. The Evolving Matrix of Environmental Federalism and Intergovernmental Relationships. *Publius: The Journal of Federalism* 36 (1): 69–86.

Schickler, Eric, and Kathryn Pearson. 2005. The House Leadership in an Era of Partisan Warfare. In *Congress Reconsidered,* 8th ed., ed. Lawrence C. Dodd and Bruce I. Oppenheimer. Washington, DC: CQ Press.

Schlesinger, Joseph A. 1966. *Ambition and Politics.* Chicago: Rand McNally.

———. 1985. The New American Political Party. *American Political Science Review* 79:1152–69.

Schlesinger, Mark. 1997. Paradigms Lost: The Persisting Search for Community in U.S. Health Policy. *Journal of Health Politics, Policy, and Law* 22:937–92.

Schlesinger, Mark, and Richard R. Lau. 2000. The Meaning and Measure of Policy Metaphors. *American Political Science Review* 94:611–26.

Schon, Donald. 1971. *Beyond the Stable State: Public and Private Learning in a Changing Society.* Hammondsworth, UK: Penguin.

Schorr, Daniel. 2003. The Best Politics Money Can Buy. *Christian Science Monitor,* Nov. 28, 11.

Schram, Sanford, and Carol S. Weissert. 1999. The State of U.S. Federalism: 1998–1999. *Publius: The Journal of Federalism* 29 (2): 1–34.

Schuler, Kate. 2004a. Challenged Estimates of Benefit's Cost Worry Medicare Drug Law Backers. *CQ Weekly,* Mar. 27, 750–51.

———. 2004b. Weighing Promise and Perils of Drug Importation. *CQ Weekly,* July 24, 1788–91.

Schuler, Kate, and Mary Agnes Carey. 2004. Estimates, Ethics and Ads Tarnish Medicare Overhaul. *CQ Weekly,* Mar. 20, 699–701.

Schull, Steven A. 1989. *The President and Civil Rights Policy: Leadership and Change.* Westport, CT: Greenwood Press.

Scott, Ruth K., and Ronald J. Hrebenar. 1979. *Parties in Crisis.* New York: Wiley and Sons.

Seelye, Katharine Q. 1994. Lobbyists Are the Loudest in the Health Care Debate. *New York Times,* Aug. 16, A1, A10.

Segal, David. 1994. A House Divided. *Washington Monthly,* Jan.–Feb., 23–32.

Shepsle, Kenneth A. 1991. Penultimate Power: Conference Committees and the Legislative Process. In *Home Style and Washington Work,* ed. Morris P. Fiorina and David W. Rohde. Ann Arbor: University of Michigan Press.

Shepsle, Kenneth A., and Barry R. Weingast. 1984. Legislative Politics and Budget Outcomes. In *Federal Budget Policy in the 1980s,* ed. Gregory Mills and John Palmer. Washington, DC: Urban Institute Press.

———. 1987. The Institutional Foundations of Committee Power. *American Political Science Review* 81:85–104.

———. 1994. Positive Theories of Congressional Institutions. *Legislative Studies Quarterly* 19:149–79.

Shields, Gerard. 2004. Tauzin Takes Pharmacy Industry Post. *Advocate* (Baton Rouge), Dec. 16, 1B.

Sigelman, Lee, and Roland E. Smith. 1980. Consumer Legislation in the American States: An Attempt at Explanation. *Social Science Quarterly* 61:58–70.

Sigelman, Lee, P. Roder, and C. Sigelman. 1981. Social Service Innovation in the American States: Deinstitutionalization of the Mentally Retarded. *Social Science Quarterly* 62:503–15.

Silver, George A. 1991. The Route to a National Health Policy Lies through the States. *Yale Journal of Biology and Medicine* 64:443–53.

Simon, Herbert. 1945. *Administrative Behavior: A Study of Decision-Making Processes in Administration Organization.* New York: Free Press.

———. 1960. *The New Science of Management Decision.* New York: Harper and Row.

———. 1976. *Administrative Behavior: A Study of Decision-Making Processes in Administration Organization,* 2d ed. New York: Free Press.

Sinclair, Barbara. 1989. *The Transformation of the U.S. Senate.* Baltimore: Johns Hopkins University Press.

———. 1997. *Unorthodox Lawmaking: New Legislative Processes in the U.S. Congress.* Washington, DC: CQ Press.

———. 2005. The New World of U.S. Senators. In *Congress Reconsidered,* 8th ed., ed. Lawrence C. Dodd and Bruce I. Oppenheimer. Washington, DC: CQ Press.

Skocpol, Theda. 1992. *Protecting Soldiers and Mothers: The Political Origins of Social Policy in the United States.* Cambridge, MA: Harvard University Press.

———. 1996. *Boomerang: Health Care Reform and the Turn against Government.* New York: W. W. Norton.

Skrzycki, Cindy. 2000a. The Regulators: Paying by the Rules, OMB's Cost Analyses Questioned. *Washington Post*, Feb. 4, E1.

———. 2000b. The Regulators: System Overhaul? Business Groups Hope for a New Era. *Washington Post*, Dec. 19, E1.

Smith, David G. 2002. *Entitlement Politics: Medicare and Medicaid 1995–2001.* New York: Aldine de Gruyter.

Smith, Hedrick. 1988. *The Power Game: How Washington Works.* New York: Random House.

Smith, R. Jeffrey. 2003. GOP's Pressing Question on Medicare Vote: Did Some Go Too Far To Change a No to a Yes? *Washington Post*, Dec. 23, A01, final edition.

Smith, Richard A. 1995. Interest Group Influence in the U.S. Congress. *Legislative Studies Quarterly* 20:89–139.

Smith, Steven, and Christopher Deering. 1990. *Committees in Congress*, 2d ed. Washington, DC: Congressional Quarterly Press.

Snyder, James M., Jr., and Tim Groseclose. 2000. Estimating Party Influence in Congressional Roll-Call Voting. *American Journal of Political Science* 44:193–211.

Sonner, Molly W., and Clyde Wilcox. 1999. Forgiving and Forgetting: Public Support for Bill Clinton during the Lewinsky scandal. *PS* 32 (554–57): 294.

Spake, Amanda. 2004. A Sick Agency in Need of a Cure? *U.S. News and World Report*, Dec. 13, 32–36.

Sparer, Michael. 1996. *Medicaid and the Limits of State Health Reform.* Philadelphia: Temple University Press.

Sparer, Michael, and Lawrence D. Brown. 1993. Between a Rock and a Hard Place: How Public Managers Manage Medicaid. In *Revitalizing State and Local Public Service*, ed. Frank J. Thompson. San Francisco: Jossey-Bass.

Spitzer, Robert J. 1983. *The Presidency and Public Policy: The Four Arenas of Presidential Power.* Tuscaloosa: University of Alabama Press.

Starr, Paul. 1982. *The Social Transformation of American Medicine.* New York: Basic Books.

StatePublicHealth.org. 2005. State Health Agency Profile Database. www.statepublichealth.org

Stein, M. Robert, and N. Kenneth Bickers. 1995. *Perpetuating the Pork Barrel: Policy Subsystems and American Democracy.* New York: Cambridge University Press.

Steinmo, Sven, and Jon Watts. 1995. It's the Institutions Stupid! Why Comprehensive National Health Insurance Always Fails in America. *Journal of Health Politics, Policy, and Law* 20:329–72.

Stevenson, Richard W. 2005. For This President, Power Is There for the Taking. *New York Times*, May 15, 3.

Stolberg, Sheryl Gay. 1998. A Surge in Herbal Remedies Pulls Drug Regulators' Gaze. *New York Times*, June 10, A1, A18.

———. 2002a. After Impasse, F.D.A. May Fill Top Job. *New York Times*, Sept. 25, A18.

———. 2002b. Bush Urges a Cap on Medical Liability. *New York Times*, July 26, A16.

———. 2003a. Drug Lobby Pushed Letter by Senators on Medicare. *New York Times*, July 30, A13.

———. 2003b. An 800-Pound Gorilla Changes Partners over Medicare. *New York Times*, Nov. 23, 4–5.

———. 2003c. Vaccine Liability Compromise Collapses. *New York Times*, Apr. 10, A17.

Stolberg, Sheryl Gay, and Milt Freudenheim. 2003. AARP Support Came as Group Grew "Younger." *New York Times*, Nov. 26, A1, late edition, East Coast.

Stone, Deborah A. 1988. *Policy Paradox and Political Reason*. Glenview, IL: Scott Foresman.

———. 1989. Causal Stories and the Formation of Policy Agendas. *Political Science Quarterly* 104:281–300.

———. 1993. The Struggle for the Soul of Health Insurance. *Journal of Health Politics, Policy, and Law* 18:287–317.

Stone, Peter H. 1994. Back Off! *National Journal* 26 (Dec. 3): 2840–44.

Sullivan, Terry. 1987. Presidential Leadership in Congress: Security Commitments. In *Congress: Structure and Policy*, ed. Mathew McCubbins and Terry Sullivan. Cambridge: Cambridge University Press.

———. 1991. The Bank Account Presidency: A New Measure and Evidence on the Temporal Path of Presidential Influence. *American Journal of Political Science* 35:686–723.

Suro, Robert. 1992. Report of AIDS Unsettles a Town. *New York Times*, Feb. 19, A15.

Swoboda, Frank, and Martha M. Hamilton. 1994. The War on Workplace Smoke Goes Nationwide. *Washington Post*, Sept. 18, H1.

Tackett, Michael. 2005. The Business of Influence in Washington. *Chicago Tribune*, Apr. 10, 1, 17.

Tannenwald, Robert. 1998. Implications of the Balanced Budget Act of 1997 for the "Devolution Revolution." *Publius: The Journal of Federalism* 28 (1): 23–48.

Tanner, Robert. 2005. Legislatures to Teenagers: Hang Up and Drive. *Tallahassee Democrat,* June 26, 6A.

Taylor, Andrew J. 1998. Domestic Agenda Setting 1947–1994. *Legislative Studies Quarterly* 23:373–97.

———. 2003. Medicare Bill's True Cost a Study in Guesswork. *CQ Weekly.* Oct. 25. http://library.cqpress.com/index.php

———. 2004. Denied Their Smoke and Mirrors, Appropriators Hold to Limits. *CQ Weekly,* Nov. 27, 2778–80.

———. 2005a. Chambers Spar over Spending Panels. *CQ Weekly,* Feb. 7, 306–7.

———. 2005b. Deficit Hues Still Grim and Grimmer. *CQ Weekly,* Jan. 31, 245.

———. 2005c. GOP's Tough Talk on Deficit up against Costly Realities. *CQ Weekly,* Jan. 17:106–11.

Thaemert, Rita. 1994. Twenty Percent and Climbing. *State Legislatures* 20:28–32.

Thomas, Helen. 1999. *Front Row at the White House: My Life and Times.* New York: Scribner.

Thompson, Frank J. 1983. *Health Policy and the Bureaucracy.* Cambridge, MA: MIT Press.

———. 2001. Federalism and Health Care Policy: Towards Redefinition? In *The New Politics of State Health Policy,* ed. Robert Hackey and David Rochefort. Lawrence: University Press of Kansas.

Thorpe, Kenneth E. 2000. A Comparison of Vice-President Gore's Medicare Drug Proposal and Governor Bush's Immediate Helping Hand Medicare Prescription Drug Proposal. Emory University. Sept. 22. www.sph.emory.edu/hpm/gore-bradley/gorebush6.htm (1 of 4)

Tierney, John T. 1987. Organized Interests in Health Politics and Policy-Making. *Medical Care Review* 44:89–118.

Toner, Robin. 1994. Gold Rush Fever Grips Capital as Health Care Struggle Begins. *New York Times,* Mar. 13, 1, 10.

———. 2003. An Imperfect Compromise. *New York Times,* Nov. 25, A1.

Toner, Robin, and Robert Pear. 2003. Bush Seeks Medicare Drug Bill That Conservatives Oppose. *New York Times,* June 23, A18.

Torres-Gil, Fernando. 1989. The Politics of Catastrophic and Long-Term Care Coverage. *Journal of Aging and Social Policy* 1:61–86.

Truman, David B. 1951. *The Governmental Process: Political Interests and Public Opinion.* New York: Knopf.

U.S. Census Bureau. 2005. *Statistical Abstract of the United States 2004–2005.* Washington, DC: Government Printing Office.

Ullman, Frank, Ian Hill, and Ruth Almeida. 1999. *CHIP: A Look at Emerging State Programs.* Washington, DC: Urban Institute.

VandeHei, Jim, and Juliet Eilperin. 2003. Drug Firms Gain Church Group's Aid: Claim about Import Measure Stirs Anger. *Washington Post,* July 23, A01. www.washingtonpost.com

Vergari, Sandra. 2001. Morality Politics and the Implementation of Abstinence-Only Sex Education: A Case of Policy Compromise. In *The Public Clash of Private Values: The Politics of Morality Politics,* ed. Christopher Z. Mooney. New York: Chatham House.

Von Drehle, David. 2003. New Ground for GOP, with Kennedy's Unlikely Aid. *Washington Post,* Dec. 9, A08, final edition.

Wald, Matthew L. 2005. Senate Version of Bill Pushes States to Adopt Stiff Drunken Driving Penalties. *New York Times,* June 17, A11.

Wald, Matthew L., and Steve Greenhouse. 2000. E.P.A. Institutes Water Regulations before a Bill Blocking Them Becomes Law. *New York Times,* July 12, A14.

Waldo, Dwight. 1955. *The Study of Administration.* New York: Random House.

Walker, David B. 2000. *The Rebirth of Federalism: Slouching toward Washington,* 2d ed. New York: Chatham House.

Walker, David M. 2004. GAO Answers the Question: What's in a Name? *Roll Call,* July 19. http://rollcall.com

Walker, Jack. 1969. The Diffusion of Innovations among the American States. *American Political Science Review* 63:880–99.

———. 1991. *Mobilizing Interest Groups in America.* Ann Arbor: University of Michigan Press.

Wawro, Gregory. 2000. *Legislative Entrepreneurship in the U.S. House of Representatives.* Ann Arbor: University of Michigan Press.

Wehr, Elizabeth. 1984. House Passes Drug Bill That Could Cut Costs. *CQ Weekly,* Sept. 8, 2184–88.

Weingast, Barry, and Mark Moran. 1983. Bureaucratic Discretion or Congressional Control? Regulatory Policymaking by the Federal Trade Commission. *Journal of Political Economy* 91:765–800.

Weise, Elizabeth. 2002. FDA Tries to Remove Genetic Label before It Sticks. *USA Today,* Oct. 9, D7.

Weisman, Jonathan. 2003. Prescription Bill Fuels Lobbying Blitz on Hill: Competition Fierce for $400 Billion Pot. *Washington Post,* June 13, A6.

Weisman, Jonathan, and Jim VandeHei. 2005. Road Bill Reflects the Power of the Pork. *Washington Post,* Aug. 11, A1.

Weissert, Carol S. 1992. Medicaid in the 1990s: Trends, Innovations, and the Future of the "PAC-Man" of State Budgets. *Publius: The Journal of Federalism* 22 (3): 93–109.

———. 1994. Beyond the Organization: The Influence of Community and Personal Values on Street-Level Bureaucrats' Responsiveness. *Journal of Public Administration Research and Theory* 4:225–54.

Weissert, Carol S., and Malcolm L. Goggin. 2000. *Fire, Ready, Aim: The Politics and Implementation of Michigan's Medicaid Managed Care Program.* Albany, NY: Rockefeller Institute of Government.

Weissert, Carol S., Jack H. Knott, and Blair S. Stieber. 1994. Education and the Health Professions: Explaining Policy Choice. *Journal of Health Politics, Policy, and Law* 19:361–92.

Weissert, Carol S., and William G. Weissert. 2002. *Governing Health: The Politics of Health Policy,* 2d ed. Baltimore: Johns Hopkins University Press.

Weissert, William G., and Edward Alan Miller. 2005. Punishing the Pioneers: The Medicare Modernization Act and State Pharmacy Assistance Programs. *Publius: The Journal of Federalism* 35 (1): 115–142.

Weisskopf, Michael. 1995. To the Victors Belong the PAC Checks. *Washington Post National Weekly Edition,* Jan. 2–8, 13.

Weisskopf, Michael, and David Maraniss. 1995. In on the Takeoff. *Washington Post National Weekly Edition,* Mar. 20–26, 13–14.

Welch, W. P., and Lisa Dubay. 1989. The Impact of Administratively Necessary Days on Hospital Costs. *Medical Care* 27:1117–32.

West, Darrell M., and Richard Francis. 1995. Selling the Contract with America: Interest Groups and Public Policymaking. Paper presented at the annual meeting of the American Political Science Association, Chicago, Aug. 3–Sept. 3.

———. 1996. Electronic Advocacy: Interest Groups and Public Policy Making. *PS,* Mar., 25–29.

West, Darrell M., and Burdett A. Loomis. 1998. *The Sound of Money: How Political Interests Get What They Want.* New York: W. W. Norton.

West, William. 1984. Structuring Administrative Discretion: The Pursuit of Rationality and Responsiveness. *American Journal of Political Science* 28:340–60.

West, William, and Joseph Cooper. 1989–90. Legislative Influence v. Presidential Dominance: Competing Models of Bureaucratic Control. *Political Science Quarterly* 104:581–606.

White, Joseph. 1995. The Horses and the Jumps: Comments on the Health Care Reform Steeplechase. *Journal of Health Politics, Policy, and Law* 20:373–83.

White House. 2002. President Takes Action to Lower Prescription Drug Prices by Improving Access to Generic Drugs. Oct. 21. www.whitehouse.gov/news/releases/2002/10/20021021-4.html

Whiteman, David. 1987. What Do They Know and When Do They Know It? Health Staff on the Hill. *PS* 20:221–25.

Wilcox, Clyde. 1999. The Dynamics of Lobbying the Hill. In *Interest Group Connection: Electioneering, Lobbying, and Policymaking in Washington,* ed. Paul S. Herrnson, Ronald G. Shaiko, and Clyde Wilcox. Chatham, NJ: Chatham House.

Wildavsky, Aaron. 1966. The Two Presidencies. *Trans-Action* 4:7–14.

———. 1979. *Speaking Truth to Power.* Boston: Little, Brown.

Wilkerson, John D., and David Carrell. 1999. Money, Politics, and Medicine: The American Medical PAC's Strategy of Giving in U.S. House Races. *Journal of Health Politics, Policy, and Law* 24:335–55.

Wilson, James Q. 1989. *Bureaucracy: What Government Agencies Do and Why They Do It.* New York: Basic Books.

Wilson, Rick. 1992. Review of *Parties and Leaders in the Postreform House* by David Rohde. *American Political Science Review* 86:806–7.

Wilson, Woodrow. [1885] 1913. *Congressional Government.* Boston: Houghton Mifflin.

Wines, Michael. 1994. Clinton Puts Onus for Health Care on Republicans. *New York Times,* Aug. 4, A1, A9.

Winn, Mylon. 1987. Competitive Health Care: Assessing an Alternative Solution for Health Care Problems. In *Health Care Issues in Black America: Policies, Problems, and Prospects,* ed. Woodrow Jones, Jr., and Mitchell F. Rice. Westport, CT: Greenwood Press.

Wood, Bruce. 1999. The Politics of Disease-Related Patients' Associations: An Anglo-American Comparison. Paper presented at the annual meeting of the American Political Science Association, Atlanta, Sept. 3.

Woodward, B. 1994. *The Agenda: Inside the Clinton White House.* New York: Simon and Schuster.

Wright, John R. 1985. PACs, Contributions, and Roll Calls: An Organizational Perspective. *American Political Science Review* 79:400–414.

———. 1990. Contributions, Lobbying, and Committee Voting in the U.S. House of Representatives. *American Political Science Review* 84:417–38.

———. 1996. *Interest Groups and Congress.* Boston: Allyn and Bacon.

Zachary, G. Pascal. 1994. How Some Schools Get Fat with Federal Pork. *Wall Street Journal,* Apr. 29, B1, B2.

Zielbauer, Paul. 2000. States and Cities Flout Law on Underground Fuel Tanks. *New York Times,* Aug. 8, A1, A27.

Zuckman, Jill. 2003. Medicare Drug Bill Nears Passage: Senate GOP Leaders Overcome Efforts to Block Measure. *Chicago Tribune,* Nov. 25, 1, final edition, Chicago.

Index